Haematology Nursing

Haematology Nursing

Marvelle Brown MA (Ed.), Post-Graduate Cert.
LMCC, Post-Graduate Dip. (Ed.) Post-Grad Dip.
(Health Research) BA (Hons) Social Policy

*Macmillan Senior Lecturer (Haematology)/Work Based Fellow
RN, RM, RHV, RNT*

Tracey J. Cutler BSc (Hons) Clinical Nursing
Studies (Specialist Practitioner Oncology), MA Education and
Professional Development

Senior Lecturer, Birmingham City University RN Adult

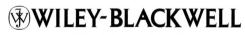**WILEY-BLACKWELL**

A John Wiley & Sons, Ltd., Publication

This edition first published 2012
© 2012 by Blackwell Publishing Ltd.

Chapter 4 is adapted from Chapter 4 of *The Biology of Cancer*, First Edition. Janice Gabriel.
© 2007 John Wiley & Sons, Ltd. Used with permission.

Blackwell Publishing was acquired by John Wiley & Sons in February 2007. Blackwell's publishing program
has been merged with Wiley's global Scientific, Technical and Medical business to form Wiley-Blackwell.

Registered Office
John Wiley & Sons, Ltd, The Atrium, Southern Gate, Chichester, West Sussex, PO19 8SQ, UK

Editorial Offices
9600 Garsington Road, Oxford, OX4 2DQ, UK
The Atrium, Southern Gate, Chichester, West Sussex, PO19 8SQ, UK
2121 State Avenue, Ames, Iowa 50014-8300, USA

For details of our global editorial offices, for customer services and for information about how
to apply for permission to reuse the copyright material in this book please see our website at
www.wiley.com/wiley-blackwell.

Library of Congress Cataloging-in-Publication Data

Haematology nursing / [edited by] Marvelle Brown, Tracey J. Cutler.
    p. ; cm.
  Includes bibliographical references and index.
  ISBN 978-1-4051-6996-7 (pbk. : alk. paper)
I. Brown, Marvelle.   II. Cutler, Tracey J.
[DNLM: 1. Hematologic Diseases–nursing.   WY 152.5]
  616.1′50231–dc23
                                            2011048152

A catalogue record for this book is available from the British Library.

This book is published in the following electronic formats: ePDF 9781118276112; ePub 9781118276129;
Mobi 9781118276105

Set in 10/12.5pt Times by SPi Publisher Services, Pondicherry, India
Printed in Singapore by Ho Printing Singapore Pte Ltd

1   2012

Contents

Contributors

Editors

Marvelle Brown has been in the NHS and nurse education for over 30 years. In 1991, she developed the first professionally and academically recognised haematology course in England. She went on to further develop this into both a diploma and degree. She was a member of one of the working groups, which led to the development of the NICE Guidance in Haemato-oncology.

She was Chair of the RCN Haematology/BMT Forum and is currently Chair of the Acute Nurses Forum for Sickle Cell and Thalassemia.

Marvelle was a non-executive director for a north-west London hospital trust and is currently a non-executive director for Milton Keynes PCT. She became a work based fellow in 2009. Marvelle is a senior lecturer in haematology and her role expanded to lead on international nursing education.

Marvelle has written a number of articles and chapters on haematology.

She is an invited speaker nationally and internationally on a wide number of issues in haematology nursing and is completing her PhD.

Tracey Cutler began nursing in haematology in 1987, first in Bristol with children undergoing bone marrow transplant and receiving chemotherapy for haematological and oncological conditions. She then moved to Birmingham into the adult setting.

The majority of her nursing experience is in haemopoietic stem cell transplant and she progressed to a clinical nurse specialist as the transplant coordinator.

Tracey was on the working committee for the NICE (2003) Improving Outcomes in Haemato- oncology and has presented nationally and internationally.

Tracey now works as a senior lecturer in education and ran the specialist degrees in haematology, cancer care and chemotherapy for ten years. Her role has now developed to assist practitioners in their ongoing professional and academic development.

Contributors

Janice Gabriel has worked in cancer nursing for over 30 years and has had an interest in vascular access devices since the early 1980s. In 1993 she received a Nightingale Scholarship to visit the USA to independently assess the use of PICCs for patients undergoing chemotherapy. In 1994 she placed her first PICC here in the UK. Janice is currently Nurse Director for the Central South Coast Cancer Network, based in Portsmouth.

Jackie Green qualified as an RGN in 1989 and very quickly realised her passion was in cancer nursing. In 1990 she trained as an oncology nurse and went on to set up a haematology day care unit and developed the clinical haematology service. In 2001 she moved to Kings College Hospital as a lead cancer nurse and senior nurse in haematology and cancer.

In 2002 she returned to Mayday University Hospital in the role of a nurse consultant for haematology and cancer, as well as a lead cancer nurse.

Jan Green completed her nurse training in 1988 and went on to specialise in adult haematology nursing, becoming a Macmillan Haematology CNS in 1997. During her career she has set up a satellite chemotherapy unit, a venesection service for patients diagnosed with Haemochromatosis and a day case blood transfusion service for patients with Myelodysplastic Syndrome. In 2003 she became a Transfusion Liaison Nurse, supporting hospitals across the London region in the education of safe and appropriate use of blood.

Louise Knight has worked in the Translational Oncology Research Centre, Portsmouth for 10 years and gained her PhD in Modulating sensitivity and response to DNA damaging cytotoxic drugs in 2004. Her current post is Cellular Pathology Quality, Risk and Governance Manager.

Gwyneth Morgan in 1997 Gwyneth became an education and research coordinator at the West Midlands regional genetics unit and has been involved with the development of genetic programmes of study for HCPs She has since worked in higher education for a number of years, and is currently working as a senior lecturer at Birmingham City University.

Jane Richardson is a Senior Lecturer in Allied Health Sciences, she work at Worcester University in the Institute of Health and Society.

Her interests are in Genetics and Nutrition and she is a member of the British Association for Applied Nutrition and Nutrition Therapy (BANT) and the Nutrition Society.

Alison Simons has worked in oncology since qualifying almost 20 years ago. She worked within an in-patient setting looking after patients with a wide variety of cancers, undergoing chemotherapy, radiotherapy, brachytherapy, symptom management, emergency care and end of life care. She then took up the post of professional development sister responsible for oncological and haematological education and training. For the last two years she has worked at Birmingham City University as a senior lecturer in cancer care, leading the cancer care and chemotherapy programmes.

Dion Smyth has worked in cancer nursing care and education for 25 years, during which time he developed his interest and clinical service provision around the palliative, supportive and end of life care needs of patients with blood disorders. He is currently a lecturer-practitioner at Birmingham City University, UK.

Samantha Toland has worked in the field of Haematology and oncology for the last 11 years, initially working in the acute setting of a Haematology and bone marrow transplant unit, then as a specialist nurse and trainer in chemotherapy. She is currently working as a Leukaemia Nurse specialist, and also as a Senior Lecturer practitioner in Haematology at Birmingham City University.

Audrey Yandle is a Lecturer at Kings College University; she is a registered nurse with a clinical background in haematological-oncology nursing practice and has a particular interest in the nursing contribution to patient outcomes in the haematological-oncology and stem cell transplantation settings.

Foreword

Haematology is a fascinating field of clinical practice, and the developments in our understanding of haematological conditions have made this specialty a highly dynamic and exciting field in which to work. As such, it has been an area that has generated a great interest for nurses and there are now career progression opportunities to become a specialist nurse in both malignant and non-malignant haematology.

Haematology Nursing plugs a significant gap, being the first book published in the United Kingdom that addresses both these disciplines, thereby making it a valuable reference tool for all nurses managing patients with a haematological condition.

This groundbreaking textbook provides an understanding of pathology and then relates this to nursing practice. The layout of the book makes it easy for readers to navigate.

It is a comprehensive and key resource for nurses practising in haematology.

Professor Dame Sally C Davies
Chief Medical Officer and Chief Scientific Adviser,
Department of Health

Section 1

Introduction to haematology

Chapter 1

Understanding haemopoiesis

Marvelle Brown

> *This chapter aims to provide an overview of the haemopoiesis process and by the end of reading this chapter you should:*
> - Have a detailed knowledge of all marrow cell development and function
> - Be aware of the different sites of haemopoiesis
> - Be aware of the role of stem cells and how they function
> - Understand growth factors and how they function

Introduction

Blood is not immediately thought of as an organ, but it is one of the largest in the body. The volume of blood in adults is approximately 4.5–5 litres and marrow cells form about 40% of this volume.

Haemopoiesis is the production of marrow cells and it is a fascinating process involving a diverse range of cytokinetic interactions, which produce cells responsible for gaseous exchange, fighting infections and haemostasis. Haemopoiesis is a complex process of proliferation, differentiation and maturation, with an intricate balance between demand and supply of marrow cells. Through ongoing research of haemopoiesis and the behaviour of stem cells, their relationship with growth factors, the microenvironment of the bone marrow and regulatory mechanisms are increasing knowledge of our haematological pathologies and informing therapeutic interventions.

Haemopoiesis is the name given to the production of marrow cells and this is further subdivided into erythropoiesis (production of red blood cells), leucopoiesis (production of white blood cells) and thrombopoiesis (production of platelets). In humans there are various haemopoietic sites, starting with the blood islands in the yolk sac, which forms the basis of marrow cell production for up to two months of gestation. Red blood cells are the first to be produced, with leucopoiesis and thrombopoiesis occurring from six weeks (Pallister 1997).

Haematology Nursing, First Edition. Marvelle Brown and Tracey J. Cutler.
© 2012 Blackwell Publishing Ltd. Published 2012 by Blackwell Publishing Ltd.

During this early period the main haemoglobin being produced is Gower 1 ($\zeta2\epsilon2$). The liver and spleen become the main sites for marrow cell production from about two months through to seven months' gestation and here the haemoglobin is now foetal haemoglobin, Hb F ($\alpha2\gamma2$). From six months' gestation the skeletal system becomes the prime source of marrow cell production and with this change in site is also a gradual change in the haemoglobin from haemoglobin F (HbF) to haemoglobin A (HbA) ($\alpha2\beta2$). The liver and spleen continue to produce marrow cells for at least two weeks after birth, but in much reduced quantities (Hoffbrand *et al.* 2004). The significance of the liver and spleen being sites of early marrow cell production is significant as they can revert (back) to producing marrow cells (known as 'extramedullary' haemopoiesis) when the bone marrow is unable to do so or is inefficient in production due to disease, such as haemato-oncological malignancies, sickle cell disease and thalassaemia syndromes (haemoglobinopathies).

During infancy and up to three years of age the entire skeletal system produces marrow cells. Progressively, there is replacement of marrow with yellow fatty tissue in the long bones and by the early twenties the distinct skeletal sites of the vertebrae, ribs, sternum, skull, proximal end of the humerus and femur, sacrum and pelvis become the only sites for haemopoiesis. In addition, similarly to the liver and spleen, the fatty tissue in the bone marrow can also reconvert to active haemopoiesis in times of increased demand.

The bone marrow has three types of stem cells, haemopoietic stem cells responsible for the production of marrow cells, endothelial tissues, which form the sinusoids, and, finally, mesenchymal stem cells. Mesenchymal stem cells differentiate into osteoblasts (bone tissue), chondrocytes (cartilage tissue) and myocytes (muscle tissue) (Litchtman *et al.* 2005). The existence of stems cells other than haemopoietic stem cells found in the bone marrow has generated great interest in researchers and scientists in their potential use in treating neurological and muscular diseases in the future.

All marrow cells start their development from haemopoietic stem cells, known as multipotent or pluripotent stem cells. The terms multipotent and pluripotent refer to the fact that these cells have the ability to become any type of marrow cell. These primitive progenitor cells are unrecognisable by their cell morphology but have been identified through immunological testing as being CD34+ cells. The identification of these progenitor cells as CD34+ involves the use of a monoclonal antibody (Guo *et al.* 2003; Yasui *et al.* 2003). The term CD means cluster of differentiation and relates to what are known as surface markers on a cell which are unique to that cell.

Stems cells constitute approximately 4% of the haemopoietic cells in the bone marrow and one stem cell can produce 10^6 cells after 20 divisions (Hoffbrand *et al.* 2004). The committed progenitor cells form approximately 3% and the maturing/mature cells approximately 95% of the haemopoietic stem cells (HSC) (Traynor 2006). Stem cells also have the capacity to self-renew, which is important as this means there is always a constant supply of stem cells to respond quickly to demand such as infection, haemorrhage and anaemia. Under normal circumstances, mature marrow cells are lost through normal activities and aging.

Once the HSC has been triggered all marrow cells are produced along two lines: myeloid and lymphoid. Erythrocytes, granulocytes, myelocytes and megakaryocytes are produced along the myeloid line, and lymphocytes and natural killer cells (NK) are produced along the lymphoid line. To start the differentiation process, the pluripotent stem cells can differentiate into either the precursor, colony-forming unit – granulocyte, erythrocytes, myelocytes, megakaryocytes (CFU-GEMM), or lymphoid stem cell. Differentiation of these lines produces committed cell lines. The exception is the progenitor cell, CFU-GM, which gives rise to monocytes and neutrophils. As a cell goes through its stages of development, it progressively loses its capacity to self-renew and once matured is unable to do so at all (terminal differentiation) (see Figure 1.1).

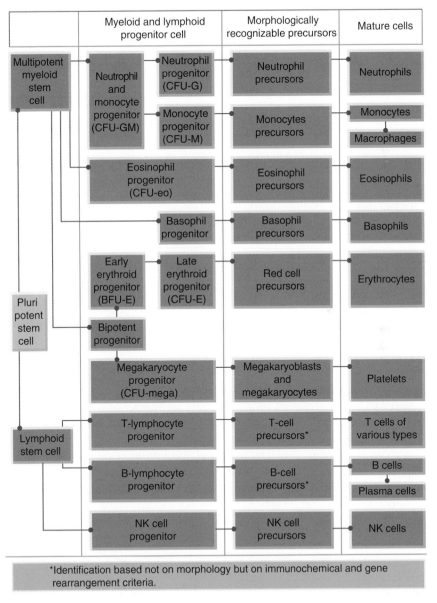

Figure 1.1 Relationships between the various types of cell involved in haemopoiesis (from Hughes-Jones *et al.* 2009). Reprinted with permission of John Wiley & Sons, Inc.

Growth factors are naturally occurring glycoproteins and determine the behaviour of the stem cell. They are produced from a number of sources: macrophages, fibroblasts, endothelial cells, monocytes, T-cells, the kidneys and the liver (Pallister 2005). Growth factors can work solely on a committed line such as erythropoietin. Others are synergistic, whilst others can influence both early progenitor cells and later committed cells. Granulocyte colony stimulating factor (G-CSF) and thrombopoietin (TPO) enhance the activities of stem cell factor (SCF), interleukin-3 (IL-3), granulocyte monocyte-colony stimulating factor (GM-CSF). In addition, G-CSF and GM-CSF enhance the function of mature cells (Hoffbrand *et al.* 2004; Metcalf and Nicola 1995). Our understanding of the activities of growth factors has aided in the pharmacological production of erythropoietin used in renal disease and recombinant granulocyte stimulating factor, (rHG-CSF), used in stem cell transplantation to reduce the period of neutropenia. Table 1.1 provides an overview of growth factors, their sources and functions.

The microenvironment of the bone marrow is known as bone marrow stroma and is a unique environment which forms the structural base, allowing stem cells to grow and develop. The stroma is made up of a structural base of cells which are macrophages, reticular connective tissue, osteoclasts, osteoblasts, adipocytes, fibroblasts and endothelial cells which form the sinusoids. The structure also enables the generation of the mesenchymal tissue providing vessels and bones to support stem cell development. The HSC form the parenchyma cells (functioning cells) of the stroma and their close proximity with the stromal layer is essential for proliferation (Kronenwett *et al.* 2000). Stromal cells produce growth factors, SCF, (kit ligand, steel factor) to ensure self-renewal of those cells. In addition, the stromal cells produce adhesive proteins such as fibronectin, forming an extra-cellular matrix. These adhesive proteins allow growth factors to become attached to receptor sites on the stem cell and once attached, set off intracellular chemical reactions to prepare the stem cell to respond to the growth factor instruction, which could be to become quiescent, proliferate, become committed, differentiate or mature. The adhesive interactions between stem cells and stromal layers are key to migration, circulation and proliferation.

It has been identified that HSCs have their own 'space' within the bone marrow (Traynor 2006). Erythrocyte precursors lie adjacent to venous sinus in erythroblast islands and each has its own macrophage. Megakaryocytes are found next to the venous sinus and their cytoplasmic projections extend directly into the lumen. Cytoplasmic granules, which are to become platelets, congregate at the edges of the projection, making holes in the megakaryocytes (known as platelet budding) and flow into the circulation. The precursors for monocytes and granulocytes are found deep within the cavity and when they mature are very motile and migrate to the venous sinus to enter into circulation (Pallister 1997).

Stem cells' primary home is the bone marrow, but a small percentage enter circulation. The recognition of this has led to the development of being able to collect peripheral stem cells via apheresis for 'harvesting' and transplantation. Circulating progenitor cells form part of the self-renewal process and are able to re-populate stem cells in the bone marrow. Peripheral stem cells are known to be more mature than those in the bone marrow; when used for haemopoietic stem cell transplantation, they generally engraft earlier, leading to less time for the patient being neutropenic and hence reducing the potential for infections. See Chapter 2 and Chapter 20 for more details.

Table 1.1 Overview of growth factors, source and activities (adapted from Pallister 2005 and Hoffbrand et al. 2004).

	Growth factors	Activity	Where produced
Growth factors that influence early progenitor cells	IL-3	Stem cell production	Stromal cells T-cells
	TPO	Stimulates myeloid cell production Influences CFU$_{MEG}$	Liver and kidneys
	GM-CSF	Stimulates production of erythrocytes, thrombocytes and phagocytic cells; neutrophils, eosinophils, monocytes	T-cells, fibroblasts, endothelial cells
	IL-7	Stimulates proliferation of all cells in the lymphoid lineage (B and T-lymphocytes and NK cells)	Fibroblasts, endothelial cells, thymus
Growth factors that act on committed cell lines	G-CSF	Stimulates production of neutrophils	Monocytes, fibroblasts
	M-CSF	Stimulates production of monocytes	Macrophages, endothelial cells
	IL-5	Influences CFU$_{EO}$ and differentiation of activated B-cells	T-cells
	Erythropoietin	Stimulates erythrocytes production	Kidneys, limited production in the liver
	IL-7	B-cell maturation,	As above
Growth factors released from activated T-cell, macrophages	IL-1	Stimulates T-cell, macrophages, fibroblast, endothelial cells to produce GM-CSF, IL-6, G-CSF, M-CSF	IL-1
	Tumour necrosis factor (TNF)		Tumour necrosis factor (TNF)

Key: SCF, stem cell factor; IL-3, interleukin-3; TPO, thrombopoietin; GM-CSF, granulocyte macrophage colony stimulating factor; IL-7, interleukin-7; G-CS, F granulocyte colony stimulating factor; M-CSF, monocyte colony stimulating factor; IL-5, interleukin-5; IL-1, interleukin-1.

Table 1.2   Down-regulators of haemopoiesis.

Transforming growth factor β (TNF-β)
Prostaglandin E
Macrophage inflammatory protein 1a (MIP-1a)
α and γ interferon
Leukaemia inhibitory factor
Tumour necrosis factor -α (TNF-α)
Lactoferrin
Inhibin

Adapted from Queensberry and Colvin (2001).

We do not as yet have the entire picture of the regulatory mechanism of HSC to under-stand how homeostasis is maintained within the bone marrow. Growth factors clearly up-regulate bone marrow activity but down-regulation is less well understood. The known regulatory factors are listed in Table 1.2. Ultimately, the actions of the regulators are to maintain haemopoiesis in a steady state, inhibiting mitosis or preventing apoptosis.

Apoptosis is a key factor in maintaining homeostasis of haemopoiesis. Apoptosis is programmed cell death (PCD), equated to 'cellular suicide'. It is regulated by a number of physiological processes leading to biochemical activities of intracellular proteins known as capases, taking place within the cell, resulting in a change in cell morphology. The morphological changes primarily are: changes to the cell membrane which cause loss of attachment, cell shrinkage, loss of membrane symmetry and blebbing. In addition, nuclear changes also occur, which include chromatin condensation, nuclear fragmenta-tion and chromosomal DNA fragmentation (Charras *et al.* 2008). All these activities will ultimately lead to the death of the cell (see Figure 1.2).

Myeloid lineage bone marrow cells

Erythropoiesis

Erythropoiesis is the name for red blood cell production. Red blood cells are the most numerous of all marrow cells, as indicated in Table 1.3. Their production is triggered by hypoxia. When the blood enters the kidneys, hypoxia triggers erythropoietin (EPO) release. It is a glycoprotein synthesised by the peritubular interstitial cells of the kidneys, and chromosome 7 carries the gene for its coding (Pallister 1997).

Erythrocytes develop and mature in the bone marrow and Figure 1.3 is a schematic representation of the stages of their development. Receptor sites for EPO are found on BFU_E, CFU_E and pronormoblasts. Erythropoietin shortens the pronormoblast phase, enabling faster production of red blood cells.

Development starts from the CFU-GEMM to BFU_E, progressing to CFU_E, which develops into the first recognisable erythroid precursor, the pronormoblast. Under Ramonsky staining the pronormoblast appears blue due to RNA ribosomes (Turgeon 2005). It has a very large nucleus to cytoplasm ratio. As it continues through stages of development, it becomes increasingly smaller in size, the haemoglobin concentration increases, giving the cell a pink colour. The nucleus is eventually ejected at the late normoblastic phase when it then becomes known as the marrow reticulocyte. The reticulocyte stage continues for a further 1–2 days in the marrow, losing its RNA, further increasing the concentration of the haemoglobin. Reticulocytes circulate in the blood for a further 1–2 days to mature into erythrocytes. The process of maturation from pronormoblast to erythrocyte can take approximately five days and the lifespan for a normal red blood cell is 120 days (Lewis *et al.* 2001). Reticulocytosis tends to be an indication of either excessive haemolysis (as seen, for example, in sickle cell disease and thalassaemia) or excessive haemorrhage.

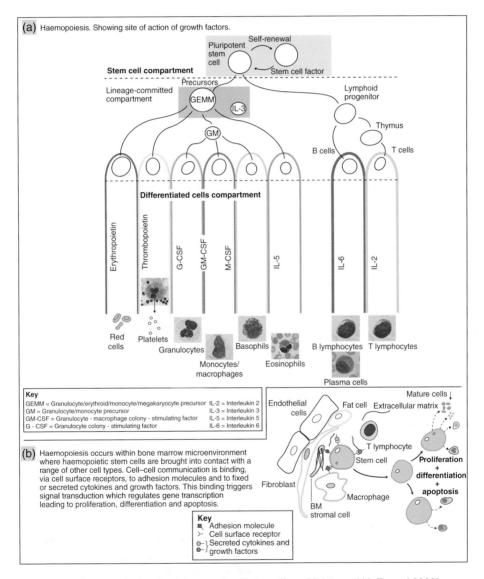

Figure 1.2 Haemopoiesis, physiology and pathology (from Mehta and Hoffbrand 2009). Reprinted with permission of John Wiley & Sons, Inc.

Table 1.3   Normal values and functions of cells.

Marrow cell	Normal count	Overview of function
Red blood cells	Women 4–5 x 10^{12}/L Men 5–5.5 x 10^{12}/L	Gaseous exchange
White cell count (WCC)	4–11/10^9/L	Fight infections
Platelets	150–400^9/L	Instigates haemostasis

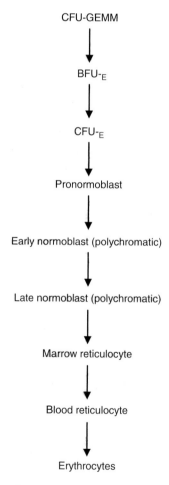

CFU-GEMM

BFU-$_E$

CFU-$_E$

Pronormoblast

Early normoblast (polychromatic)

Late normoblast (polychromatic)

Marrow reticulocyte

Blood reticulocyte

Erythrocytes

Figure 1.3   Development of erythrocytes.

Erythrocytes are anucleated, biconcave in shape, which provides a greater surface area for their function of gaseous exchange: taking oxygen (O_2) from the lungs to the tissues and carbon dioxide (CO_2) from the tissues to the lungs. The ability of the erythrocyte to carry out its function is made possible by the haemoprotein, haemoglobin, and each erythrocyte has approximately 600 million haemoglobin molecules. The lack of nuclei and organelles also contributes to increased haemoglobin content and gas-carrying capacity. Approximately one half of the CO_2 is directly bound to haemoglobin. The rest is converted by the enzyme carbonic anhydrase, which is found in erythrocytes, into bicarbonate ions that diffuse back out into the plasma and hydrogen ions (H^+) that bind to the protein portion of the haemoglobin, thereby keeping the pH of the erythrocyte, relatively neutral.

Erythrocytes are able to make energy from breaking down glucose, known as glycolysis. This process involves enzymatic activity, which occurs along two chemical pathways known as the Embden-Meyerhof pathway (EMP) (95% of glycolysis takes place along this pathway) and pentose phosphate pathway (PPP).

Erythrocytes have structural and contractile proteins which make up the cytoskeleton. These proteins are α and β spectrin, ankyrin, actin protein 4.1 and enable erythrocytes to be deformable and flexible (Lewis *et al.* 2001). Erythrocytes have a diameter of 6–7 μm approximately and they have to pass through microvessels, which can have a diameter of 3 μm. Therefore deformability is crucial to their ability to travel to tissues. Defects of any of these proteins compromise the erythrocyte's function. The most abundant of the proteins is spectrin and a lack of it leads to a condition known as hereditary spherocytosis. The surface of erythrocytes also has antigens, some of which denote the blood group an individual has inherited (see Chapter 17).

In addition to erythropoietin, erythrocytes also require nutrients and some hormones which help to influence their development. Protein is required for the cell membrane as well as being a component of haemoglobin. Iron is an essential component of haemoglobin and vitamin B_{12} is required for nucleic synthesis. Vitamin C increases the absorption of iron and copper acts as a catalyst for iron to be taken up by haemoglobin. Vitamin B6 is required for haemoglobin synthesis and folic acid aids in maturation. Lack of the hormone thyroxin compromises EPO production and the 'sex' hormones have opposing influences on erythrocyte's development. Testosterone stimulates erythrocyte production; conversely oestrogen decreases red blood cell production. This explains why the red blood cell count is higher in men than women and why androgenic drugs are used in conditions like Fanconi's anaemia.

The reticulo-endothelial system (RES), comprising the liver, spleen, lymph nodes and bone marrow is responsible for the destruction of senescent red blood cells. Aging red blood cells are recognised by macrophages in the RES due to a number of changes which take place. The changes are caused by a reduction in the glycolytic activity, leading to reduced activities of its essential enzymes. This has the effect of making the chemical pumps (sodium pump and magnesium pump) inside the red blood cell inefficient, allowing an increased intake of water, making it unable to deform easily. The abnormal spherical shape is detected by the macrophages, particularly in the spleen, and the red blood cell is then phagocytosed.

During this process the haemoglobin molecule is removed and the globin component is broken down into amino acids to be reused for new erythrocytes. The iron is separated from the haem and is transported by apopferritin for storage as ferritin for future use in

Table 1.4   Normal values of Granulocytes and
agranulocytes.

Neutrophils *	$2.5–7.5 \times 10^9$/L
Basophils	$0.01–0.1 \times 10^9$/L
Eosinophils	$0.04–0.4 \times 10^9$/L
Monocytes	$0.2–0.8 \times 10^9$/L
Lymphocytes	$1.5–3.5 \times 10^9$/L

Adapted from (Hoffbrand *et al*. 2004).
There may be some variations on the above results depending on
the population the hospital laboratory serves.
*It is well known the WCC count is lower in blacks than
Caucasians, but it is not clearly understood why that occurs.

Table 1.5   Granulocytes and Agranulocytes.

Granulocytes	Agranulocytes		
Neutrophils Eosinophils Basophils	Monocytes Lymphocytes Natural killer cells (NK cells)	T-lymphocytes	B-lymphocytes

production of erythrocytes. When iron is required for erythrocyte production, the plasma protein transferrin transports the ferritin to the bone marrow where developing erythroblasts have receptor sites for transferrin. The haem forms biliverdin, which converts to bilirubin and is stored as bile in the gall bladder.

Leukocytosis

The entire process of leukocyte production is not fully understood, although it is known that there are specific growth factors involved in their development (see Table 1.1 on growth factors) and the production is increased during periods of infection and inflammation.

A leukocyte's prime function is to defend the body against and react to infective organisms and toxins. They are less numerous than erythrocytes and are nucleated. Leukocytes are divided into granulocytes (also known as polymorphonuclear cells because they are multi-nucleated and agranulocytes as indicated in Table 1.5). Granulocytes populate three environments, marrow, blood and tissues (Bainton 2001). Their movement is unidirectional, meaning they do not return to a previous environment, for example once they have left the marrow and entered circulation, they do not return to the marrow; similarly once in tissues, they do not return to circulation.

Granulocytes and monocytes provide innate immunity, meaning it is present from birth, is non-specific, for example attacks many pathogens and does not require sensitisation. Lymphocytes provide acquired immunity, meaning they need to be sensitised by a specific antigen, either from an infection or vaccination and produce memory cells.

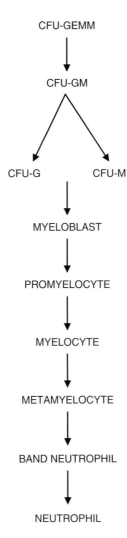

Figure 1.4 Neutrophil development.

The total white cell count (WCC) can be seen in Table 1.3, but to establish the numbers of each type of white cell a differential count is required. Table 1.4 indicates the normal differential counts.

Granulocytes

Neutrophils are the most numerous of white cells and they are produced on the myeloid line in the bone marrow, from the CFU-GM committed progenitor cell, as illustrated in Figure 1.4. Both neutrophils and monocytes share the CFU-GM which is developed from the CFU-GEMM. When the CFU-GM differentiates to CFU-G this becomes committed to producing neutrophils. The production of CFU-G progenitor cell is triggered by the growth factor, G-CSF.

The myeloblast is a large cell with a high nucleus to cytoplasm ratio, which undergoes several stages of division (as illustrated in Figure 1.4) and is the first granulocyte precursor which is recognised by cell morphology. At the promyelocyte stage primary granules are found and they contain myeloperoxidase, cathepsin G and other acid hydrolases. Secondary granules, such as lactoferrin, lysozyme and collagenase, are first seen at the myelocyte stage and in abundance in the mature neutrophil (Babior and Golde 2001).

The penultimate stage of neutrophil development is a band neutrophil. These are non-proliferating cells, and proceed to full maturation as neutrophils. Mature neutrophils are denoted by having a 3–4 lobe nucleus, held together by a thin chromatin strand and stain pink on Ramonsky staining. The whole maturity process can take up to five days, but where there is an infection, this process can be sped up to completing maturation in 48 hours. Once matured, neutrophils enter the bloodstream, making up to 60% of circulating white blood cells. Half the neutrophils will circulate and the others will loosely attach themselves to the endothelial lining of blood vessels, known as margination. This ensures there is a ready access of neutrophils to fight infections and inflammation. Neutrophils circulate for about 4–10 hours in the blood before entering tissues, where they remain for about 2–3 days, taking on the role of being non-specific against bacteria and other microbes. The daily production of neutrophils is 0.85–1.6 x 10^9/cells/kg/day (Babior and Golde 2001).

Neutrophils are microcytic, phagocytic cells; they are highly motile and act rapidly at the site of tissue injury and are the hallmark of acute inflammation. When active they have a limited lifespan of a few hours. They have the ability to respond to an invading organism in two critical ways: diapedesis and chemotaxis. Diapedesis is amoeboid movement. Neutrophils are able to elongate forming a pseudopodium, taking on a 'hand-mirror' shape to squeeze through the blood vessels and enter the interstitial tissue space. Chemotaxis is the neutrophils' ability to detect chemicals released by pathogens and from inflammatory cytokines such as interleukin-8 (IL-8), interferon-gamma (IFN-gamma), tumour necrosis factor (TNF) and opsonins, namely the complement proteins, C3a, C5a and C6. To function efficiently neutrophils rely on being presented with the antigens and they have receptor sites for IgG and complement proteins complement C3, which coats the organism (a process known as opsonisation), making it easier for the neutrophil to engulf coated organisms (Rich *et al.* 2009).

When being phagocytic, the neutrophil will engulf the organism, forming a vacuole, and the secondary granules' degranulation, releasing lysozyme, lactoferrin into the vacuole. These produce hydrogen peroxide and a highly active form of oxygen (superoxide) which ultimately leads to the death of the ingested organism.

Eosinophils

Eosinophils develop and mature in the bone marrow, being produced from the CFUeo, and go through phases of development as illustrated in Figure 1.5. The development of eosinophils is triggered in response to interleukin 3 (IL-3), interleukin-5 (IL-5) and granulocyte macrophage colony stimulating factor (GM-CSF). Mature eosinophils stain red with eosin dye using Ramonsky technique.

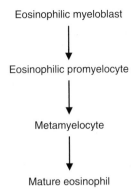

Eosinophilic myeloblast

Eosinophilic promyelocyte

Metamyelocyte

Mature eosinophil

Figure 1.5 Development of eosinophils.

Following maturation they have large cytoplasmic granules and less than 1% circulate in blood, approximately 50% marginate like neutrophils and the rest enter tissues such as the skin and lower gastrointestinal tract. Eosinophils circulate in the blood for 8–10 hours and if not stimulated can survive for approximately 10–12 days. They are phagocytic, but not as aggressive as neutrophils. They are approximately the same size as neutrophils, but have large granules and respond to parasitic infections. They have a major role in controlling inflammatory responses, by neutralising histamine produced by basophils and mast cells. Along with mast cells they have a role to play in mechanisms involved in allergic reactions and asthma. Eosinophil count can vary with age, exercise and environmental stimuli such as allergens.

Basophils

Basophils are the least numerous of circulating white blood cells, forming 1% of their total and are non-phagocytic cells. They are produced from the CFU-baso and differentiation from basophilic promyelocyte → to myelocyte → to metamyelocyte and → final maturation. Their development takes place in the bone marrow and the growth factor, interleukin-5 (IL-5) initiates their development. Basophils are given their name because of their capacity to stain with base dyes and have a bluish-purple colouring on Ramonsky staining. They are the least understood of the white cells, but it is known that they are involved in hypersensitivity and have a role in instigating inflammatory response since they have granules containing substances such as heparin, histamine and platelet activating factor (Roitt 2001). Basophils also have receptor sites for antibody IgE and when bound to basophils, they aid the release of the above chemicals leading to inflammation and vascular permeability, enabling phagocytic cells to leave the circulation and enter interstitial tissue space to engulf and digest organisms.

Basophils are involved in hypersensitivity reactions and anaphylaxis. By binding to IgE this is thought to be a significant factor in the selective response of these cells to environmental stimuli such as pollen and and the clinical symptoms of an allergic reaction: watery eyes, runny nose and difficult breathing.

Platelets

The production of platelets starts with the CFU-$_{meg}$ in the bone marrow. The stage of development then proceeds from megakaryoblast to megakarocyte. The process of the development of platelets is different to that of other marrow cells as it is based on endomitotic replication (Coleman *et al.* 2005). Endocytosis is the doubling of chromosomes within a nucleus, but there is no nuclear division and the cytoplasm does not divide. Instead, the cytoplasm increases in volume. The replication of the chromosome within the nucleus can occur several times. As a consequence, with each cell cycle division of endomitosis the cell becomes larger. Once mitotic division has been completed, the nucleus within the megakaryocyte becomes lobulated and the cytoplasmic granules are formed to make the platelets. The control and production of platelets is regulated by the glycoprotein thrombopoietin, which is produced by the liver and kidneys. Platelets have receptor sites (C-MPL) for thrombopoietin, which removes it from circulation (Pallister 2005).

The megakaryocyte by its name indicates this is a very large cell, almost ten times the size of other marrow cells in the bone marrow, and each megakaryocyte can produce 2000–4000 platelets. Platelets are non-nucleated, disc-like structures which are formed from fragmentation of the megakaryocytic cytoplasm. They form holes in the megakaryocyte, known as platelet budding, to enter into circulation and are the second most numerous of all circulating marrow cells, as indicated in Table 1.3. Once in circulation, approximately one third are stored in the spleen, which acts as a reservoir and is able to be responsive to emergency demand. Platelets have a lifespan of 10–14 days in circulation.

Platelets are essential for maintaining haemostasis and critical in instigating the clotting cascade to stop haemorrhagic episodes. Platelets have glycoproteins on the surface which enable them to become adhesive following vascular injury and to allow aggregation and enable them to form a platelet plug. When activated, platelets release the contents of their granules into their canalicular system and into the surrounding blood, providing a reactive surface to enable plasma coagulation proteins to be absorbed. The platelets produce two types of granules: dense granules and α-granules. They are listed in Table 1.6.

Thromboxane A2 is a powerful vasoconstrictor and aggregator. It is produced by the platelets and plays a key role in activating other platelets. The actions of the above enable the formation of the platelet plug, which instigates action from the clotting factors.

Table 1.6   Types of granules produced by platelets.

Dense granules	α-granules
Adenosine diphosphate	Platelet factor IV
Adenosine triphosphate	Platelet derived growth factor (PDGF)
Calcium	Von Willebrand factor (vWF)
Serotonin	Heparin antagonist
	Fibrinogen
	Fibronectin
	Coagulation factors V and X111
	β-thromboglobulin

Adapted from (Harrison and Cramer 1993 and George 20υ0).

Through a cascading action clotting factors are activated and along with other substances form a fibrin clot.

Disorders or abnormalities of platelets are known as thrombocytopathy: an increase in platelets is thrombocytosis, a decrease is called thrombocytopenia and a decrease in function is thrombasthenia.

Lymphoid lineage marrow cells

Agranulocytes

Lymphocytes are the second most common white blood cell, with T-lymphocytes constituting approximately 60–80% of circulating lymphocytes, B-lymphocytes making approximately 10–30% and NK cells making up 2–10% (Hughes-Jones *et al.* 2009). Most lymphocytes are generally small, having a diameter of about 10–20 μm, making them larger than erythrocytes but much smaller than monocytes. In lymphocytes the nucleus is round and takes up most of the cell space.

Lymphocytes are found in large numbers in the lymph nodes, spleen, thymus, tonsils and in the Peyer's patches of the gastrointestinal tract. Unlike other blood cells which are unidirectional, some lymphocytes may leave and re-enter the circulation, surviving for about one year or more. The principal paths of re-circulating lymphocytes are through the spleen or lymph nodes (Delves and Roitt 2000). Lymphocytes enable the body to remember antigens and to distinguish self from non-self.

Lymphocytes are derived from the lymphoid multipotent stem cells in the bone marrow and provide acquired immunity. Lymphoid stem cells can divide into T or B-lymphocytes, each carrying out specific functions to defend the body against infections. Both T and B-cells travel between blood and tissues, enabling them to kill invading organisms. Differentiation between T and B-lymphocytes is based on gene rearrangements, cluster differentiation, cell membrane markers and antibody receptors (Kircher and Marquardt 2002).

T-lymphocytes

T-lymphocytes provide cellular mediated immunity and start their development in the bone marrow, continuing their maturity in the thymus gland under the influence of thymosin. T-lymphocytes develop from pro-thymocytes to mature T-lymphoblasts, becoming immunological competent. T-lymphocytes leave the thymus gland and circulate in the bloodstream to the lymph nodes and the spleen. T-lymphocytes, further subdivide into four sub-classes:

- T helper cells (CD4+)
- T suppressor cells (CD8+)
- Cytotoxic T-cell (Tc)
- Natural killer cells (NK cells)

T-lymphocytes recognise and respond to antigens that appear on cell membranes in association with other molecules, known as the major histocompatibility complex (MHC).

They are glycoproteins that present antigens in a form that is recognised by T-lymphocytes. (See Chapter 2 on Immunology and Chapter 20 Haemopoietic stem cell transplant.)

CD4+ helper cells and CD8+ suppressor cells have the responsibility of orchestrating the specific immune response. CD4+ (helper cells) help B-cells to differentiate and mature. They also recognise (MHC) molecules, class II (HLA-D, HLA-DR). CD8+ suppressor cells turn off the immune response, suppress other lymphocyte function and they recognise MHC class I antigens (HLA-A, HLA-B, HLA-C).

Cytotoxic T-cells (Tc) have a number of roles:

- Kill virally infected cells
- Destroy dysfunctional cells
- Destroy malignant cells
- Are responsible for organ rejection in transplantation

Tc cells have receptor sites (T-cell receptors) which recognise MHC class I antigen which are bound to CD8+.

Natural killer cells (NK), as their name suggest, rid the body of any harmful organism. They are cytotoxic and the granules contain proteins such as perforin and proteases (Roitt *et al.* 2001). The difference between Tc and NK cells is that Tc need to recognise antigens and MHC molecules in order to mount an immunological response to get rid of the organism (Papamichail *et al.* 2004). NK cells do not require sensitisation; they are able to lyse antibody coated cells, hence NK cells are also called antibody dependent cytotoxic cells (ADCC) but are also capable of destroying tumour and virally infected cells without presentation by an antibody. Tc and NK cells kill on contact by undergoing blast transformation releasing highly potent lymphokines such as IL-2 which destroys the organism and attract other lymphocytes, thereby increasing killing potential (Symth *et al.* 2001).

Natural killer cells can also become activated in response to interferon, a macrophage derived cytokine, and they 'hold' the virus while the adaptive immune response is generating antigen-specific cytotoxic T-cells that can clear the infection. Ultimately, T-lymphocytes are responsible for continuous surveillance of cell surfaces for the presence of foreign antigens.

B-lymphocytes

B-lymphocytes provide humoral immunity and start and complete their development in the bone marrow. They undergo several stages of development from pre-B progenitor cells to B-lymphoblast. The name B-cell was originally derived from the bursa of Fabricius, an outpouching organ in the gastrointestinal tract found in birds. CD4+ helper cells assist in the differentiation of B-cells aiding in their maturity. Once matured, B-cells migrate in the blood and then enter organs such as the lymph nodes, spleen, marrow, tonsils and appendix. The fundamental function of B-cells is to produce antibodies against antigens. Mature B-cells produce plasma cells which secrete antibodies. B-lymphocytes have many surface receptors enabling them to bind to many antigens. When mature B-cells become sensitised they not only produce plasma cells which secrete distinct antibodies (immunoglobulins) to a specific antigen, they also produce memory cells which are the basis of immunological memory and lead to a more rapid response in the future.

Antibodies are 'Y' monomer structures and there are five classifications: IgG (gamma), IgA (alpha), IgE (Epsilon), IgM (Mu) and IgD (delta). Antibodies can live for many years and carry out a variety of functions including:

- Attacking viruses and bacteria directly
- Activating the complement system
- Inactivating toxic substances
- Helping phagocytic cells

Monocytes

Monocytes are the largest of the marrow cells when matured, almost twice the size of red blood cells, (averaging 15–18 micrometres), and they make up about 7% of the leukocytes. The cytoplasm contains large numbers of fine granules, and they are macrocytic phagocytic cells. In the bone marrow, monocytes develop from CFU-$_M$, differentiating into promonocytes and then to monocytes. The nucleus is relatively big and tends to be indented or folded rather than multilobed. Monocytes leave the bone marrow and circulate in the blood for a few hours and they migrate to tissues, continuing their development. Once in tissues they are then called tissue macrophages. Unlike erythrocytes, macrophages have the capacity for cell division and therefore have a reasonably long life.

Monocytes are highly motile and capable of ingesting infectious agents, red blood cells and other large particles. They usually enter areas of inflamed tissue later than the granulocytes and often they are found at sites of chronic infections.

Macrophages are sited in parts of the body in a strategic manner to fight infection and have particular names and form the reticulo-endothelial system (RES).

Apart from being (see table 1.7) part of the above organs, macrophages are also free wandering cells, providing non-specific immunity and are able to regulate immune responses. Through their ability to phagocytose, they prepare antigens for presentation to T-lymphocytes and enable the antigen-antibody complex which can stimulate B memory cells. They have the ability to produce chemicals known as monokines (Kircher and Marguard 2002).

Table 1.7   Sites of macrophages.

Site	Name
Skin	Langerhans cells
Spleen	Lattoral cells
Liver	Kupffer cells
Lungs	Alveolar macrophages
Brain	Microglia
Bones	Osteoclasts
Kidneys	Glomerulus mesanahgial cells
Lymphoid	Medullary sinus

Apart from their role as scavengers, macrophages play a key role in immunity by ingesting antigens, old faulty cells, microscopic particles and processing them so that they can be recognized as foreign substances by lymphocytes, thereby taking on the role of antigen presenting cells (APC). Macrophages have the ability to ingest not only other cells but also many other microscopic particles.

Conclusion

Haemopoiesis is a fascinating system, involving many complex processes to produce marrow cells. The process takes place within quite narrow margins and it is therefore not surprising that any fault within the system can in some conditions, like acute leukaemia, manifest symptoms quickly.

The continual growth in our understanding of the behaviour and action of stem cells and growth factors will impact on therapeutic modalities.

References

Antonchuk, J., Hyland., C.D, Hilton, D.J. and Alexander, W.S. (2004) Synergistic effects on erythropoiesis, thrombopoiesis and stem cell competitiveness in mice deficient in thrombopoietin and stem cell factor receptors. *Blood*, 104 (5), 1306–1313.

Bain, B. (2004) *A Beginners Guide to Blood Cells*. Blackwell Publishing Ltd, Oxford.

Bainton, D.F. (2001) Morphology of neutrophils, eosinophils and basophils. In: *Williams Hematology*. (eds E. Beutler, M.A. Litchtman, B.S. Coller, T.J. Kipps and U. Seligsohn). 6th edition. pp. 723–743. McGraw Hill, USA.

Beutler, E. (2001) Production and destruction of erythrocytes. In: *Williams Hematology* (eds E.Beutler, M.A.Litchtman, B.S. Coller, T.J. Kipps and U. Seligsohn), 6th edition. McGraw Hill, USA.

Babior, B.M. and Golde, D.W. (2001) Production, distribution and fate of neutrophils. In: *Williams Hematology* (eds E.Beutler, M.A.Litchtman, B.S. Coller, T.J. Kipps and U. Seligsohn), 6th edition. pp. 753–759. McGraw Hill, USA.

Coleman, R.W., Marder, V.J., Clowes, A.W., George, J.N. and Goldhaber, S.Z. (2005) *Hemostasis and Thrombosis; Basic Prinicples and Clinical Practice*, 5th edition. Lipincott. Williams & Wilkins, Hagerstown.

Charras, G.T., Coughlin, M., Mitchison, T.J. and Mahadevan, L. (2008) Life and times of a cellular bleb. *Biophys J.*, 94 (5), 1836–1853.

Delves, P.J. and Roitt, I.M. (2000) The immune system. *New England Journal Medicine*, 343, 37–49, 108–117.

George, J.N. (2000) *Platelets. Lancet.* 355, 1531–1539.

Guo, Y., Lubbert, M. and Engelhardt, M. (2003) C34-haempoietic stem cells: current concepts and controversies. *Stem Cells*, 21, 15–20.

Harrison, P. and Cramer, E. (1993) Platelet alpha-granules. *Blood Rev*, 7 (1), 52–62.

Hoffbrand, A.V., Pettit, J.E. and Moss, P.A.H. (2004) *Essential Haematology*. Blackwell Publishing Ltd, Oxford.

Hughes-Jones, N.C., Wickramasinghe, S.N. and Hatton, C.S.R. (2009) *Lecture Notes – Haematology*, 8th edition. Wiley-Blackwell, Oxford.

Kircher, S. and Marquardt, D. (2002) Introduction to the immune system. In: *Manual of Allergy and Immunology* (eds D.C. Adelman, T.B. Casale and J. Corren), 4th edition. pp. 1–24. Williams & Wilkins, Baltimore.

Kronenwett, R., Martin, S. and Haas, R. (2000) The role of cytokines and adhesion molecules for mobilization of peripheral blood stem cells. *Stem Cells*, 18, 320–330.

Lewis, S.M., Bain, B.J. and Bates, I. (2001) ABC haematology. In: *Practical Haematology* (ed. S.M. Dacie Lewis). Churchill Livingstone, Edinburgh.

Litchtman, M.A., Beutler, E., Kaushansky, K., Kipps, T.J., Seligsohn, U. and Prchal, J. (2005) *Williams Hematology*, 7th edition McGraw-Hill. New York.

Mehta, A.B. and Hoffbrand, V. (2009) *Haematology at a Glance*. Wiley-Blackwell, Oxford.

Metcalf, D. and Nicola, N.A. (1995) *The Hemopoietc Colony – Stimulating Factors: from Biology to Clinical Applications*. Cambridge University Press, Cambridge.

Pallister, C. (1997) *Blood. Physiology and Pathophysiology*. Butterworth-Heinemann, Oxford.

Pallister, C. (2005) *Haematology*. Edward Arnold, Oxford.

Papamichail, M., Perez, S.A., Gritzapis, A.D. and Baxevanis, C.N. (2004) Natural killer lymphocytes: biology, development and function. *Cancer Immunology Immunotherapy*, 53, 176–186.

Queensberry. P.J. and Colvin, G.A. (2001) Hematopoietic stem cells, progenitor cells and cytokines. In: *Williams Hematology* (eds E.Beutler, M.A.Litchtman, B.S. Coller, T.J. Kipps and U. Seligsohn), 6th edition. pp. 153–174. McGraw Hill, USA.

Rich, R.R. Fleisher, T.A., Shearer, W.T., Schroeder, H.W., Frew, A.J. and Weyand, C.M. (2009) *Clinical Immunology: Principles and Practice*. Elsevier, Phildelphia.

Roitt, I.M. (2001) *Essential Immunology*, 10th edition. Blackwell Science, Oxford.

Roitt, I., Brostoff, J. and Male, D. (2001) *Immunology*, 6th ed. p. 480. Mosby, St Louis.

Symth, M.J, Godfrey, D.I. and Trapani, J.A. (2001) A fresh look at tumour immunosurveillance and immunotherapy. *Nature Immunology*, 2 (4), 293–299.

Traynor, B. (2006) Haemopoiesis. In: *Nursing in Haematological Oncology* (ed. M. Grundy). pp. 3–28. Baillière-Tindall Elsevier, London.

Turgeon, M.L. (2005) *Clinical Hematology: Theory and Procedures*, 4th edition. Lippincott Williams and Wilkins, Philadelphia.

Young, B., Lowe, J.S., Stevens, A. and Heath, J.W. (2006), *Wheater's Functional Histology*, 5th edition. Elsevier Limited, Edinburgh.

Yasui, K., Matsumuto,Y., Hirayama, F., Tani, Y. and Nakano,T. (2003) Differences between peripheral blood and cord blood in kinetics of lineage-restricted hematopoiteic cells: implocations for delayed platelet recovery following cord blood transplantation. *Stem Cells*. 21, 143–151.

Chapter 2

Immunology

Jane Richardson and Tracey Cutler

The aim of this chapter is to discuss the physiology of the immune system and how it can be applied in haematology nursing. By the end of reading this chapter you will:

- Have an overview of the immune system
- Be able to consider the impact treatment has on the normal immune response
- Be able to consider the importance of early recognition of infection

---

What does the immune system do?

The internal environment of the body is maintained by homeostasis so that it is warm and moist, with a good supply of nutrients. This is an ideal environment for body cells to grow and to perform their specialist functions efficiently. However, this can also provide suitable conditions in which many types of microorganism are also able to grow and multiply. The immune system acts to resist infection by disease-causing (pathogenic) microorganisms including bacteria, viruses, parasites, fungi and yeast. The immune system may also act to maintain useful bacteria in their appropriate locations.

Friendly bacteria

The human body contains many useful microorganisms (sometimes known as 'friendly' bacteria). In fact, it has been estimated that a typical adult body contains ten times more bacterial cells than body cells (Manas *et al.* 2003). Most of these are symbiotic bacteria that benefit from living in or on the human body, but are also beneficial to it. Most of these bacteria are either on the outside of the body where they colonise the skin surface, oral mucosa and the vaginal mucosa, or in the gut where they colonise the lower intestine, particularly the colon. The gut may contain more than a trillion bacteria from around 400 different species (Hammerman *et al.* 2006). In these locations the friendly bacteria form a

---

Haematology Nursing, First Edition. Marvelle Brown and Tracey J. Cutler.
© 2012 Blackwell Publishing Ltd. Published 2012 by Blackwell Publishing Ltd.

complex ecosystem or microflora which has a variety of health benefits (O'Hara and Shanahan 2006). One major benefit is that the presence of the friendly bacteria inhibit colonisation by pathogenic species. This may be achieved by preventing pathogenic bacteria from attaching to the gut wall or by producing substances that act as local antibiotics (Berger 2002). Resident bacteria may also inhibit pathogens by competing more successfully for space or nutrients, or by producing acid conditions which inhibit the growth of many other species. *Lactobacillus* bacteria on the vaginal mucosa produce acid conditions that inhibit the growth of other microorganisms (Gould and Brooker 2000). Some of the friendly gut bacteria in particular are also helpful as they ferment undigested or partially digested food in the colon, producing useful products such as vitamin K and short chain fatty acids which are absorbed and used (O'Hara and Shanahan 2006).

The use of antibiotics in a patient to kill or inhibit bacteria causing an infection may also kill some of the friendly bacteria. This is likely to disturb the delicate resident bacterial ecosystem. Until the microflora is able to re-establish itself, this is likely to lead to an increased susceptibility to infections in these locations (Berger 2002).

Friendly bacteria are usually only friendly if they remain in the appropriate location in the body. If gut bacteria are able to migrate through the gut wall, for example, they may be able to cause systemic infection. The gut wall is usually protected from invasion by gut bacteria by the single cell layer of the mucosal epithelium (O'Hara and Shanahan 2006) and by the presence of gut-associated lymphoid tissue (GALT) in nodules within the mucosa and submucosa layers (Gibney *et al.* 2003; Stagg *et al.* 2003) (see Figure 2.1).

This is particularly relevant to patients who are undergoing radiotherapy and/or chemotherapy for haematological malignancies as two of the side effects (of radiotherapy and chemotherapy) are bone marrow suppression and mucositis (Chapel *et al.* 2007). Damage to the mucosal epithelial barrier can lead to mucositis. If mucositis occurs in the gastrointestinal mucosa there may be an increased risk of infection by normal gut flora passing through the usually intact barrier (Sonis 2004). For this reason many treatment protocols advocate the use of broad spectrum antibiotics as prophylactic cover against infection whilst the patient is neutropenic (NICE 2003). However, this will also disturb the normal bacterial microflora.

Friendly bacteria are present in many food products such as yogurt and are widely eaten. Some studies have shown that yogurt consumption is beneficial to gut health (Adolfsson *et al.* 2004). Many new food products also contain prebiotics and probiotics to enhance gut health. Prebiotics are food ingredients that pass through the small intestine and into the colon where they provide a nutrient source to enhance the growth and development of friendly bacteria species such as *Bifidobacteria* and *Lactobacillus*. This boosts the natural populations of gut bacteria and may help to re-establish the microflora if it has become disturbed during an infection or following treatment. Probiotics are foods containing friendly bacteria. They may be useful to reduce diarrhoea associated with antibiotic use (Adolfsson *et al.* 2004) by enhancing natural immunity and accelerating the recolonisation of the gut after antibiotic therapy.

This is an important issue to consider when patients are undergoing chemotherapy or radiotherapy as there is some debate whether patients who are receiving broad spectrum antibiotics need to have a restricted (low microbial) diet. The opinion is that the broad spectrum antibiotics will also affect the 'friendly' bacteria, lowering the

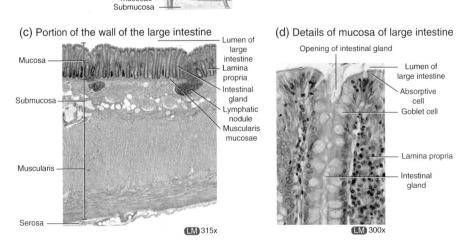

(a) Three-dimensional view of layers of the large intestine

Lumen of large intestine

Openings of intestinal glands

Simple columnar epithelium

Intestinal gland

Lamina propria

MUCOSA

Lymphatic nodule

Muscularis mucosae
Lymphatic vessel
Arteriole
Venule
Circular layer of muscle
Myenteric plexus
Longitudinal layer of muscle

SUBMUCOSA

MUSCULARIS

SEROSA

(b) Sectional view of intestinal glands and cell types

Openings of intestinal glands

Lamina propria

Microvilli

Intestinal gland

Absorptive cell (absorbs water)

Goblet cell (secretes mucus)

Lymphatic nodule

Muscularis mucosae
Submucosa

(c) Portion of the wall of the large intestine

Mucosa

Submucosa

Muscularis

Serosa

Lumen of large intestine
Lamina propria
Intestinal gland
Lymphatic nodule
Muscularis mucosae

LM 315x

(d) Details of mucosa of large intestine

Opening of intestinal gland

Lumen of large intestine

Absorptive cell

Goblet cell

Lamina propria

Intestinal gland

LM 300x

Figure 2.1   Diagram to show the structure of the gut wall in the large intestine (from Tortora and Grabowski 2000). Reprinted with permission of John Wiley & Sons, Inc.

body's natural defences. Foods which are thought to be an issue are the ones avoided during pregnancy, for example live yoghurts and soft cheeses.

Many friendly bacteria are also present on the skin surface, where they may protect it from pathogens. The resident microflora may include species that are harmless when carried on the surface of healthy skin, but may cause infection if they are able to penetrate the skin surface, for example through a wound (Chiller *et al.* 2001). The skin surface can also support the growth of pathogens such as *Staphylococcus aureus* and *Streptococcus pyogenes*.

Haematology patients will require regular blood tests, bone marrow aspiration and trephine biopsies. If they require treatment, cannulation will be a necessity and, if treatment is long term, central venous access devices (CVAD) may be inserted. All of these procedures will break the intact skin barrier and therefore all require strict aseptic technique to prevent the entry of pathogens (Wilkes and Barton-Burke 2008). CVADs also increase the risk of infection as they are often *in situ* long term, which provides the potential for entry of pathogens directly into the bloodstream.

Innate immunity

There are two types of immunity that interact to protect the body. These are:

- Innate (natural) immunity
- Acquired (specific) immunity

Innate (inborn) immunity, as its name suggests, is present from birth. It is genetically determined and is due to a number of non-specific mechanisms that interact to protect the body from a variety of threats from the environment, including microorganisms. It consists of two lines of defence: the barriers and cellular mechanisms.

The barriers to infection

The body is protected by a system of physical and chemical barriers that prevent microorganisms from entering into its interior. The most important of these is healthy intact skin as there are very few microorganisms that are able to penetrate through this physical barrier. Skin cells are protected by the presence of the protein keratin and their continuous loss by shedding at the surface removes microorganisms (Chiller *et al.* 2003). Sebaceous and sweat glands in the skin produce acid secretions which can inhibit bacterial growth, while the skin surface microflora inhibits the growth of pathogens (see previous section) (see Figure 2.2).

At openings through the skin such as the oral cavity, the vagina, the urethra and the respiratory openings, body surfaces are protected by mucous membranes. Epithelial cells line these openings and cells divide rapidly to repair any damage and to maintain the integrity of the barrier. In addition, mucus traps debris including microorganisms and can be removed, for example by swallowing, or by the action of cilia sweeping it up to the throat where it is swallowed, or by the cough reflex. The body is also protected by the antibacterial enzyme lysozyme which is present in saliva, sweat, tears and nasal secretions.

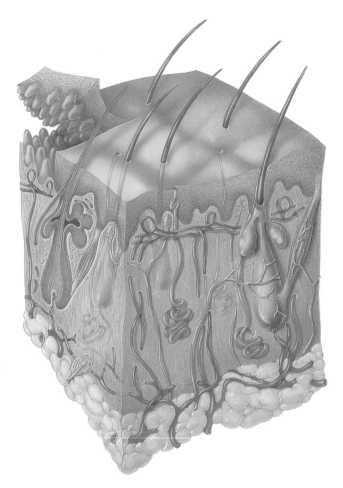

Figure 2.2   The structure of the skin (from Tortora and Grabowski 2000). Reprinted with permission of John Wiley & Sons, Inc.

Saliva also continuously washes food debris and bacteria from the oral cavity to limit pathogen growth and prevent oral infection. The presence of digestive enzymes and low pH of gastric acid secretions in the stomach, and high pH of bile in the small intestine provide environments that protect the intestines from bacterial contamination in food and drink.

Radiotherapy and chemotherapy can reduce saliva production. This side effect affects the natural defence causing dryness and soreness as the natural lubrication is reduced and the acidity of the oral cavity increases. It is important to assess the oral cavity regularly for the amount of saliva and early signs of mucositis as this can cause ulceration of the mucosa and also entry of pathogens.

Proton pump inhibitors are used within treatment regimes to reduce the gastric reflux often experienced by patients. These medications will reduce the amount of gastric secretions, which will also reduce the protection.

Cellular mechanisms

If microorganisms penetrate the external surface of the body, the second line of innate defence occurs due to the activities of various immune cells to limit the spread to prevent widespread or systemic infection. The immune response is often enhanced by an increased body temperature, which may inhibit the growth of microorganisms while it enhances the activity of the immune system (McCance and Huether 2005).

The second line of defence involves many types of leucocyte (see Chapter 1) and some plasma proteins including:

- Neutrophils and mast cells
- Monocytes and macrophages
- Natural killer (NK) cells
- The complement system

Neutrophils, monocytes and macrophages (see Chapter 1) are able to destroy microorganisms by ingesting and killing them by phagocytosis (see Figure 2.3). This process is more efficient if the microorganisms are coated with antibodies or complement proteins.

Neutrophils   are the most numerous leucocytes in the blood and are important phagocytes, especially during the initial stages of an infection. They are usually the first type of white blood cell to arrive at the site of an infection, where they may be able to limit its spread by removing pathogens by phagocytosis. Neutrophils then die and the resultant mixture of dead bacteria and neutrophils forms pus (McCance and Huether 2005). Neutrophils are very short-lived (7–48 hours) and are constantly replaced by division of stem cells in the bone marrow. Rapidly dividing cells are vulnerable to chemotherapy damage and so this process may be impaired following chemotherapy. Therefore fewer neutrophils are produced and this results in neutropenia (a white count of less than $1.5 \times 10^9/L$ (Chapel *et al.* 2006). Patients with neutropenia are unable to protect themselves effectively against microorganisms and so infections are common. The infection site will not resolve and pus will not form until the neutrophils are replenished. This is commonly seen in practice when CVADs become infected; pus will not be present until the neutrophil count recovers.

Mast cells   are found in the tissues and are derived from basophils in the blood (see Chapter 1). Mast cells are involved in the initiation of the inflammatory response as they release inflammatory mediators following infection or tissue damage.

Monocytes   are present in the blood and can destroy microorganisms by phagocytosis. They can also migrate into the tissues where they may mature to form fixed resident macrophages in tissues such the liver, alveoli, spleen and bone marrow. Monocytes circulate in the blood and arrive more slowly than neutrophils at sites of infection, where they mature into macrophages.

Macrophages   are the main phagocytes present during the later stages of inflammation. They are able to survive and divide at the infection site for long periods of time (McCance and Huether 2005).

(a) Phases of phagocytosis

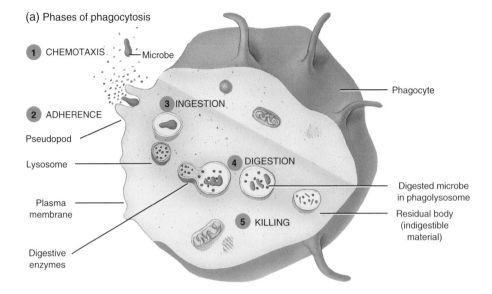

(b) Phagocyte (white blood cell) engulfing a microbe.

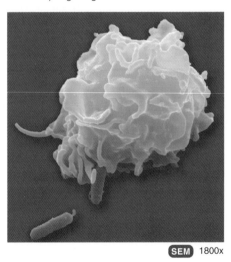

SEM 1800x

Figure 2.3   Phagocytosis (from Tortora and Grabowski 2000). Reprinted with permission of John Wiley & Sons, Inc.

Natural killer (NK) cells   are large granular white blood cells that resemble lymphocytes and are mainly found in the peripheral blood and spleen. As the name suggests, they have an innate ability to recognise and kill cells that have become altered, such as infected cells, especially virus infected cells, and some tumour cells (Martini and Nath 2009). They are 'natural' killer cells as they are able to do this without prior exposure to them (in contrast to the actions of lymphocytes below). Natural killer cells are responsible for constant checking of body cells for abnormalities; this is known as immune surveillance.

Natural killer cells release cytokines such as gamma interferon (IFN-γ) which stimulates macrophages (Martini and Nath 2009).

The complement system is a system of plasma proteins that contribute to inflammation and bacterial killing. The name refers to the way they *complement* the activities of antibodies. There are two main ways to activate the complement cascade: the classical and alternative pathways (Coico and Sunshine 2009).

The classical pathway is activated by an antibody attached to an antigen on a bacterial cell wall. This activates the first component C1. This activates a series of other complement proteins (C4, C2, C3 and C5) and promotes inflammation. During this process, bacteria also become coated with complement protein fragments that enhance their removal by phagocytosis. This is known as opsonisation (McCance and Huether 2005).

The alternative pathway is activated by the polysaccharides on bacterial cell walls and results in activation of components C3 and C5. Once C5 is activated, this activates C6, C7, C8 and C9, forming a complex that can puncture bacterial cell walls causing bacterial death (Martini and Nath 2009).

Inflammation

Inflammation is a major component of the second line of defence. It is a local response that occurs immediately after tissue damage or infection. The four signs of inflammation are redness, heat, swelling and pain. The main stages of inflammation may be summarised as:

- Trauma causes the degranulation of mast cells in the tissues, which releases histamine and other inflammatory mediators.
- Histamine promotes vasodilation and increased permeability of blood vessels in the area.
- Initially, neutrophils are attracted to the area of trauma and remove micro-organisms by phagocytosis resulting in pus formation.
- Later, macrophages arrive at the area and continue to remove microorganisms and damaged tissue by phagocytosis.

Neutropenic patients will have a delayed inflammatory response; this delay can allow the pathogens time to replicate and colonise an area which means that local infections can very easily become systemic and life threatening.

Pyrexia of unknown origin is often the first sign of a systemic inflammatory response in neutropenic patients; it is important to consider the neutropenia policy (DoH 2004) in practice areas as this will highlight diagnostic procedures and the use of antipyretics in the home setting. These medications are often avoided as they will prevent the early identification of a systemic infection.

Acquired (specific) immunity

Acquired or specific immunity is immunity that is gained after birth by exposure to foreign antigens that provoke a specific immune response. This initial response leads to immunological memory. This means that a person may have to become infected with a disease first in order to become immune to it.

This type of immunity is mediated by a particular type of white blood cell, the *lymphocyte*. Lymphocytes are long-lived white blood cells (see Chapter 1) which are found in the blood, spleen, lymph and in lymph nodes. They originate in the bone marrow but can subsequently mature into one of two main types depending on the final site of their maturation: *B-lymphocytes* and *T-lymphocytes*. These two types of lymphocyte are responsible for the two main types of acquired immunity: *humoral immunity* (antibody mediated immunity) and *cellular immunity* (cell mediated immunity) respectively.

B-lymphocytes probably remain in the bone marrow while they mature and are subsequently released into the blood and lymph system. B-lymphocytes (or B-cells) are responsible for the production of antibodies in response to antigens and are therefore responsible for *humoral immunity* which is immunity due to the presence of specific antibodies (or immunoglobulins) in body fluids.

Each B-lymphocyte is able to recognise and respond to one specific antigen. When it encounters this antigen it is stimulated to divide and mature further. The resultant clone of cells either differentiates into plasma cells or memory cells. Plasma cells each produce the same specific antibody to the original stimulating antigen, while memory cells remain ready to respond quickly if the same antigen is encountered again (Coico and Sunshine 2009).

T-lymphocytes (T-cells) are initially produced in the bone marrow, but subsequently move to the thymus gland to complete their maturation and develop their specificity (Coico and Sunshine 2009). T-lymphocytes are each specific for a particular type of antigen present on a body cell surface. When they encounter the specific antigen they can also multiply to form a clone and some are able to directly kill the body cell with the altered antigen. This is known as *cellular immunity*.

Both types of lymphocyte are able to respond to specific *antigens*. Antigens are molecules that can bind specifically to lymphocytes. Lymphocytes are able to distinguish between molecules that are normally present within that individual's body (self-antigens) and those that are 'foreign'. Self-antigens do not provoke an immune response as lymphocytes usually only respond to foreign antigens (Coico and Sunshine 2009).

Autoimmune conditions are those in which the lymphocytes mistakenly respond to self-antigens. Several haematological diseases are thought to be at least partly due to autoimmunity, including:

- Autoimmune haemolytic anaemia
- Autoimmune neutropenia
- Immune thrombocytopenia purpura

Antigens are usually large, complex, 'foreign' molecules and are often present on the surface of microorganisms such as bacteria. When microorganisms enter body cells they may be phagocytosed by macrophages. The bacterial antigens are then processed and attached to the surface of the macrophages where they are able to stimulate an immune response in both B and T-lymphocytes. These macrophages are known as antigen-presenting cells (APC).

Mature lymphocytes are thought to be produced by *clonal selection*. According to this theory, a rearrangement of genes occurs during maturation of individual lymphocytes giving them individual antigen specificity. Therefore each mature lymphocyte is able to reproduce rapidly in response to one specific antigen. Lymphocytes that can respond to self-antigens are thought to be inactivated during this process (Coico and Sunshine 2009).

Humoral immunity

During B-lymphocyte maturation, rearrangement of antibody genes occurs so that each cell only produces one specific type of antibody. When a B-lymphocyte is first released from the bone marrow it displays this specific type of antibody on its membrane surface as an antigen receptor; but antibody is not released from the cell at this stage. The antigen receptor is shaped so that only a specific type of antigen is able to attach to it. The receptor has antigen-binding sites that have a specific shape that is complementary to that of the antigen. Specific antigen is able to slot into the antigen-binding sites, like a key fits into a lock.

Antigens on the surface of infecting microorganisms may meet a B-lymphocyte with a specific receptor for their antigens in a lymph node. The attachment of the specific antigen onto the antigen receptor stimulates the B-cell to undergo further cell divisions forming a clone of cells that develop into *plasma cells* that are able to produce and release specific antibody.

As the number of specific B-lymphocytes multiplies, this may make the lymph gland feel enlarged and painful. During this time, the infecting microorganisms, may also have multiplied and could cause disease symptoms. After a few days plasma cells are able to produce and release the same specific antibody into the plasma. The released antibodies circulate around the body and are able to attach to any specific antigens on the microorganisms and this leads to their clearance and recovery occurs. Antibodies attach onto antigens on the surface of microorganisms and this eliminates them in a number of ways; it enhances phagocytosis (opsonisation), it may immobilise them, it may stick them together (agglutinate them) and it may neutralise toxins released by certain bacteria. After recovery, the antigen is removed from the body and some of the plasma cells become *memory cells* which remain in the body primed and ready to respond rapidly should the antigen be encountered again.

Scientists are able to stimulate *individual* B-lymphocytes in the laboratory to multiply and produce antibodies. As each B-lymphocyte is able to produce one specific type of antibody, these multiply to form a clone of identical B-cells that mature to produce the same specific single type of antibody. These can be tested clinically and growth of particular clones can be used to produce therapeutic *monoclonal antibodies* such as rituximab, used in the treatment of B-cell lymphoma (see Chapter 19).

Antibodies (or immunoglobulins) circulate around the body in the plasma and are a major part of a group of plasma proteins known as *gamma globulins*. Some patients have an X-linked inherited condition in which they are unable to produce B mature lymphocytes and therefore do not have plasma antibodies or gammaglobulins. This condition is known as Bruton's agammaglobilinaemia (Coico and Sunshine 2009). This condition is more common in boys as it is carried on the X chromosome, while girls tend to be carriers. Without circulating antibodies these patients are prone to recurrent infections and may be treated with IV immunoglobulin (Ig) and antibiotics.

Other children may have recurrent infections such as sinusitis or tonsillitis due to a deficiency of antibodies. This results in low levels of antibody in the plasma or hypogammaglobulinaemia. In children this may present as a failure to thrive. If the same microorganism with the same antigens on its surface is encountered again, its antigens will be immediately recognised by the large number of circulating memory cells. They are able to respond quickly by multiplying and antibody levels rise rapidly, eliminating the infectious organism before symptoms develop. The person is then said to be immune to that specific type of infection.

Immunisations are used to provoke the body into producing specific plasma cells and memory cells without the person having to have a disease. Immunisations usually involve introducing antigens into the body to provoke an immune response, but they are introduced in a form that cannot cause disease. Vaccines may include weakened (attenuated) microorganisms that are no longer pathogenic, dead microorganisms or sometimes purified cell walls that also include the antigens.

Cell-mediated immunity

This type of immunity is carried out by T-lymphocytes which are released from the thymus gland. When T-lymphocytes mature in the thymus, gene rearrangements occur that are responsible for the formation of a specific cell surface receptor. Each T-cell is able to respond to one specific type of foreign antigen present on a body cell surface. Body cells may have foreign antigens on their surface if they are infected, cancer or transplanted cells. If the antigens are recognised as foreign, then the T-cells will mount an immune response and the body cells may be killed.

T-lymphocytes are usually able to distinguish normal body cells from infected, cancer or transplanted cells. They are able to do this as everybody's cells have proteins on their surface that identify them. These are known as MHC proteins (major histocompatibility complex) or HLA proteins (human leucocyte antigens) and they give cells their tissue type.

Major Histocompatibility Complex (MHC)

There are two main types of MHC proteins present on the surface of body cells:

- MHC class I proteins are present on all body cells except red blood cells (all cells with nuclei) and are involved in rejection of foreign tissue.
- MHC class II proteins are present on lymphocytes, macrophages, monocytes and antigen presenting cells.
- The MHC class I and class II proteins allow the cells to distinguish self from non-self and probably influence the immune response of an individual (Coico and Sunshine 2009).

MHC proteins are determined by a cluster of at least six genes that are present close together on the short arm of chromosome 6. Each gene exists in many different versions (alleles). This means that no two people have exactly the same combination of MHC genes and therefore no two people have the same tissue type (except identical twins); though close relatives are more likely to have a similar tissue type that two people from the general population (Martini and Nath 2009).

Haematology patients often receive transfusions of blood, platelets, clotting factors, monoclonal antibodies and in some cases haemopoietic stem cells from a donor. These treatments can all be recognised as foreign, therefore potential for rejection and risk of anaphylaxis is carried out prior to infusion.

Graft versus host reactions can occur where a patient has had an allogeneic haemopoietic stem cell transplant (HSCT) especially if the graft is not fully HLA matched, as the immune cells in the *transplant* can become activated and mount an immune response against the body cells of the patient that has received the transplant.

Prior to allogeneic haematopoietic bone marrow transplant the patient and donor are tissue typed and the donor will be a matched donor. This means that the donor is chosen as they have similar MHC antigens to that of the patient. This reduces the ability of the new marrow's T-lymphocytes to recognise the patient's cells as foreign and therefore reduces the immune reaction against them. However, patients and transplanted bone marrow can never be a perfect match (unless the donor and patient are identical twins!) and therefore the patient will also require immunosuppressant therapy to reduce the risks of rejection.

While they are maturing and differentiating in the thymus, T-cells also produce membrane proteins called cluster of differentiation (CD) receptors. There are many different types of CD receptors found on T-cell surfaces and they are often associated with different types of T-lymphocyte. For example, CD4 protein is found on helper T-cells (see below) where it allows the cells to adhere to class II MHC antigens. CD8 protein is found on cytotoxic T-cells and suppressor T-cells (see below), where it allows binding to class I MHC molecules (Martini and Nath 2009).

T-cells are activated by specific antigens when they are found on the surface of body cells in combination with MHC antigens. When stimulated, activated T-cells enlarge and proliferate to form a clone of T-cells which can then differentiate into a number of different subtypes: cytotoxic T-cells (T_C), helper T-cells (T_H), suppressor T-cells (T_S) and memory T-cells. The different subtypes of T-cell each have a different role in the immune response.

Role of T-cell subtypes in the immune response

Cytotoxic T-cells (or killer T-cells) have a CD8 receptor on their surface and when activated can release toxins that can kill body cells. *Helper T-cells* have protein CD4 on their surface. They release factors that stimulate T and B-cells to multiply once they have been activated by antigen. There are two types of T helper cell: T_H1 and T_H2. T_H1 cells interact with Tc cells and macrophages and enhance their activity. T_H2 cells stimulate the antibody formation by activated B-lymphocytes. *Suppressor T-cells* have CD8 on their surface and when activated release factors that slow the immune response to control and contain it. *Memory T_C cells* remain in the body for long periods of time and are responsible for immunological memory. When they are activated by antigen on body cells they immediately differentiate into killer T-cells (Martini and Nath 2009).

Helper T-cells can themselves become infected by HIV (human immunodeficiency virus) as it is able to bind to the CD4 receptor and then enter the cells. Like all viruses, HIV uses its host cell to multiply itself; in the process the helper T-cells are weakened and may die. HIV is released into the plasma and can infect surrounding helper T-cells. If the infection is not controlled by drug therapy, numbers of helper T-cells decline, as the cell is no longer able to stimulate other activated lymphocytes. The whole immune system is weakened and the patient becomes prone to recurrent infections (Coico and Sunshine 2009).

Some patients may be born with SCID (severe combined immunodeficiency diseases). These patients have an inherited deficiency in both antibody production and cell-mediated immunity and are therefore prone to develop all types of infection and are unable to develop immunity (Coico and Sunshine 2009). These patients need to be maintained in a sterile environment and may be treated with HLA-matched haemopoietic stem cell transplant.

The immune response

Few antigens can initiate an immune response in isolation: in most cases immune responses occur due to interactions between a variety of cell types. Microorganisms with antigens on their surface are ingested by often interacting first with a phagocyte. This could occur in the spleen or regional lymph node, depending on the route of entry of the pathogen, or it could also occur in the skin or mucous membranes. As a result of this, some of the pathogen's antigens appear on the surface of the macrophage, which then acts as an *antigen-presenting cell (APC)*. The antigens presented on the APC may then stimulate a helper T-cell (T_H) which in turn stimulates specific B-cells to multiply and produce antibodies. The T_H cell may also stimulate cytotoxic T-cells (Tc) to mount a cell mediated response. The immune response therefore involves a great deal of communication between cells and this is mediated by cell signals called *cytokines* (Coico and Sunshine 2009).

Cytokines produced by lymphocytes are known as *lymphokines*, those produced by monocytes are *monokines* (see Table 2.1 of common cytokines in use). Interleukins (IL) are cytokines produced by lymphocytes or macrophages in response to antigens.

The activity of the immune system is affected by a wide variety of factors and it tends to decrease with increasing age. T-cell and B-cell functions decline, while the production of autoantibodies may increase. This is also an important consideration when searching for a haemopoietic stem cell donor as older donors and females who have given birth may

Table 2.1 Common cytokines in use.

Interferon α	Antiproliferative and immunomodulatory	Used in CML, MM and ALL
Interleukin 2	Amplify the immune response to an antigen	Trialled in AML
G-CSF	Naturally occurring glycoproteins, which stimulate proliferation, differentiation and maturation of cells	Reduction of neutropenic episodes Collection of haemopoietic stem cells

increase the risk of graft versus host disease. The immune response is also affected by stress as it is inhibited by stress hormones such as cortisol. Nutrition plays a key role in immunity. Patients who are undernourished or lack key nutrients such as protein in the diet are likely to produce a less robust and less efficient immune response. For this reason it is important to consider the nutritional status of the patient at time of diagnosis. Proliferative disorders can cause hypermetabolic cell production which has an impact on weight loss especially affecting protein/muscle loss. Referral to a dietician is imperative to monitor and increase dietary protein intake.

Conclusion

Any disease or treatment which affects the production or function of the haemopoietic system will also cause an effect on the immunological process. Whether this is the proliferation of immature cells, use of broad spectrum antibiotics, insertion of CVADs or the destruction of cells. The nurse caring for these patients will need an understanding of the immunological effect so that action can be taken to identify the first signs of infection, and treatment can be initiated before life-threatening sepsis occurs.

References

Adolfsson, O., Meydani, S.N. and Russell, R.M. (2004) Yogurt and gut function. *American Journal of Clinical Nutrition*, 80 (2), 245–256.

Berger, A. (2002) Science commentary: probiotics. *British Medical Journal*, 324, 8.

Chapel, H., Haeney, M., Misbah, S. and Snowden, N. (2006) *Essentials of Clinical Immunology*, 5th edition. Blackwell Publishing Ltd, Oxford.

Chiller, K., Selkin, B. and Murakawa, G. (2001) Skin microflora and bacterial infections of the skin. *Journal of Investigative Dermatology Symposium Proceedings*, 6, 170–174.

Coico, R. and Sunshine, G. (2009) *Immunology: a Short Course*. Wiley-Blackwell, New Jersey.

Department of Health (2004) *Manual of Cancer Standards*. DoH, London.

Gibney, M.J., MacDonald, A. and Roche, H.M. (2003) *Nutrition and Metabolism*. Blackwell, Oxford.

Gould, D. and Brooker, C. (2000) *Applied Microbiology for Nurses*. Macmillan, Basingstoke.

Hammerman, C., Bin-Nun, A. and Kaplan, M. (2006) Safety of probiotics: comparison of two popular strains. *British Medical Journal*, 333, 1006–1008.

Manas, M., Martinez de Victoria, E., Gil, A., Yago, M. and Mathers, J. (2003) The gastrointestinal tract. In: *Nutrition and Metabolism* (eds M.J. Gibney, A. MacDonald and H.M. Roche). Blackwell Publishing Ltd, Oxford.

Martini, F. and Nath, J. (2009) *Fundamentals of Anatomy and Physiology*. Pearson, San Francisco.

McCance, K. and Huether, S. (2005) *Pathophysiology: the Biologic Basis of Disease in Adults and Children*. Mosby, St Louis.

McCarthy, H. (2001) Childhood immunisation. *Nursing Standard*, 15, 44, 39–44.

National Institute for Clinical Excellence (2003) *Guidance on Cancer Services: Improving Outcomes in Haematological Cancers. The Manual*. NICE, London.

O'Hara, A. and Shanahan, F. (2006) The gut flora as a forgotten organ. *EMBO Reports*, 7 (7), 688–693.

Sadler, J.E. (2006) Update on the pathophysiology and classification of von Willebrand disease: a report of the subcommittee on von Willebrand Factor. *Journal of Thrombosis and Haemostasis*, 4, 2103–2114.

Sonis, S. (2004) The pathobiology of mucositis. *National Review of Cancer*, 4 (4), 277–284,

Stagg, A., Hart, A., Knight, S. and Kamm, M. (2003) The dendritic cell: its role in intestinal inflammation and relationship with gut bacteria. *Gut*, 52, 1522–1529.

Tortora, G. and Grabowski, S. (2000) *Principles of Anatomy and Physiology*, 9th edition. John Wiley and Sons, Chichester.

Wilkes, G.M. and Barton-Burke, M. (2008) *Oncology Nursing Drug Handbook*. Jones and Bartlett, London.

Chapter 3

Genes and haematology

Gwyneth Morgan

This chapter is a broad overview of genetic concepts and their application in haematology. The aim of this chapter is to provide an introduction to basic genetics and genetic mutations in haematological disease. By the end of reading this chapter you will:

- Have an overview of genetics
- Be familiar with DNA replication and the formation of proteins
- Understand the mode of inheritance patterns
- See how genes play a major role in haematology

---

23 pairs of chromosomes, 3.2 billion base pairs and 31,000ish genes, the completion of the first draft of the human genome sequence announced in June 2000 confirmed our existing knowledge, but also introduced many new facts and some surprises (Dennis and Gallagher 2001).

The human genome is our genetic make-up; it is the information inherited from our parents which in part shapes our life. Activities such as fighting infection require elaborate patterns of gene interaction in order to start the inflammatory process. Our genes do not work in isolation but are highly coordinated controllers of information which enable our cells to function. A startling result of the human genome project was that our genome is 99.9% identical to everyone else's. This 0.1% of uniqueness influences our individual behaviour, vulnerability to disease and response to medication, and of course within families even this 0.1% has similarities (Dennis and Gallagher 2001).

Although all cells of the human body have similar basic structures there are a range of differences, for example skin, muscle and liver cells, and yet each of the 200 different human cells contains the same genetic information. It is the selective expression of this information through the switching on and off of genes that provides the variety or differentiation (Jones *et al.* 2001). Changes in this mechanism can result in cells not functioning properly, for example losing their differentiation and/or taking on inappropriate functions, which may occur in cells that are malignant.

Haematology Nursing, First Edition. Marvelle Brown and Tracey J. Cutler.
© 2012 Blackwell Publishing Ltd. Published 2012 by Blackwell Publishing Ltd.

Overview of chromosomes, genes and DNA

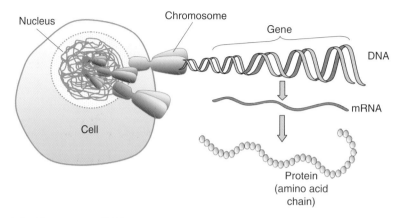

Figure 3.1   Chromosome DNA genes. Reproduced from an original by Roger McFadden.

The normal human chromosome complement or karyotype consists of 46 chromosomes made up of 44 autosomes and 2 sex chromosomes XX in normal females and XY in normal males. Most cells of the human body contain these 46 chromosomes which are two matched sets of chromosomes, one set from each parent known as the diploid number, whilst gametes contain only 23, the haploid number, a single set of unpaired chromosomes (see Figure 3.1).

By convention the number of chromosomes is given first, followed by the types of sex chromosomes, followed by the types of any additional missing or abnormal chromosomes (see Figure 3.2). For example:

46XX (normal female)
46XY (normal male)
47XY +21 (male with trisomy 21 example: 3 number 21 chromosomes)

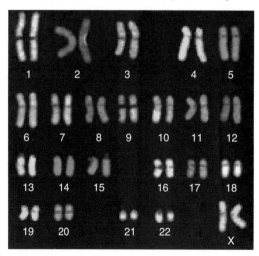

Figure 3.2   Normal female karyotype (Brown 2003). Reprinted with permission of John Wiley & Sons, Inc.

Each chromosome is divided into long and short arms by a specialised area of the chromosome known as the centromere. The short arm is abbreviated to *p* and the long arm to *q* (see Figure 3.3).

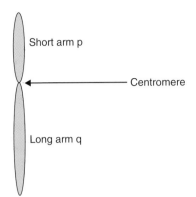

Short arm p

Centromere

Long arm q

Figure 3.3 A chromosome. normal female karyotype in – Strachan T & Read AP (2001) Human Molecular genetics (2nd edition) John Wiley & Sons, Inc.

Every chromosome in a cell is now known to contain many genes, but rather less in number than was first thought. Initially it was thought that because of the complexity of humans the human genome would contain a vast number of genes, but the number of human genes amounts to just twice the number of genes of the fruit fly, one of the surprises from sequencing the human genome (Dennis and Gallagher 2001).

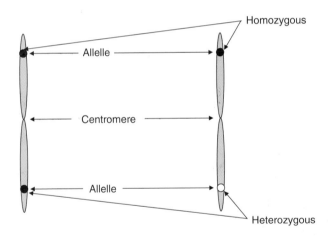

Homozygous

Allele

Centromere

Allele

Heterozygous

Figure 3.4 Chromosome alleles.

Because chromosomes are paired, everyone carries two copies of each gene, with the exception of genes carried on the sex chromosomes in males. Each gene is located at a particular site known as the locus on the chromosome. Genes on the same locus are known as alleles. If two alleles at a locus are identical the individual is said to be homozygous at that locus. If the two alleles are non-identical then the individual is said to be heterozygous (see Figure 3.4).

A person's genetic make-up, that is whether one is homozygous or heterozygous for the various gene pairs is referred to as their genotype. Genes influence our physical characteristics—such as eye colour, height and hair colour, as well as our susceptibility to some illnesses. These visible characteristics are known as the person's phenotype (Marieb and Hoehn 2007).

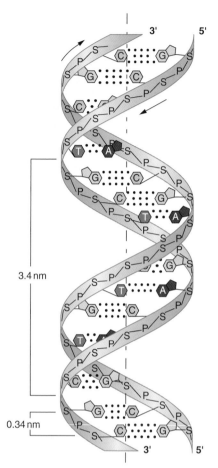

3.4 nm

0.34 nm

Figure 3.5   Double Helix structure of DNA (Snustad 2012). Reprinted with permission of John Wiley & Sons, Inc.

Each gene is composed of sections of deoxyribonucleic acid (DNA) strands, presented in a double helix arrangement (see Figure 3.5). The basic unit of DNA is composed of a sugar molecule, a phosphate molecule and a nitrogenous base. The base is the information carrying element and there are four of them: thymine, adenine, guanine and cytosine, abbreviated to T, A, G, C the four letters of the genetic alphabet. An important aspect of DNA is the way in which the pairs of bases are held together: A only pairs with T, and C only with G. These arrangements are known as base pairs. The base pairs are held together by hydrogen bonds this is the weakest of the chemical bonds.

Human genes vary in size, ranging from 1606 base pairs for genes coding for β globin and 2.4 million base pairs coding for dystrophin. Dystrophin is a protein found in muscle that is missing in people with muscular dystrophy.

DNA carries the instructions for making particular proteins. Proteins are the building blocks of cells, providing their structure, enzymes and signalling molecules to coordinate cellular activity. When a cell is making a protein the gene is said to be 'switched on' or 'expressed' or 'active'. What makes each cell function differently is which genes are switched on or off.

From DNA to protein

The four letters of the DNA alphabet are translated into the 22 different amino acids. How these amino acids are arranged determines which protein is made (see Figure 3.6). DNA bases are grouped into three, called a codon. For example the sequence GAG codes for the amino acid glutamic acid and GTC for valine. The genetic code is therefore a series of three base codons that provide information for the order in which to string amino acids together and the order of the amino acids on the string makes a particular protein. Changing the order of the bases changes the order of the amino acids and therefore the protein. Just like any language where several words mean the same thing so there is more than one codon for an amino acid. For example GTT, GTC, GTA and GTG all code for valine.

The process of making proteins is not quite as simple as DNA to protein; there is an intermediary messenger ribonucleic acid (mRNA) (please see Chapter 4 for further information). RNA is very similar to a single strand of DNA, except that it has one different base; instead of thymine the base is uracil, abbreviated as U. DNA is therefore transcribed into RNA like a photocopier making lots of copies but keeping the original safe; RNA is then translated into strings of amino acid which is the specific protein.

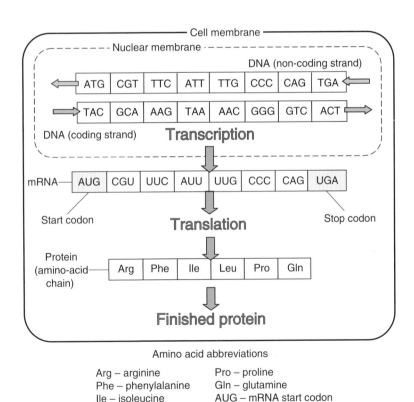

Amino acid abbreviations

Arg – arginine
Phe – phenylalanine
Ile – isoleucine
Leu – leucine

Pro – proline
Gln – glutamine
AUG – mRNA start codon
UGA – mRNA stop codon

Figure 3.6 From DNA to protein. Reproduced from an original by Roger McFadden.

Not all these DNA codons are transcribed. Just like a sentence in English there are punctuations that if not used would not change the sentence. Some codons are start commands like a capital letter and some are stop codons like a full stop, the sequence of DNA is therefore much longer than the sequence of mRNA. Some genes make more than one protein. This can be done by splicing together different lengths of base pairs, so there are many more proteins than there are genes (see Figure 3.7).

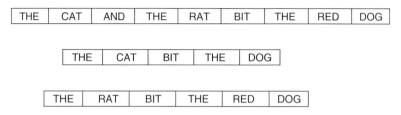

By including different words in the sequence many sentences can be made; this is similar to how one gene can code for many different proteins.

Figure 3.7 One gene, many proteins. DNA in Strachan T & Read AP (2001) Human Molecular genetics (2nd edition) – John Wiley & Sons, Inc.

Gene mutations

Any change to the sequence of the base pairs on the strand of DNA is a mutation in that gene. Fortunately these typographic errors are harmless if they do not occur in parts of the DNA that contain instructions for making proteins, or because they make no difference to the eventual amino acid sequence. Sometimes, however, a mutation in a gene affects the structure or function of the protein and this can result in disease. A mutation is described as germline; if it is present in a gamete involved in a fertilization event leading to the conception of an individual, it is then present in every cell. Alternatively it is described as somatic if it occurs after conception and is therefore present only in a proportion of body cells.

Point mutations

Alterations of a single base are called point mutations. A sentence in English is used to illustrate this point

THE CAT BIT THE DOG.

If there is a change in one of the letters the way the sentence reads is affected. A point mutation would be the substitution of one letter for another.

THE RAT BIT THE DOG

This change still allows the sentence to be read although the sense is changed slightly. This is equivalent to a miss-sense point mutation which may or may not cause an alteration in the final protein structure.

THE CAT B**IT** THE DOG

This change has disrupted the sense of the sentence and is classed as a non-sense muta-tion. These mutations usually have a serious effect on the protein structure.

Other changes in the DNA sequence are insertions or deletions which may be one or more of the bases.

THE CAT **AND THE RAT** BIT THE DOG

THE BIT THE DOG

If the number of bases inserted or deleted are not multiples of three then the whole sen-tence is disrupted.

THE **C**CA TBI TTH EDO G

THE CAB ITT HED OG

These are known as frameshift insertions and deletions and usually have a serious effect on the protein structure (Skirton *et al.* 2005).

Haemoglobin and the haemoglobinopathies

Sickle cell anaemia

Sickle cell anaemia (SCA) was the first human disease to be successfully understood at the molecular level. In 1975 Ingram demonstrated that the difference between HbA normal haemoglobin and HbS sickle cell haemoglobin lay in a single point mutation of the β globin gene on chromosome 11p at position 6. The normal residue at this position is glutamic acid, whereas in SCA valine is present instead (Sudbury 2002).

Since then more than 300 Hb variants have been described (see Box 3.1).

Box 3.1   Haemoglobin variants.

DNA

5	6	7	
CCT	GAG	GAG	β a
CCT	G**TG**	GAG	β s
CCT	**A**AG	GAG	β c

PROTEIN

	5 6	7	
Pro	Glu	Glu	β a
Pro	Val	Glu	β s
Pro	Lys	Glu	β c

Thalassaemia

Thalassaemia, first described by Cooley in 1925 as a rare form of anaemia, exists in two forms. The α thalassaemias are primarily caused by deletions. Chromosome 16 carries two functioning α globin genes, leading to a total of four genes in the normal situation. The α thalassaemias involve inactivation of anywhere from one to four genes and therefore, depending on the number of genes lost, will lead to a range of disorders. If three of the four genes are functioning the clinical abnormalities are subtle, denoted as the silent carrier state. If two of the four genes are inactivated this is denoted as α thalassaemia trait. A more severe situation occurs if only one of the four α genes is functioning and most severe in which there are no functioning genes, leading to stillbirth or early neonatal death.

A β thalassaemia is usually the result of more subtle mutations, which either reduce or completely abolish β-globin synthesis. There are more than one hundred different mutations that have been shown to cause β thalassaemia.

Hereditary (primary) haemochromatosis

When functioning normally genes play an important role in body function as in the HFE gene that produces HFE protein, which amongst other minor things regulates the absorption of iron through the intestinal wall. When this gene mutates iron absorption is uncontrolled. HFE gene on chromosome 6 was identified in 1996 and the mutation that occurs in this gene (most affected people have two copies of a mutation called C282Y) leads to accumulation of body iron stores over time (Young 2005). This is another example of a point mutation; instead of the base pair guanine, adenine is substituted. This results in a cysteine to tyrosine substitution at codon 282, a different amino acid, which means the protein responsible for iron uptake control is not produced (see Boxes 3.2 and 3.3).

Box 3.2   Wild type HFE sequence.

DNA	AGA	TAT	ACG	TGC	CAG	GTG	GAG
Amino acid	arg	tyr	thr	cys	gin	val	glu
	279			282			285

Box 3.3   HFE sequence with C282Y mutation.

DNA	AGA	TAT	ACG	TAC	CAG	GTG	GAG
Amino acid	arg	tyr	thr	tyr	gin	val	glu
	279			282			285

Key: Arg – arginine; Try – tyrosine; Thr – threonine; Gin – glutamine; Val – valine; Glu – glutamic acid

---

Chromosomal abnormalities

These can be described on the basis of whether they are numerical, involving the presence of an additional chromosome, or structural, involving a change or changes to a chromosome (Strachan and Read 2001). The outcome of chromosomal abnormalities depends on whether there is any loss or gain of chromosomal material.

Numerical chromosomal abnormalities

Numerical abnormalities include loss (monosomy) or gain (trisomy) of a single chromosome.

Examples are:

Trisomy 21 Down's syndrome
Monosomy XO Turner's syndrome

Structural abnormalities include translocations, deletions or insertions. Translocations are a transfer of a segment of chromosome from one to another chromosome. Deletions are a loss of chromosome material. Insertions are a gain of chromosomal material.

It is now well recognised that chromosomal abnormalities show a strong causal association with malignancy. These acquired chromosomal abnormalities and rearrangements result in changes in the DNA sequences of genes and in particular genes such as proto-oncogenes, tumour suppressor genes and DNA repair genes.

Chromosomes, genes and malignancy

In the majority of cases cancer is a multifactorial disorder in which genetics and environmental factors interact to initiate carcinogenesis. In a minority, about 5–10%, the genetic mutation is in the germline and therefore can be inherited. Studies of these cancers has helped in our understanding of the more common multifactorial cancers that occur as an interaction of environment on somatic cell DNA. Carcinogenesis requires the accumulation of many mutations in oncogenes, tumour suppressor genes and DNA repair genes. Proto-oncogenes are normal genes that act to promote cell growth, programmed cell death (apoptosis), regulation of angiogenesis and cell adhesion. When a mutation occurs in these genes (there are many of them scattered throughout the genome) they are called oncogenes. Activation of these genes results in tumour growth, migration and metastasis.

Activation of oncogenes occurs by: Translocations

The hallmark of chronic myeloid leukaemia is the Philadelphia chromosome (Ph+) which was the first consistent chromosomal aberration to be associated with human malignancy (Hodgson *et al*. 2007). It involves a translocation of chromosome 9 and 22 t(9,22) (q34q11). The breakpoint on chromosome 9 involves the Abelson oncogene c-abl and on chromosome 22 the breakpoint involves bcr gene (Guilhot and Roy 2005). This resultant translocation produces a new or hybrid gene, this new bcr-abl fusion gene codes for a protein tyrosine kinase, with the ability to transform white blood cell precursors in bone marrow (see Figure 3.8).

In Burkitts lymphoma the translocation involving t(8:14) (q24:q32), t(2:8) (p12:q24) or t (8:22) (q24:q11) moves the c-myc proto-oncogene to a region of the genome where immunoglobulin genes are actively transcribed (Hagenbeek and Kluin 2005). This results in the over expression or gene amplification of c-myc, which appears to be a key step in the development of the tumour.

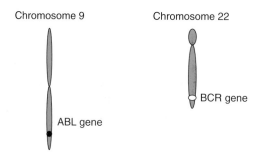

The translocated ABL gene inserts into the BCR gene. The two genes fuse. The altered ABL gene functions improperly, resulting in CML

Figure 3.8　Philadelphia chromosome.

Karyotyping is a method of diagnosing chromosomal abnormalities and one of the most commonly known chromosomal abnormalities is trisomy 21 (which means having three number 21 chromosomes) or Down's syndrome. It is important in leukaemias and lymphomas because this aids diagnosis, prognosis and indicates which patient might benefit or not benefit from specific treatments.

Tumour suppressor genes

Inactivation of a tumour suppressor gene, called PRDM1, could be a major cause of diffuse large B-cell lymphoma (Pasqualucci *et al.* 2006). This tumour suppressor gene is abnormally switched off which results in the mature B-cells getting stuck in a loop where they proliferate and fail to differentiate and die as they should.

DNA repair genes

The complexity of the human genome is such that during cell division when 3.2×10^9 DNA bases have to be faithfully replicated it is almost inevitable that errors will occur. There is, though, a repair system consisting of two pathways: one that repairs single base errors and the other responsible for the replacement of a length of DNA (Jones *et al.* 2001). A small number of rare conditions the chromosome breakage syndromes are associated with are inherited abnormalities of these repair mechanisms and they convey increased susceptibility to cancer (see Table 3.1).

Table 3.1

Chromosome breakage syndrome	Associated risk
Ataxia telangiectasis	Lymphomas
Fanconi's syndrome	Leukaemia
	Acute lymphoblastic leukaemia
Bloom's syndrome	Lymphoreticula tumours

(Jones *et al.* 2001; Young 2005)

Inheritance patterns

Genetic information is inherited from our parents, errors in single genes can have different patterns of inheritance depending on the chromosome on which the relevant gene is located and whether the disorder is caused by a mutation in one or both copies of the gene. 'Mendelian' is often applied to the pattern of inheritance in single gene disorders in recognition of the huge contribution made by the monk Gregor Mendel.

Single gene inheritance patterns are one of the following:

- Autosomal dominant
- Autosomal recessive
- Sex linked

Autosomal dominant inheritance

A disorder which shows autosomal dominant inheritance is caused by an error in a single copy of a gene located on one of the 22 autosomes. An individual will be affected if one gene is normal (wild type allele) and the other copy is faulty (mutant allele). When this individual has children there is one chance in two that each child will inherit the mutant allele and therefore be affected. An example of a haematology condition which is inherited as an autosomal dominant inherited condition is hereditary spherocytosis (HS).

Autosomal recessive inheritance

A disorder that shows autosomal recessive inheritance can only occur if both copies of the gene are faulty, for example the individual is homozygous, having two mutant alleles. This individual has inherited the mutated genes, one from each parent. The parents having only the one mutated gene are not affected but are known as carriers. When both parents are carriers the probability of each child having the disease is 1 in 4 (Marieb and Hoenn 2007). For example, sickle cell anaemia is a recessive condition. A child who inherits two copies of the faulty gene is said to have sickle disease, if they inherit one normal and one mutated gene they are said to have sickle cell trait. Thalassaemia is another example of recessive inheritance.

X-linked recessive inheritance

This is caused by a mutation in a gene on the X chromosome. Females have two X chromosomes, males have only one. Females are therefore not usually affected but are carriers. A carrier female transmits the mutated gene on average to half of her daughters, who will be carriers, and to half of her sons who will be affected. An affected male transmits the mutated gene to all of his daughters and to none of his sons. Glucose-phosphate-dehydrogenase deficiency (G6PD) and haemophilia A and B are examples of X-linked inheritance. The gene which causes G6PD deficiency is found on the long arm of the X chromosome, locus (position of the gene on the chromosome is 28) Xq28.

The factor VIII gene is located at the tip of the long arm of the X chromosome; this is a large gene and a number of mutations have been detected, including large and small deletions, point mutations and small insertions. Factor IX gene is located below the factor VIII gene and is also associated with a large number of mutations (Strachan and Read 2001). Haemophilia A and B are examples of X-linked inheritance. There are defects in other clotting factors in the cascade but the relevant genes are located on autosomes and so inheritance is autosomal recessive and most of these disorders are rare.

X-linked dominant inheritance and Y-linked inheritance

Although possible in clinical practice these are rarely encountered. X-linked dominant inheritance results in females having the disorder as the presence of just one copy of the mutant allele is sufficient to cause the condition. In males this X-linked dominant condition is often incompatible with life. In Y-linked genes, the condition can only be expressed in males, and although it used to be thought that there were no significant diseases causing gene mutations associated with the Y chromosome, the recognition of Y-linked genes necessary for spermatogenesis has implications for procedures such as IVF. This subfertility, if caused by a mutated gene on the Y chromosome, would be transmitted to all male children (Skirton *et al.* 2005).

Clinical application

DNA testing

In haemochromatosis, for example, DNA testing will result in detecting the disease before iron overload occurs, which allows ideal management of this preventable and potentially curable disease. On the other hand, the rapid progress of molecular genetics in the sickle cell diseases may prove difficult to translate into improving therapy for these conditions and raises issues of treatment options.

In 2001 the UK government introduced universal neonatal screening for the haemoglobinopathies. This has been fully established in England (but not in the other three national countries). The screening involves the use of Guthrie bloodspot sampling at around seven days after birth.

There are a number of issues that need to be taken into account:

- If DNA-based technology is used, carriers of these recessive genes will be detected as well as affected individuals, should parents be informed of their carrier status?
- The haemoglobinopathies are more prevalent in specific ethnic groups; should screening be universal or targeted?

The increasing knowledge of genetic alterations and their link to clinical correlations may raise moral dilemmas for HCP in whom to treat.

Conclusion

This chapter has included some basic information and concepts, but the face of genetics is constantly advancing, resulting in increasing knowledge in diseases and treatments. The sequencing of the human genome has created the opportunity to identify, treat and prevent disease, but has also raised ethical issues for society and moral dilemmas for health care professionals.

Websites of interest

http://www.genome.gov/10001618
http://www.ornl.gov/sci/techresources/Human_Genome/publicat/hgn/hgn.shtm
http://www.genetests.org

References

Brown, S.M. (2003) *Essential of Medical Genomics*. John Wiley & Sons, Ltd, Oxford.

Cooley, T.B. and Lee, P. (1925) Series of cases of splenomegaly in children with anaemia and peculiar bone change. *Trans Am Pediatr Soc*, 37, 29–30.

Degos, L., Linch, D.C. and Lowenberg, B. (eds) (2005) *Textbook of Malignant Haematology*. Thompson Publishing Services, Hampshire.

Dennis, C. and Gallagher, R. (eds) (2001) *The Human Genome*. Palgrave Publishers Ltd, New York.

Guilhot, F. and Roy, L. (2005) Chronic myeloid leukaemia. In: *Textbook of Malignant Haematology* (eds L. Degos, D.C. Linch and B. Lowenberg). Thompson Publishing Services, Hampshire.

Hagenbeek, A. and Kluin, P.M. (2005) Non-Hodgkin Lymphomas. In: *Textbook of Malignant Haematology* (eds L. Degos, D.C. Linch and B. Lowenberg). Thompson Publishing Services, Hampshire.

Harper, P.S. (2004) *Practical Genetic Counselling*, 6th edition. Edward Arnold Ltd, London.

Hodgson, S.V., Foulkes, W., Eng, C. and Maher, E.R. (2007) *A Practical Guide to Human Cancer Genetics*, 3rd edition. Cambridge University Press, Cambridge.

Jones, R.N., Karp, A. and Giddings, G. (2001) *The Essentials of Genetics*. John Murray Ltd, London.

Marieb, E.N. and Hoehn, K. (2007) *Anatomy and Physiology*. The Benjamin/Cummings Publishing Company Inc., California.

Pasqualucci, L., Compagno, M., Houldsworth, J. *et al.* (2006) Inactivation of the PRDM1/BLIMP1 gene in diffuse large B cell lymphoma. *Journal of Experimental Medicine*, 20 February, 203 (2), 311–317.

Skirton, H., Patch, C. and Williams, J. (2005) *Applied Genetics in Health Care: a Book for Specialist Practitioners*. Taylor & Francis Group Cromwell Press, Wiltshire.

Snustad, D.P., Simmons, M.J. (2012) *Priniciples of Genetics* (6th Edition) John Wiley & Sons, Inc., New York.

Strachan, T. and Read, A.P. (2001) *Human Molecular Genetics*, 2nd edition. John Wiley and Sons Inc., Oxford.

Sudbury, P. (2002) *Human Molecular Genetics*, 2nd edition. Pearson Education Ltd, UK.

Young, I.D. (2005) *Medical Genetics*. Oxford University Press, UK.

Chapter 4

The cell*

Louise Knight

This chapter aims to introduce the cell and its component parts (organelles), describe how a cell develops and replicates, and how this is controlled. By the end of this chapter you:

- Will have an understanding of normal cell replication and the different types of cell that the human body is composed of
- Will have an overview of cellular processes that can transform a cell from normal to malignant
- Will have an understanding of cellular and molecular events that can lead to malignancy
- Understand what growth factors are and how they function

The chapter summarises four different types of leukaemia to provide an overview and understanding of the symptoms.

The human body is made up of about ten trillion cells and the ability of each of these to produce exact replicas is an essential component of life. In order to begin to understand how things might go wrong and cancer may develop it is essential to understand normal cellular processes.

What is a cell?

The cell is the basic unit of all living matter, whether it is a single celled bacterium like *Escherichia coli* (*E. coli*) or a multicelled organism like a human being. Every cell is remarkable; not only do they have the ability to carry out complex tasks, for example uptake of nutrients and conversion to energy and the ability to replicate, but they also contain all the instructions to carry out these tasks.

Cells are divided into two categories: (1) prokaryotes and (2) eukaryotes. Prokaryotes lack a nuclear membrane (the membrane that surrounds the nucleus) and the best-known examples of prokaryotic organisms are bacteria. They are comprised of a cell envelope within which the cytoplasmic region is contained. This region contains cytoplasm, which is a fluid made up of about 70% water, the remainder is composed of enzymes that the cell has manufactured,

*Adapted from Chapter 4 of *The Biology of Cancer*, First Edition. Janice Gabriel.
© 2007 John Wiley & Sons, Ltd. Used with permission.

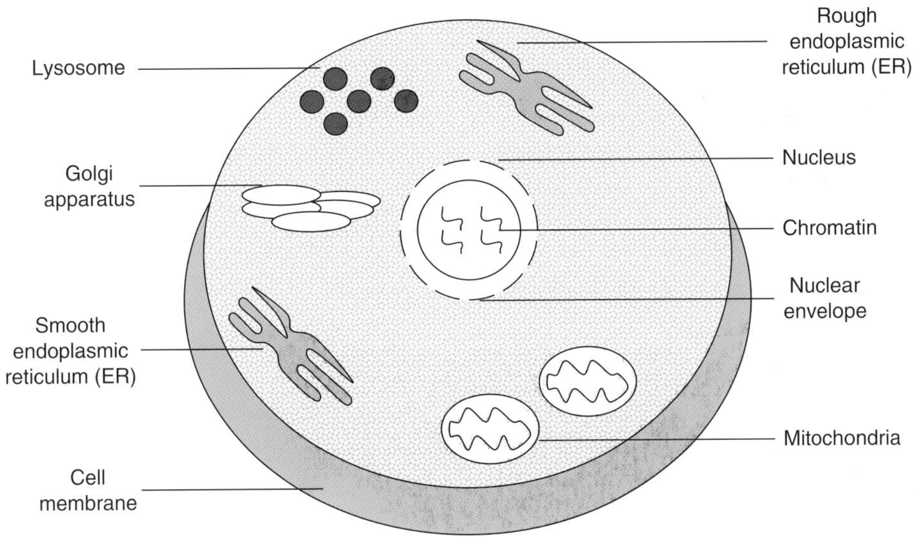

Figure 4.1   A typical eukaryotic cell and some of the components that are found within it.

amino acids, glucose molecules and adenosine triphosphate (ATP). At the centre of the cell is its DNA, which due to the lack of a nuclear membrane floats within the cytoplasm.

In comparison, eukaryotes contain cell organelles; similar to organs within the body, each organelle has its own structure and specific function or metabolic process to carry out. Figure 4.1 illustrates some of the organelles that are found within the eukaryotic cell; among these structures is the nucleus, which is composed of three main parts:

* *Nucleolus*   This is the most prominent part of the nucleus and its function is to produces ribosomes.
* *Nuclear envelope*   This is a double-layered membrane, which protects and separates the nucleus from the cytoplasm and molecules that could cause damage.
* *Chromatin*   This is a DNA/protein complex containing our genes; during replication it condenses into chromosomes.

It is the nucleus that gives the eukaryotye (meaning 'true nucleus') its name. Other important components that are illustrated in the diagram include:

* *Cell membrane*   This is comprised of a double layer of lipid molecules, which gives the cell support and protection, letting nutrients in and waste molecules out. It is able to alter its shape and receive signals from the outside environment.
* *Mitochondrion*   These are often thought of as the 'power houses' of cells as this is where energy is produced. The mitochondria break down sugar molecules in the presence of oxygen to produce energy in the form of ATP.
* *Rough/smooth endoplasmic reticulum (ER)*   These are a series of interconnecting tubular tunnels, which are continuous with the outer membrane of the nucleus. The membrane structure of both types is identical but the rough ER has *ribosomes* attached to it as opposed to smooth ER, which does not. The rough ER is involved in protein

synthesis, allowing proteins made on the ribosomes to fold into their three-dimensional shape; the smooth ER is the site of steroid production.

- *Lysosomes*   These are spherical bodies containing many digestive enzymes that are used to break down large molecules.
- *Golgi apparatus*   This is a stack of flattened sacs, which is associated with the ER. The golgi apparatus modifies proteins and fats, for example the addition of sugar molecules forming glycoproteins.

It is important to remember that not all cell organelles have been described within this text. For a more detailed description of cell organelles you could read Alberts *et al.* (1994).

How does the cell develop and replicate?

Eukaryotic cells divide to produce two identical daughter cells, each containing exact copies of the DNA from the parent cell; in this way multicellular organisms are able to replace damaged or worn out cells. These processes are called interphase and mitosis and together they make up the cell cycle (Figure 4.2). To the naked eye interphase appears to be a period of rest for the cell, but in fact much activity is taking place. During this time RNA is constantly being synthesised, protein is produced and the cell is growing in size. Scientists have determined at a molecular level that the interphase can be divided into the following four steps:

- *Gap 0 (G_0)*   Cells may leave the cell cycle for a temporary resting period or more permanently if they have reached the end of their development, for example neurons. Cells in this phase are often termed quiescent. In order to enter back into the cycle, cells must be stimulated by growth factors, for example platelet-derived growth factor (PDGF).
- *Gap 1 (G_1)*   Cells increase in size, produce RNA and synthesise protein. There is an important cell cycle control mechanism (checkpoint) activated during this stage (see tumour suppressor genes) that cells must pass through in order to progress to S phase.
- *Synthesis phase (S phase)*   DNA is replicated during this phase so that the two daughter cells produced following mitosis will contain a copy of the DNA from the parent cells.
- *Gap 2 (G_2)*   Cells continue to grow and produce new proteins. At the end of G_2 another important checkpoint is activated (see tumour suppressor genes).

Now the cell is ready to enter mitosis, this is further divided into the following stages:

- *Prophase*   At the beginning of prophase the nuclear membrane breaks down and chromatin in the nucleus condenses into chromosomes (these can be viewed under a light microscope). Each chromosome consists of two genetically identical chromatids. Microtubules, which are responsible for cell shape, disassemble and the building blocks of these are used to form the mitotic spindle.
- *Prometaphase*   There is now no longer a recognisable nucleus. Some mitotic spindle fibres elongate to specific areas on the chromosomes.
- *Metaphase*   Tension is applied to the spindle fibres, which aligns all the chromosomes in one plane at the centre of the cell.
- *Anaphase*   The chromosomes are pulled away from the central plane towards the cell poles.

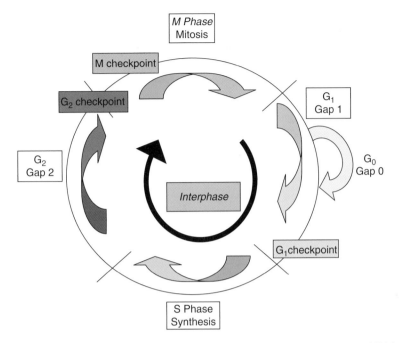

Figure 4.2 Overview of the five stages of normal mammalian cell development. Within each stage there are checkpoints which are regulated by components within the cycle.

- *Telophase* Chromosomes arrive at cell poles and decondense and the nuclear envelope reforms around the clusters at each end of the cell, thereby forming new nuclei.
- *Cytokinesis* The cell is cleaved to form two daughter cells and microtubules reform for the cells' entry into interphase. These cells are said to be diploid because they contain two sets of homologous chromosomes. Another form of cell division to be aware of is meiosis, which occurs only in reproductive cells during the formation of gametes (sex cells). A cell dividing by meiosis duplicates its DNA as with cells undergoing mitosis, but splits into four new cells instead of two and contains only one copy of each chromosome. These cells are said to be haploid.

How is the cell cycle controlled?

Cancer can be described as the uncontrolled proliferation and growth of cells into other tissues. If we can understand the normal mechanisms in place to control the cell cycle, we can begin to understand how these controls may malfunction and cause cancer to develop. Understanding the cell cycle and its controls also allows the development of specific and targeted therapies to treat the disease.

Cyclins and cyclin-dependant kinases

Many different proteins located within the cytoplasm control the cell cycle; two of the main types are cyclins (structural proteins) and cyclin-dependant kinases (CDKs).

A cyclin joins with a CDK to form a complex (cyclin-CDK). However, if a problem with the cell cycle is detected then activation of the cyclin-CDK complex is not completed. If there are no problems then activation is completed; this leads to the activation of a transcription factor by the removal of a transcription factor inhibitor. The transcription factor activates transcription of the genes required for the next stage of the cell cycle, including the cyclin and CDK genes. During the cell cycle, levels of cyclins within the cell will rise and fall but the levels of CDKs will remain fairly constant. Activation of CDKs is a central event in regulating the cell cycle and their activity is therefore regulated at many different levels.

Tumour suppressor genes

Tumour suppressor genes prevent excessive growth of a cell; the most well-known ones are p53 and the retinoblastoma (Rb) gene.

Retinoblastoma gene

The retinoblastoma gene is involved in the G_1 checkpoint (Figure 4.2) in the following way. It binds to a family of transcription factors known as the E2F family, thereby repressing their transcription of E2F-responsive genes such as thymidine kinase (TK) needed for DNA replication and cyclin E and A needed for cell cycle progression. The retinoblastoma gene is activated when cyclin D forms a complex with CDK4/6 (cyclin D/CDK4/6, hence making it active) this in turn phosphorylates Rb, which allows E2F to be released (Figure 4.3).

p53

The p53 protein is essential for protecting us against cancer, more than half of human cancers have p53 mutations and therefore no functioning p53. It works by sensing DNA damage and halting the cell cycle (Figure 4.2). This is essential because if DNA is damaged but still replicated in S phase, it could eventually manifest in the form of a protein mutation, therefore by halting the cell cycle at the G_1 checkpoint this can be prevented. So how does this process work? Again, it comes back to the involvement of CDKs. First, in response to a variety of stress signals, for example DNA damage, p53 switches from an inactive state to an active state. It then triggers transcription of the gene for p21 which is a CDK inhibitor; because active CDKs are needed to progress through the cell cycle an inactive CDK will cause the cycle to halt.

p53 is also involved at the G_2 checkpoint in cases, for example, where DNA has been synthesised incorrectly. At this checkpoint, p53 binds to E2F (see Rb section) and prevents it from triggering transcription of protooncogenes, for example c-myc and c-fos, which are required for mitosis (Figure 4.3). Protooncogenes are important promoters of normal cell growth and division; however, if they become mutated they are known as oncogenes and can have a detrimental effect. A single oncogene cannot cause cancer by itself but it can cause the cell cycle to lose its inhibitory controls, thereby increasing the rate of mitosis. When a cell loses control over mitosis, it can be the beginning of the pathway leading to the development of cancer.

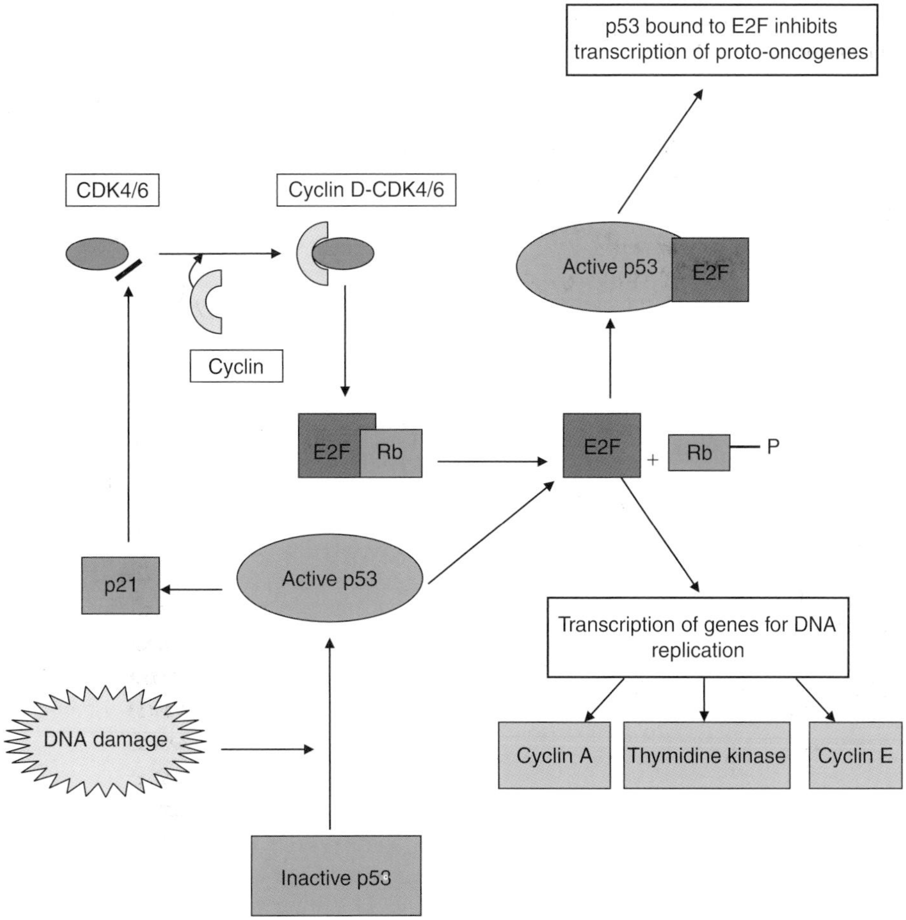

Figure 4.3 If no damage is detected at the G1 checkpoint CDK4/6 joins with cyclin D to form a cyclin-CDK complex. This phosphorylates Rb, thereby releasing E2F from its complex and making it active. E2F promotes transcription of E2F responsive genes and hence cell cycle progression. If there is DNA damage, p53 changes from its inactive state to its active state. This triggers transcription of the CDK inhibitor p21, which subsequently blocks the CDK forming a complex with a cyclin.

Apoptosis

There are six main types of DNA repair mechanisms operating in mammals; however, these are not always successful. The alternative pathway that can be activated by p53 is apoptosis or programmed cell death. This process involves a series of specific cellular changes that result in the elimination of the cell and therefore any mutations within it.

Different types of cells

The human body is made up of three types of cell: somatic, germ and stem cells. Somatic cells make up the majority of the body; they have two copies of each chromosome and are therefore diploid. Germ cells give rise to gametes and are constant throughout their

Table 4.1　Cell and tissue types found within the body and their function.

Tissue/cell type	Function
Epithelia*	
Absorptive	They have numerous hair-like structures called microvili projecting from their surface to increase the surface area for absorption.
Secretory	These are specialised cells that secrete substances onto the surface of the cell sheet. They are often collected together to form a gland that specialises in the secretion of a particular substance. Exocrine glands secrete their products, for example gastric juices into ducts, endocrine glands secrete into the blood.
Ciliated	They have cilia on their free surface that beat in synchrony to move substances, e.g. mucus, over the epithelial sheet.
Connective tissue	
Fibroblasts	They are located in loose connective tissue and secrete the extracellular matrix that fills spaces between organs and tissues.
Osteoblasts	These cells secrete the extracellular matrix in which crystals of calcium phosphate are later deposited to form bone.
Adipose	These are among the largest in the body and produce and store fat. A large lipid droplet within the cell squeezes the nucleus and cytoplasm.
Nervous tissue	
Neurons	These are specialised cells for communication, for example the brain and spinal cord are comprised of a network of neurons.
Glial	These are cells that support neurons.
Schwann/ oligodendrocytes	These wrap around the axon forming a multilayered membrane sheath. The axon is the structure that conducts electrical signals away from the neuron.
Muscle tissue	
Skeletal	These are large multinucleated cells that form muscle fibres. Skeletal muscle moves joints by its strong rapid contraction.
Smooth	Composed of thin elongated cells containing one nucleus each. Found in the digestive tract, bladder, arteries and veins.
Cardiac	An intermediate of the previous two types. Cardiac muscle produces the heartbeat, cells are linked by electrically conducting junctions.
Blood	
Erythrocytes (red blood cells)	These are very small cells usually with no nucleus or internal membrane, full of oxygen-binding protein haemoglobin.
Lymphocytes (white blood cells)	These cells protect us against infections. They are further subdivided into lymphocytes, macrophages and neutrophils.
Sensory	
Hair	Sensory cells are some of the most highly specialised cells within the vertebrate body. Hair cells of the inner ear are primary detectors of sound.
Rod	These are found in the retina of the eye and are specialised to respond to light.

*Epithelial Zcells form cell sheets called epithelia, this lines inner and outer surfaces of the body.

generations. Stem cells, on the other hand, have the ability to divide indefinitely and give rise to specialised cells. For example, blood stem cells can give rise to red blood cells, platelets and white blood cells. Table 4.1 describes some of the different types of tissues within the body and cells that they are comprised of; most tissues are made up of more than one type of cell.

What happens when the cell undergoes malignant changes?

Over the years it has been suggested that the development of cancer is a multi-step process, each step reflecting a genetic alteration that transforms a normal cell into a malignant cell. A review by Hanahan and Weinberg (2000) summarised these changes as six essential alterations to cell physiology that collectively dictate malignant growth. The alterations are as follows:

- *Self-sufficiency in growth signals*   Normal cells require growth signals to proliferate. Many cancer cells acquire the ability to produce their own growth signals, for example they can synthesise growth factors, to which they also respond. The cells begin to operate as an independent entity as opposed to functioning as part of a larger organism. An example of this is the ability of glioblastomas to produce PDGF (Hermansson *et al.* 1988).
- *Insensitivity to inhibitory (antigrowth) signals*   Cells monitor their external environment and decide whether to proliferate or not. Many anti-proliferative signals function via the Rb protein (see tumour suppressor genes); therefore if this is disrupted, control of the cell cycle is lost and cells will proliferate. This is demonstrated in retinoblastoma cancer where deletion or mutation of the Rb gene causes tumour growth in one or both eyes in early childhood.
- *Evasion of apoptosis*   Research over the past decade has determined that the apoptotic programme is present in nearly all cells in the body in a latent form. It seems that resistance towards it is a characteristic of most and perhaps all cancers. One way in which apoptosis might be avoided is the loss or mutation of p53, which acts as a proapoptotic regulator by sensing DNA damage.
- *Limitless replicative potential*   Research involving cells in culture has suggested that normal cells can only undergo 60–70 replications, after which time they stop growing and die. Cancer cells, however, have acquired the capability of endlessly replicating, in many cases due to an enzyme known as telomerase. At the end of chromosomes are telomeres, which are composed of several thousand repeats of base pairs. During each normal cell replication the telomeres shorten until they can no longer protect the chromosomal DNA, and subsequently the cell dies. However, if telomerase is up-regulated the telomeres will be maintained above a critical length, making the cells immortal.
- *Sustained angiogenesis*   Angiogenesis is the formation of new blood vessels, which is an essential process if the cells in the tumour mass are to be supplied with oxygen and nutrients. It seems that tumours are able to shift the balance of angiogenesis inducers and inhibitors by altering gene expression and, for example, increasing VEGF expression (Hanahan and Folkman 1996).
- *Tissue invasion and metastasis*   The majority of cancer deaths are caused by metastasis of the primary tumour mass to other sites of the body. It begins with the rearrangement

of the cells' cytoskeleton, which allows them to attach to other cells and move over or around them. Once they hit a blockage, for example the basal lamina, the cancer cells secrete enzymes to break it down. Included in these enzymes are matrix metalloproteins (MMP), which act as 'molecular scissors' and cut through proteins that may hinder the passage of the cancer cells. Once through the basal lamina the cells can move into the bloodstream and circulate throughout the body until they find a suitable site to settle on and regrow. A commonly observed alteration that leads to metastasis involves the cell-to-cell interaction molecule E-cadherin. Coupling of this molecule between cells results in transmission of antigrowth signals, thereby acting as a suppressor of invasion and metastasis. It appears that E-cadherin function is lost in the majority of epithelial cancers due to gene mutations.

Haematological malignancies

Haematological malignancies derive from either the myeloid cell line which normally produces granulocytes, erythrocytes, thrombocytes, macrophages and mast cells or the lymphoid cell line which normally produces B, T, natural killer (NK) and plasma cells. Different types of haematological malignancy are linked through the immune system and therefore often a disease of one can affect the others, for example leukaemia affects the blood and bone marrow and is characterised by abnormal proliferation of blood cells; lymphoma is a disease of the lymphocytes and lymph nodes but can spread to the bone marrow and affect the blood.

Leukaemia can be divided into two categories; acute leukaemia is characterised by a rapid (days or weeks) increase in immature blood cells resulting in an inability of the bone marrow to produce healthy cells and chronic leukaemia which is characterised by an excessive build up of abnormal mature blood cells and develops slowly often over a number of months or years.

The four main types of leukaemia are: acute myeloid leukaemia (AML); acute lymphoblastic leukaemia (ALL); chronic lymphocytic leukaemia (CLL); chronic myeloid leukaemia (CML) and the next section briefly describes each disease and some of the symptoms associated with it.

Acute myeloid leukaemia

Acute myeloid leukaemia (AML) is the most common acute leukaemia affecting adults and is characterised by a rapid growth of abnormal white blood cells that accumulate in the bone marrow, thereby interfering with the production of healthy blood cells. There are two classification systems for AML: the World Health Organisation (WHO) which attempts to provide a clinically useful and meaningful prognostic scheme and the French-American-British (FAB) system which categorises according to the type of cell the leukaemia has developed from and its degree of maturity (Cancer Research UK 2009).

Symptoms of AML are often non-specific and can be similar to those experienced during common illnesses such as flu. The decrease in red blood cells can cause anaemia, resulting in fatigue, paleness and breathlessness. The lack of white blood cells can cause a susceptibility to infections, resulting in fever, and the lack of platelets can cause unusual bleeding, for example bleeding gums, frequent nose bleeds, easy bruising and tiny flat red spots under the skin called petechiae.

Acute lymphoblastic leukaemia

Acute lymphoblastic leukaemia (ALL) is the most common type of leukaemia in children and is characterised by excess lymphoblasts. The symptoms are non-specific and similar to those exhibited in AML.

Chronic lymphocytic leukaemia

Chronic lymphocytic leukaemia (CLL) is the most common type of leukaemia, mainly affecting people over 60 (Cancer Research UK 2009). It involves a specific subtype of lymphocyte known as a B-cell. Often this type of leukaemia is diagnosed without symptoms as the result of a routine blood test, but as the disease progresses it can cause swollen lymph nodes, spleen, liver and anaemia. Along with AML each disease accounts for approximately a third of all leukaemias diagnosed in the UK.

Chronic myeloid leukaemia

Chronic myeloid leukaemia (CML) is characterised by an over production of abnormal granulocytes and was the first malignancy to be linked to a specific genetic abnormality, the chromosomal translocation known as the Philadelphia chromosome. As with the previous type of leukaemia, CML is often asymptomatic at diagnosis.

The disease is divided into three phases: the chronic phase during which the disease is most stable and developing slowly, approximately 90% of people are diagnosed at this stage (Cancer Research UK 2009); the accelerated phase during which there are no more obvious symptoms but sufferers may feel fatigued, lose weight and the spleen may be enlarged and blast phase (or blast crisis) during which the leukaemia behaves more like an acute leukaemia. Symptoms at this stage would be obvious and sufferers would be quite unwell.

References

Alberts, B., Bray, D., Lewis, J., Raff, M., Roberts, K. and Watson, J.D. (1994) *Internal organisation of the cell. In: Molecular Biology of the Cell*, 3rd edition. Garland Publishing, New York and London.

Andreeff, M., Goodrich, D.W. and Pardee, A.B. (2000) Cell proliferation, differentiation, and apoptosis. In: *Cancer Medicine* (eds R.C. Bast Jnr, D.W. Kufe, R.E. Pollock *et al.*), 5th edition. BC Decker Inc., Canada.

Bartleby (2000) *The American Heritage® Dictionary of the English Language*. Retrieved 3 March 2003, from http://www.bartleby.com/61/81/N0188100.html and http://www.bartleby.com/61/78/N0187800.html

British Medical Association and Royal Pharmaceutical Society of Great Britain (2002) Malignant disease and immunosuppression. *British National Formulary*.

Cancer Research UK (2008) Staging for chronic myeloid leukaemia (CML) (2008) Retrieved 8 December 2009, http://www.cancerhelp.org.uk/type/cml/treatment/staging-for-chronic-myeloid-leukaemia

Cancer Research UK (2009a) Types of myeloid leukaemia. Retrieved 8 December 2009, http://www.cancerhelp.org.uk/type/aml/about/types-of-acute-myeloid-leukaemia

Cancer Research UK (2009b) Chronic lymphocytic leukaemia (CLL) risks and causes Retrieved 8 December 2009, http://www.cancerhelp.org.uk/type/cll/about/chronic-lymphocytic-leukaemia-risks-and-causes

Colvin, M.D. (2000) Alkylating agents and platinum antitumor compounds. In: *Cancer Medicine* (eds R.C. Bast Jnr, D.W. Kufe, R.E. Pollock *et al.*), 5th edition. BC Decker Inc., Canada.

Drug Index (Professional) (2001) Retrieved February 2003, http://www.bccancer.bc.ca/HPI/DrugDatabase/DrugIndexALPro/default.htm

Hanahan, D. and Folkman, J. (1996) Patterns and emerging mechanisms of the angiogenic switch during tumorigenesis. *Cell*, 86 (3), 353–364.

Hanahan, D. and Weinberg, R.A. (2000) The hallmarks of cancer. *Cell*, 100 (1), 57–70.

Hermansson, M., Nistér, M., Betsholtz, C., Heldin, C.H., Westermark, B. and Funa, K. (1988) Endothelial cell hyperplasia in human glioblastoma: coexpression of mRNA for platelet-derived growth factor (PDGF) B chain and PDGF receptor suggests autocrine growth stimulation. *Proceedings of the National Academy of Sciences of the United States of America*, 85 (20), 7748–7752.

Section 2

Non-malignant haematology

Anaemia

Haemoglobinopathies

Haemochromatosis

Chapter 5

Aplastic anaemia: pathophysiology, care and management

Audrey Yandle

By the end of this chapter you should be able to:

- Define what is meant by bone marrow failure
- List some of the common causes of bone marrow failure
- Define the term 'aplastic anaemia'
- Discuss the pathology and treatment of acquired aplastic anaemia
- Identify and discuss the principles of management of patients with aplastic anaemia

---

Introduction

Haemopoiesis, the manufacture of our blood cells in the bone marrow, is a remarkable and complex process. The daily supply of billions of blood cells to meet our normal requirements, the capacity to rapidly respond to increased need and the coordination and regulation of complex processes involving millions of cells is truly impressive. The bone marrow is responsible for producing the cells that give us stamina and protect us and yet until something goes wrong, and this occurs with remarkable infrequency compared to other organs of the body, the bone marrow is seldom given any particular attention. Nevertheless, failure of bone marrow production is a potentially lethal event, with a number of complex causes, whose management is often challenging for both patients and health care staff.

This chapter introduces the concept of bone marrow failure and identifies some of its causes before focusing on the pathology, treatment and nursing issues of the most common primary bone marrow failure syndrome, acquired aplastic anaemia.

The bone marrow

The bone marrow is a highly structured, organised and regulated tissue that maintains the body's daily requirement for blood cells throughout life. It also has the capacity for a rapid increase of production in response to specific situations such as bleeding, injury or infection. In fact, the healthy bone marrow is a remarkable cell factory, releasing 10^{13} blood cells into the circulation every day (Gordon-Smith 2009). The bone marrow itself

---

Haematology Nursing, First Edition. Marvelle Brown and Tracey J. Cutler.
© 2012 Blackwell Publishing Ltd. Published 2012 by Blackwell Publishing Ltd.

is composed of two interrelated compartments: the cellular compartment and the bone marrow stroma. The bone marrow stroma is sometimes described as the 'soil' as it contains the cells required to support the haemopoietic stem cells and progeny (daughter cells) that make up the cellular compartment. Haemopoietic stem cells live deep within the bone marrow and serve as the 'seed' to all blood cells; although they are relatively few in numbers they are nonetheless able to maintain blood cell production throughout life. The stroma contains cells such as fibroblasts, endothelial cells, fat cells and macrophages located in an extracellular matrix that serves as a supportive framework. In addition, haemopoietic growth factors and other chemical messengers (cytokines) carefully regulate the development of blood cells and the rate of production. Just as the soil in a garden provides the appropriate environment for seeds to germinate and grow, the stromal compartment provides a structural and functional environment for the proliferation, differentiation and maturation of progenitor cells and for the long-term survival of the stem cell pool.

Bone marrow failure

In haemato-oncology practice, temporary bone marrow failure is a common though potentially life-threatening event. It is often secondary to diseases such as leukaemia, where normal haemopoiesis is replaced by the production of malignant cells or it can be an outcome of treatments such as cytotoxic chemotherapy or radiotherapy. Unlike the failure associated with pathological processes, treatment related bone marrow failure is both anticipated and time limited and the bone marrow eventually recovers from the damaging effects of the treatment. An important exception to this is the bone marrow failure induced by the conditioning therapies commonly used in haemopoietic stem cell transplantation (HSCT) which, although anticipated, is not time limited. In high doses, some cytotoxic chemotherapeutic agents and radiotherapy are capable of permanently damaging the bone marrow; this is used therapeutically as the 'conditioning' prior to transplantation. In this situation, the haemopoietic stem cells are killed off; therefore 're-seeding' the bone marrow with previously collected haemopoietic stem cells must take place in order to re-establish bone marrow function. In the case of diseases such as leukaemia, the use of repeated courses of cytotoxic chemotherapy to rid the bone marrow of the malignant cells can enable the re-establishment of normal bone marrow function.

As we have seen, failure of the bone marrow to produce sufficient blood cells can be a secondary event and may, at times, be temporary. However, it is also possible for the bone marrow to fail directly as a result of abnormalities in the cellular compartment, the stroma and/or the local regulation of bone marrow production. This is often referred to as primary bone marrow failure. This type of bone marrow failure can be seen in a few rare genetic conditions such as Fanconi's anaemia, dyskeratosis congenita and Swachman-Diamond syndrome. These are generally, though not exclusively, autosomal recessive or X-linked diseases, with unstable chromosomes and a higher incidence of cancer (Dokal and Vulliamy 2007). The diseases are also characterised by a number of somatic abnormalities such as, for example, skeletal abnormalities in Fanconi's anaemia or abnormal skin, nail and mucosa in dyskeratosis congenita. Although most individuals are diagnosed in childhood, some may initially present with primary bone marrow failure, termed aplastic anaemia, in adulthood. It is therefore essential to exclude any underlying genetic conditions prior to starting any treatment for aplastic anaemia, as treatment for these individuals differs from those of acquired aplastic anaemia. In total, these genetic conditions make up approximately 15–20% of patients with aplastic anaemia (Dokal and Vulliamy 2007). However, most cases of aplastic anaemia can be described as acquired as they are not linked to any specific inherited disease.

Acquired aplastic anaemia is the most common non-malignant primary bone marrow failure syndrome. Although in some cases the bone marrow failure can be linked to an infection such as hepatitis or can be an idiosyncratic reaction to a pharmaceutical agent such as the antibiotic chloramphenicol, the vast majority of cases of aplastic anaemia (70–80%) can be said to be idiopathic, as no definitive cause for the bone marrow failure can be identified. The remainder of this chapter will focus on acquired aplastic anaemia.

Incidence and pathophysiology

Aplastic anaemia is an uncommon disease with an incidence of approximately two per million in western countries, but with a higher incidence of 4–5 per million in South-east Asia (Young and Kaufman 2008). The geographical differences in incidence point to a possible link to environment in a proportion of cases of AA. The sex ratio is nearly 1:1 (Montane *et al.* 2008) and there are two particularly susceptible age groups: the young adult and the older person. Its causes are still not known, but it is now thought that in a large proportion of individuals there is an autoimmune component combined with a possible genetic susceptibility (Young *et al.* 2006). For example, individuals with particular HLA types appear to have a predisposition to AA; this may be a possible link to an underlying immune dysfunction (Maciejewski *et al.* 2001; Young 2006). Some patients with AA have cytogenetic abnormalities also seen in myelodysplastic syndrome (MDS), a disease which can also present as bone marrow failure. Others have abnormalities associated with paroxysmal nocturnal haemoglobinurea (PNH), a disease that arises from a mutation of a gene on the X chromosome that has strong links to acquired aplastic anaemia (de Latour *et al.* 2008).

The bone marrow failure of aplastic anaemia is now thought to be in part a result of damage to the haemopoietic stem cells and to the early offspring of the stem cells, known as progenitor cells. Experiments using bone marrow stroma from individuals with aplastic anaemia and haemopoietic cells from normal individuals have been able to show that, in general, the stroma is able to sustain haemopoietic cell growth and development (Maciejewski and Risitano 2003; Marsh 1996). On the other hand, aplastic anaemia stem cells placed in normal stroma often fail to thrive (Marsh 1996), indicating that the stem cells may in some way be deficient. AA stem cells appear to be both quantitatively and qualitatively different from their normal counterparts; there are fewer of them and they respond less well to stimulation with growth factors (Maciejewski *et al.* 1996; Maciejewski and Risitano 2003; Novitsky and Jacobs 2000).

In addition, the stem cells of a proportion of individuals with aplastic anaemia also appear to have an identifiable primary defect which may also contribute to their overall decline. In particular, these cells have shortened telomeres; these are 'tails' at the end of chromosomes that get shorter each time the cell cycles. Once the tail becomes too short then the cell is no longer able to cycle and then ages and dies. Normally human cells have telomeres that allow for approximately 30–40 cycles. However, the telomeres of stem cells are longer and can also be re-lengthened using an enzyme called telomerase, effectively extending the life of the stem cell. A proportion of individuals with AA have shorter than expected telomeres and low levels of telomerase activity which may limit the cycling potential and survival of these cells (Du *et al.* 2009; Risitano *et al.* 2007), while others have higher levels of telomerase, indicating a high rate of cell cycling, which might lead to stem cell exhaustion and failure of production (Polychronopoulou and Koutroumba 2004; Albitar *et al.* 2002). Telomeres are also shortened in inherited bone marrow failure syndromes (Dokal and Vulliamy 2008; Du *et al.* 2009) indicating a potential link between some of the genetic abnormalities of the inherited syndromes and the basis of the bone marrow failure of some individuals with acquired aplastic anaemia.

There is also evidence of an immune attack by rogue immune cells as a cause of bone marrow failure in AA. Early indicators of a possible immune pathology as the basis of AA included the spontaneous recovery of autologous (the patient's own) bone marrow function following unsuccessful allogeneic transplantation in some individuals with AA (Jeannet *et al.* 1974; Territo 1977). In those failed early transplants, the healthy transplanted cells did not survive, but then the recipient's own remaining stem cells started to grow again. This outcome led clinicians to theorise that suppressing the immune system may have given the person's own stem cells a chance to recover and that therefore the immune system itself could have been partly responsible for the bone marrow failure in the first place.

In addition, it was observed that immunosuppressive conditioning in syngeneic (identical twin) transplants was necessary. A few individuals with aplastic anaemia were fortunate enough to have a healthy identical twin. As these were assumed to be immunologically nearly identical and since the haemopoietic stem cells were also thought to be identical, it was not anticipated that there would be a need to 'knock out' the recipient's immune system in order for the new stem cells to be accepted and to grow. However, this turned out not to be the case and the transplants failed. Subsequently it was shown that suppressing the immune system with conditioning treatment did allow the transplanted stem cells to grow; this again provided evidence for an immune problem as a basis for the bone marrow failure in AA (Champlin *et al.* 1984; Hinterberger *et al.* 1997). These observations and subsequent experiments also provided the rationale for the use of immunosuppression as the primary treatment for those individuals with AA where haemopoietic stem cell transplantation is not an option.

Subsequent experiments have linked a particular type of immune cell, the T-cell (a type of lymphocyte), to the loss and suppression of stem and progenitor cells (Brodsky and Jones 2005; Young 2006; Young *et al.* 2008). These particular T-cells are involved in the destruction of abnormal cells, such as virally infected cells, and are found in larger than expected numbers in the bone marrow of AA patients. These are powerful cells that play an important role in our immune defences, but as they have the ability to destroy our own cells, they are normally tightly controlled. However, in AA it appears that they may mistakenly target bone marrow cells. These T-cells are thought to destroy stem cells by inducing apoptosis (programmed cell death) and also to inhibit haemopoiesis. This may, in part, be through the production of cytokines such as γ-interferon and tumour necrosis factor (TNF) by the rogue T-cells (Bacigalupo 2007). Auto-reactive T-cells such as these behave inappropriately by attacking the person they are meant to protect and are generally associated with the development of autoimmune disease. In addition, another type of T-cell, called regulatory T-cells, whose role it is to control or dampen down immune responses and to suppress any auto-reactive T-cells, are often deficient in AA (Solomou *et al.* 2007). Therefore AA can, in part, be viewed as an immune based condition in which the target is the haemopoietic stem cell transplant (HSCT) in the bone marrow. However, it is possible that idiopathic/acquired aplastic anaemia may also include distinct sub-groups of patients with different pathologies that ultimately lead to bone marrow failure; the exact mechanisms that result in this type of bone marrow failure have yet to be fully understood. However, when reading the scientific literature on AA, it is worth briefly reflecting on the challenges involved in researching a rare disease involving cells that are secretive at the best of times and that in addition are abnormally few in number and no longer functioning, and acknowledging the achievements to date.

The specific triggers that lead to the development of aplastic anaemia are also not yet known. Some viral infections have been implicated, for example 5–10% of patients who develop bone marrow failure present following a viral hepatitis. Certain pharmaceutical agents have also been implicated, including penicillamine, gold, sulphonamides, furo-semide, carbamazepine allopurinol, corticosteroids and anti-epileptic drugs (Focosi *et al.* 2008; Kaufman *et al.* 1996). Chloramphenicol has been strongly associated with AA in the past but is now seldom used as an oral antibiotic; chloramphenicol eye drops, which are commonly used, are not strongly associated with AA (Lam *et al.* 2002). The recreational drug ecstasy has also been linked to a few cases of AA (Richman and Ferber 2008). Pesticides, radiation, lubricating oils and solvents including benzene have also been associated with the development of AA (Muir *et al.* 2003). Aplastic anaemia can also occasionally occur in pregnancy and in this situation often requires intensive management and support as it poses a serious risk to both mother and foetus (Deka *et al.* 2004; Kwon *et al.* 2006).

Presentation

An inevitable consequence of the lack of bone marrow function is a reduction in numbers (cytopenia) of red cells (erythrocytes), platelets (thrombocytes) and white cells (leucocytes) in the peripheral blood. If the peripheral blood cytopenia can be seen in at least two or all three cell lines this is referred to as pancytopenia. Consequently, patients with AA frequently present with problems commonly associated with anaemia, neutropenia and thrombocytopenia, such as fatigue, shortness of breath, infection or abnormal bleeding. Typically, the person may present to the general practitioner with unexplained fatigue, shortness of breath during routine activities such as walking or climbing stairs, an infection that does not resolve or unexplained bruising – often this bruising is in the form of tiny pin prick bruises and is referred to as petechiae. Women may complain of unusually heavy menstrual bleeding or the person may be referred to the GP by a dentist who has observed excessive gum bleeding during routine treatment. A full blood count will indicate the need for a prompt referral to a haematologist for assessment but in itself will not be sufficient to identify the reason for the bone marrow failure.

Diagnosis

Although the diagnosis of AA can often be relatively straightforward, it is nonetheless a diagnosis of exclusion. As we have seen, bone marrow failure can be present in a number of other disease states such as haematological malignancies, myelodysplastic syndrome, paroxysmal nocturnal haemoglobinuria (PNH), Fanconi's anaemia (FA) and other conditions. Part of the diagnostic process is to rule out these other causes of marrow failure and therefore careful examination of bone marrow samples (bone marrow aspirate and trephine biopsy) taken from the person is essential for an accurate diagnosis.

In aplastic anaemia, the colonies of cells that are to become our blood cells (haemopoietic tissue) are usually scant or absent (hypocellular) and are replaced by fat cells – a normal process in inactive bone marrow. Reticulin, a network of thin connective tissue fibres that forms part of our normal bone marrow structure (McCarthy 1985), is also examined for any changes. In some pathological conditions such as in haematological malignancies, an increase in reticulin fibres or a change in the structure of the fibres can be seen (Burston and Pinninger 1963; McCarthy 1985). As reticulin is generally normal in AA (Marsh 1996), increased or altered reticulin indicates a possible alternative diagnosis. As fibrosis of the bone marrow is also generally absent in AA, its presence would also indicate another diagnosis such as a myeloproliferative disease (McCarthy 1985).

Other diagnostic tests will be performed to exclude nutritional causes for the bone marrow failure, inherited forms of the disease, PNH, and to assess for viral infections or any cytogenetic abnormalities. The peripheral blood counts are used to assess the severity of bone marrow failure; in addition, the extent of bone marrow hypocellularity is assessed. The patients are then categorised as non-severe, severe or very severe. These categories can be useful when deciding treatment options and assessing patient outcomes.

Management

It is recommended that individuals with aplastic anaemia are treated in centres familiar with the medical and nursing management of this rare disease (Marsh *et al.* 2009) and that evidence-based protocols are available to guide staff caring for these patients. Initial management of aplastic anaemia often involves managing the consequences of the cytopaenias and may include red cell and platelet transfusions, prophylactic or therapeutic antibiotics to prevent or treat infections as well as specific infection control strategies to protect the individual from exposure to potential infections. Even before the diagnosis is confirmed, when transfusing an individual with suspected AA, it is essential to consider any special requirements such as CMV negative or irradiated blood products as these could ultimately impact on long-term treatment outcomes, particularly if the person is subsequently offered HSCT as a treatment option.

When considering the most appropriate treatment options for a person with aplastic anaemia, a multidisciplinary approach to decision making is recommended (Marsh *et al.* 2009). So as to be able to answer questions that may arise while caring for the patient, nurses should have a good understanding of the available options for that individual and the factors that are taken into account in selecting the most appropriate treatment strategy. There is also evidence that minimising the delay from presentation to the start of appropriate treatment may be linked to better overall outcomes. Therefore, once the diagnosis of aplastic anaemia has been confirmed and if there is no evidence of spontaneously improving blood counts, which would indicate a transient failure of bone marrow production, prompt decisions regarding treatment are recommended. The nurse can support this process by ensuring that all of the necessary assessments and tests are completed in a timely fashion, that results are available and documented, that supportive therapies such as infection preventative measures are promptly instituted and that the patient's perspective is voiced and taken into account during the decision-making process. At this time the patient will need support in coming to terms with the diagnosis and the nurse can also be instrumental in facilitating their understanding of the disease and proposed treatment options.

Treatment options in aplastic anaemia include supportive therapies, immune suppressive therapy (IST) and haemopoietic stem cell transplantation (HSCT). As the immune attack on HSCTs results in the damage or death of those stem cells, treatment will involve suppressing the immune attack (IST) or replacing the lost/damaged stem cells with donated healthy cells (HSCT). For suppression of the immune attack to be successful, sufficient numbers of viable autologous HSC are required to ensure bone marrow recovery. On the other hand, in order to ensure the long-term growth and survival of the replacement stem cells in HSCT, a suitable donor, one who is a close immunological match, must be found. In either case, suppressing the immune system for long periods is necessary.

The treatment strategy selected for each individual will be influenced by a number of factors, including the range and severity of the cytopenias, the degree of transfusion dependence, the age and general health of the person, the availability of a matched donor and the person's quality of life. Individuals with either severe or very severe disease will generally be offered IST or HSCT; those with non-severe disease may be regularly monitored for signs of disease progression (for example falling blood counts) or be offered treatment. Younger persons may be offered transplantation as a first option, whereas immune suppressive therapy may be more appropriate for older individuals. As the two main treatment options are very different and produce different toxicities, it is important for the clinical team to take all factors into consideration prior to making a final recommendation (Armand and Antin 2007; Marsh 2006). Regardless of the decisions that are taken the patient must be helped to understand the factors that influenced those decisions and must have a clear treatment plan to help them make sense of the situation and their options.

Treatment

Immune suppression

Although the replacement of damaged stem cells via allogeneic HSCT is currently the only therapeutic strategy that affords a potential cure for aplastic anaemia, immune suppression, in particular the suppression of lymphocytes and the removal of potentially auto-reactive T-cells, can generate long-term remissions in a proportion of individuals. Remission in this context can be defined as transfusion independence and a neutrophil count above 0.5×10^9/litre (Gordon-Smith 2008). Immune-suppressive therapy includes antithymocyte globulin (ATG) and cyclosporine.

Antithymocyte globulin is composed of diverse antibodies (polyclonal immunoglobulins) of animal origin (horse or rabbit) produced following exposure to human thymocytes (early T-cells). These antibodies are primarily directed at T-cell antigens plus, to a much lesser extent, B-cells, plasma cells and natural killer (NK) cells (Mohty 2007; Zand 2006). Antibodies can be described as keys searching out particular locks. In the case of ATG, those locks are specific molecules (antigens) found on the surface of T-cells and other immune cells. Once antibodies find and connect to their corresponding locks (antigens), that cell is marked out for destruction. The antibodies that make up ATG induce T-cells to undergo apoptosis (programmed cell death) and also mediate their destruction through complement-dependent lysis. The complement cascade is a mechanism used to bore holes into the surface of targeted cells leading to their breaking open (lysis) and dying. As a consequence, the number of circulating T-cells reduces rapidly following administration of ATG. There is also some evidence that ATG may have regulatory effect on the immune system (immune modulation) and may promote regulatory T-cells (Mohty 2007) which may, in turn, help to reduce the attack of haemopoietic stem cells by the rogue T-cells. However, the exact actions of ATG on the bone marrow of AA patients are not yet fully understood. Nevertheless, it is anticipated that up to 70–80% of patients will respond to this treatment (Young *at al.* 2008). Response may be partial or temporary and the person's blood count might not return to normal. Partial responses, leading to transfusion independence can, however, improve the person's quality of life and reduce the risk of infection or haemorrhage. As relapse is common, further courses of ATG treatment can be an option (Gupta *et al.* 2005; Tichelli *et al.* 1998).

As ATG formulations differ in composition and in the capacity to suppress immunity, the appropriate therapeutic doses will vary accordingly (Mohty 2007; Zand 2006); it is therefore imperative that nurses are familiar with the formulations commonly used in their clinical setting. Antithymocyte globulin is infused in an in-patient setting usually over a period of 4–5 days; the duration of each infusion is 12–18 hours. Antithymocyte globulin can cause severe damage to veins; it therefore must be administered via a central venous catheter (CVC). As ATG is derived from animals, there is a risk of type 1 hypersensitivity (allergic) reactions. It is therefore recommended that a test dose be given prior to the start of the first infusion (Marsh *et al.* 2009).

During the test dose, patients may suddenly experience symptoms including flushing, shortness of breath, bronchospasm and tachycardia and these may progress to frank anaphylaxis and severe hypotension. The patient should therefore be closely monitored throughout the test dose; oxygen, bronchodilators, IV antihistamine/anti-inflammatory agents as well as resuscitation equipment must be readily available. The test dose and the first ATG infusion should be administered during normal working hours when members of the medical team in charge of the patient are present. If the person does exhibit a hypersensitivity response to the ATG test dose, re-challenging with ATG is not recommended (Marsh *et al.* 2009) due to the risk of anaphylaxis on subsequent exposures. Desensitisation has been attempted but carries inherent risks and has not been shown to be particularly successful (Bielory *et al.* 1988; Ferdman *et al.* 2004; Millar and Grammer 2000).

Prior to ATG infusions, the person's full blood count should be assessed. Antithymocyte globulin has anti-platelet activity (Greco *et al.* 1983) and therefore patients regularly require platelet transfusions prior to each ATG infusion; for the same reason platelets should not be given simultaneously with the ATG infusion. It is also advisable to ensure that the platelet increment is satisfactory; current BCSH guidelines (Marsh *et al.* 2009) for the management of aplastic anaemia recommend a platelet count of $>30 \times 10^9/L$. Red cell transfusions may also be required during treatment to maintain an adequate haemoglobin count. The use of irradiated blood products is currently recommended during and in the months following treatment with ATG in order to reduce the risk of transfusion associated graft versus host disease (Marsh *et al.* 2009). Intravenous (IV) antihistamines and anti-inflammatory agents such as chlorphenamine and methylprednisolone plus paracetamol are also necessary prior to each ATG infusion in order to reduce the risk of reactions.

Despite prophylaxis, many patients will nevertheless experience side effects during the infusion. Rigors and fever are very common; these often occur a few hours into the first or subsequent infusions and can be very distressing for the patient. It is therefore important to advise them of this prior to starting the ATG and to reassure them that it is an anticipated side effect. If the person does develop a fever during the infusion, it is still necessary to follow the standard procedures for neutropenia-associated fever, including blood cultures and first-line, broad-spectrum antibiotics as stipulated in local trust policies. Other side effects may include flushing, rashes, hypertension or hypotension, and fluid retention. Regular monitoring is therefore essential and includes vital signs (temperature, pulse, blood pressure and respirations), O_2 saturations, daily weights, a strict fluid input/output chart and a skin assessment. If the side effects persist and/or are difficult to tolerate, it may also be possible to reduce the infusion rate; this should not impact on the overall efficacy of the therapy.

Following ATG therapy, up to 75% of patients develop serum sickness. Serum sickness is an immune mediated reaction to protein in antiserum derived from animal sources. Serum sickness is thought to be a consequence of the development of immune complexes and is classed as a type 3 hypersensitivity response (Bielory *et al.* 1985; 1988). Signs and symptoms include fever, malaise, arthralgia, myalgia, gastro-intestinal disturbances, rashes and other skin eruptions, proteinuria and occasional lymphadenopathy. Following treatment with ATG, the person's skin should be assessed for any changes or a developing rash. Areas such as the palms of the hands or soles of the feet, and between the fingers or toes are often targets and may become erythematous (reddened) or the person may develop a rash on the trunk, back or extremities (Bielory *et al.* 1985; Lawley *et al.* 1985). As the patients are often thrombocytopaenic, the rash may become purpuric (bleeding into the rash) and the person may require additional platelet support. Following ATG therapy steroids such as prednisolone are initially given to prevent or minimise serum sickness, though these are generally quickly tailed off. In the context of established serum sickness, IV methylprednisolone will be given to control the reaction.

Response to ATG therapy is usually not seen for weeks or months and evidence supports enhancing the immune suppression with cyclosporine in addition to ATG to improve the overall response to treatment (Young *et al.* 2008). Cyclosporine is usually taken for a year following ATG treatment and is tailed off slowly as there is a risk of relapse when immunosuppression is reduced. However, it is important to remember that these profoundly immunosuppressed patients are at long-term risk of serious infections. Cyclosporine (CsA) is also a potentially toxic agent with a number of side effects, including hypertension, kidney and liver toxicities. Cyclosporine also causes hair growth which can be problematic for women in particular and can also cause gum overgrowth and fragility, leading to bleeding gums. Patients require regular oral and blood pressure assessments plus regular blood tests to monitor CsA levels, renal and liver function. In addition, patients need to report any headaches as the hypertension can occur at night, or any unusual sensations such as tingling or numbness as CsA is also neurotoxic (Rezzani 2004).

Haemopoietic stem cell transplantation

In AA, haemopoietic stem cell transplantation (HSCT) involves the replacement of damaged or absent haemopoietic stem cells with healthy donated allogeneic (which means coming from another) stem cells and offers the potential for cure. The long-term survival of an allogeneic graft involves the manipulation of complex immunological processes and also requires a healthy bone marrow microenvironment and stroma in order to ensure the long-term survival of the new pool of stem cells and to support the production of blood cells. For the transplant to be successful, the patient's own immune system must be 'knocked out' with cytotoxic chemotherapy, immune suppressive agents and perhaps also radiotherapy in order for the donated healthy stem cells to replace the damaged or absent stem cells. As the recipient's immune system is programmed to recognise these new stem cells as foreign and to destroy them, 'knocking it out' creates a window of opportunity for the transplanted cells to survive, establish themselves and grow. Once established, these transplanted stem cells will generate new immune cells and replace the rogue T-cells with healthy ones.

Unfortunately, HSCT is a treatment option for the minority of individuals with AA fortunate enough to have a closely matched donor. Donors can either be siblings or matched unrelated donors (MUD), who are volunteers on national and international donor panels. In the UK the Anthony Nolan Trust provides donor stem cells. Other factors, such as age, general state of health and co-morbidities, may also preclude HSCT as a viable option. Evidence suggests that using HSCT earlier leads to better overall outcomes (Armand and Antin 2007), therefore HSCT may be the first treatment option for the younger healthy person with a matched donor. For others, HSCT may be considered once it is clear that immune suppressive treatment has failed. Haemopoietic stem cells can be obtained in a number of ways: directly from the bone marrow, via the peripheral blood (PBSC) following donor stem cell mobilisation with G-SCF and from the umbilical cord blood immediately following delivery. In AA, bone marrow collection is currently recommended as the method of choice as there is some evidence of poorer outcomes following PBSC transplants, including graft rejection (Marsh *et al.* 2009). Umbilical cord stem cell collections currently have a limited role because of lower stem cell numbers and the risk of graft rejection following transplantation (Aki *et al.* 2009; Marsh *et al.* 2009).

Early and late graft rejection is a significant problem in HSCT for aplastic anaemia. An important risk factor for graft failure is a high number of transfusions prior to HSCT; this is one of the reasons for electing early transplantation in suitable candidates. Prior to HSCT, the irradiation of blood products, which kills off most of the lymphocytes, reduces sensitisation to others' 'self' markers and therefore reduces the risk of rejection. Irradiation of blood components during and after transplant is also essential in order to reduce the risk of transfusion-associated graft versus host disease. Conditioning regimes which include powerful immune suppressants such as ATG also reduce the incidence of graft rejection (Aki *et al.* 2009). Following HSCT, immune suppression continues a year or more with the use of cyclosporine. Blood levels of cyclosporine must be closely monitored and maintained to ensure graft survival and to minimise the risk of graft versus host disease and, at the same time, to minimise the risk of serious drug-related side effects. Tailing off the cyclosporine is often started at about nine months post-transplant and is gradually reduced over a period of three months (Marsh *et al.* 2009). If blood counts start to fall or if other tests indicate the potential for rejection, then cyclosporine doses are once again increased and the patient is closely monitored.

Recovery following HSCT is a long process; infection, fatigue, graft versus host disease, concordance with medication regimes and regular hospital attendance can be particular challenges for patients and can impact on quality of life. Nurses have an important role to play in supporting patients at this time; helping them to manage the physical, psychological and social impact of HSCT.

Supportive care

As AA patients are often pancytopenic and are also receiving immunosuppressive agents, they are invariably vulnerable to a range of bacterial, fungal and viral infections and require protection from colonisation with pathogenic organisms, reactivation of viruses and the emergence of opportunistic infections. Infections pose a particular threat to individuals with aplastic anaemia because of the persistent neutropenia and infection remains a major cause of death in AA. Aplastic anaemia patients are particularly susceptible to invasive fungal infections including candida and aspergillus and these infections are often associated with a high mortality rate (Torres *et al.* 2003; Valdez *et al.* 2009). Gram positive infections are also common; staphylococcal infections in particular are associated with central venous catheters (Torres *et al.* 2003; Wolf *et al.* 2008) and are common in this group of patients. In addition, Gram negative infections such as pseudomonas can also prove challenging, particularly as resistant bacterial strains are now regularly emerging (Valdez *et al.* 2009). Common viral infections in the context of aplastic anaemia include herpes simplex, herpes zoster and community associated respiratory tract infections (Torres *et al.* 2003; Valdez *et al.* 2009). Due to the risk of serious respiratory tract infections, it is advisable that staff with upper respiratory tract infections should avoid caring for these immune-compromised individuals.

Strategies used to protect patients from infections include the use of prophylactic antiviral, antibiotic and antifungal agents, protective isolation when hospitalised and the use of a clean food diet in order to minimise patients' exposure to potential harmful organisms. It is important to remember that AA patients are often discharged home with a low neutrophil count and many experience long-term neutropenia. They may therefore need to implement infection prevention strategies in their home environment and undertake self-monitoring with regards to infection. It is also important to remember that the single most important infection control strategy involves regular and effective hand washing by all. Staff, patients and relatives should therefore be taught to wash their hands thoroughly and at the appropriate time in order to minimise the risk of cross infection. Particular care should also be taken with central venous access devices (CVADs) as they are a direct entry point for microbes into the bloodstream. Staff must therefore be trained to access these catheters using an appropriate no-touch technique and close monitoring of the incidence and type of CVAD infections must be part of the clinical area's routine auditing strategy. In addition, ongoing monitoring of general infection control standards should be undertaken in units caring for these vulnerable individuals.

Encouraging the person to maintain optimal oral hygiene may help to reduce the incidence of oral infections. This includes regular oral cleansing during the day and after meals, the use of soft toothbrushes to minimise injury to the gums and reporting any changes in their oral health, which may include such things as pain or discomfort in the mouth or when swallowing, ulceration or gum bleeding. A daily visual assessment by a member of the health care team trained to identify oral infections such as candida is also necessary. Patients (or carers if appropriate) can also be shown how to inspect their own mouths, enabling them to continue daily inspections following discharge. It is important to remember that, unlike patients undergoing treatment with cytotoxic chemotherapy, AA patients do not generally experience the severe mucositis associated with treatment for haematological malignancies (Valdez *et al.* 2009), except during HSCT. However, as a result of the chronic neutropenia, the often low platelet counts (thrombocytopenia) and the immune-suppressive therapies, they are at risk of serious oral infections and gum bleeding; therefore regular oral care with agents that may reduce infection risk and excellent long-term oral hygiene is essential in this patient group. Once established, infection can be very distressing and painful for the person, limiting nutritional and fluid intake as well as the ability to talk and sometimes even the ability to swallow their own saliva. At these times oral care may need to be offered half-hourly or hourly and strong analgesics may well be necessary to offer relief and to enable sleep and rest.

Ongoing vigilance through close monitoring for early signs of infection is an important role of the health care professionals caring for persons who are immunocompromised. While hospitalised, daily assessments of the oral cavity, CVC exit site, urine, bowels and skin are required to identify early signs of infection. Patients should also be actively encouraged to report any symptoms as these can often serve as valuable early warning signs. As the imflammatory response is often diminished in the context of neutropenia, fever is often the only warning sign of a possible infection and the presence of fever necessitates prompt action to minimise the risks of sepsis or severe sepsis. Increased respirations and heart rate, even in the absence of fever, can also indicate a systemic infection. A falling blood pressure is indicative of sepsis and must be treated as an emergency.

Evidence indicates that starting broad-spectrum antibiotic therapy promptly (within one hour) if sepsis is suspected, improves overall survival (Dellinger *et al.* 2008). It is therefore imperative to monitor the person on a regular basis and, if infection is suspected, avoid any delay in contacting the medical team, taking appropriate blood cultures and septic screen and starting therapy. In prolonged infections, GCSF (granulocyte colony stimulating factor), a growth factor that increases the production of neutrophils, may be given in an attempt to increase the neutrophil count (Marsh *et al.* 2009).

Appropriate blood product support is a key element in the management of AA as patients may be dependent on both red cells and platelets for months or years. Patients often have special requirements such as CMV negative, irradiated or HLA matched blood products so systems must be in place to ensure that all staff are aware of patients' specific requirements and that they understand their importance. Other possible consequences of long-term transfusion requirements in aplastic anaemia include platelet refractoriness and iron overload.

Platelet refractoriness is a consequence of the immune system responding to foreign antigens associated with the transfused platelets. Once recognised, platelets are targeted for destruction and subsequent transfused platelets are destroyed. In this situation the person's platelet increment, the anticipated rise in the count, will not be achieved and there will be a quick return to the baseline platelet count. If this is suspected then a blood count is taken one hour following the transfusion to assess its effect on the platelet count. If it has not risen to the anticipated level, then the person may require either single donor platelets or HLA matched platelets to ensure an appropriate incremental rise in the platelet count following transfusion.

Iron overload occurs as a result of multiple red cell transfusions. As the body has very limited capacity to rid itself of excess iron, normally the iron released from destroyed red cells is recycled and used again in the manufacture of new red cells. Individuals who do not make their own red cells, as is the case in AA, and are dependent on transfusions to maintain normal haemoglobin levels may have large amounts of spare iron that they are unable to either use or excrete. Some of the iron can be stored but once the stores are full iron is deposited in tissue such as the skin and liver. Iron deposition is harmful to tissue and can cause organ failure. Patients with iron overload often have an unusual colouring to their skin and may, for example, have evidence of liver, renal or cardiac insufficiency. Individuals with aplastic anaemia who require regular red cell transfusions must be monitored for iron overload and may require iron chelating therapy which helps bind the iron, prevents deposition and makes it easier to excrete.

Accessible day-care facilities are an important element of the service provision for aplastic anaemia patients, as regular appointments for assessment, blood tests and red cell and platelet transfusions are required at all stages of the disease, and nurses in this clinical setting must be familiar with the specific needs of these patients. Patients often attend on a regular basis for extended periods of time and therefore become very familiar with procedures and processes. Nevertheless, it is important that the care offered should not in itself become routine and that regular re-assessments are made of their needs since their situation and their ability to cope may substantively change over time. It is also important to remember that, although they may appear to be familiar with procedures and with the terms commonly used, patients still need explanations and opportunities to ask questions.

Nurses also need to be aware of the anxiety and frustration that this chronic illness can engender. Waiting for a response to treatment is often a long and naturally anxious time for patients. Blood results often become a focus for patients, with hopeful expectation often followed by disappointment if the results do not show the hoped for improvement. It is also important to remember that the cells produced by the bone marrow give us vitality and a feeling of wellness and that their long-term absence can be very debilitating and will impact on most aspects of daily life and the person's overall quality of life. Nurses caring for these individuals cannot hope to make it 'all alright' but can help by providing a clean, flexible and inviting clinical environment, by providing knowledgeable and consistent nursing care, by offering clear and accurate explanations in a timely way and by offering emotional support through listening. It is also important that staff support the person to accept the often chronic nature of this complex disease as the bone marrow in aplastic anaemia requires long-term management and thoughtful care in the hope of making it productive once again.

References

Akı, S.Z., Sucak, G.T., Özkurt, Z.N., Yeğin, Z.A., Yağcı, M. and Haznedar, R. (2009) Allogeneic stem cell transplantation for severe aplastic anaemia: Graft rejection remains a problem. *Transfusion and Apheresis Science*, 40, 5–11.

Albitar, M., Manshouri, T., Shen, Y. *et al.* (2002) Myelodysplastic syndrome is not merely preleukaemia. *Blood*, 100 (3), 791.

Armand, P. and Antin, J. (2007) Allogeneic stem cell transplantation for aplastic anaemia. *Biology of Bone and Marrow Transplantation*, 13, 505–516.

Bacigalupo, A. (2007) Aplastic anaemia: pathogenesis and treatment. *Hematology*, 23–28.

Bielory, L., Yancey, K.B., Young, N.S., Frank, M.M. and Lawley, T.J. (1985) Cutaneous manifestations of serum sickness in patients receiving antithymocyte globulin. *Journal of the American Academy of Dermatology*, 13 (3), 411–417.

Bielory, L., Gascon, P., Lawley, T.J., Young, N.S. and Frank, M.M. (1988) Human serum sickness: a prospective analysis of 35 patients treated with equine anti-thymocyte globulin for bone marrow failure. *Medicine*, 67 (1), 40–57.

Brodsky, R. and Jones, R. (2005) Aplastic anaemia. *The Lancet*, 365, 1647–1656.

Burston, J. and Pinninger, J.L. (1963) The reticulin content of bone marrow in haematological disorders. *British Journal of Haematology*, 9, 172–184.

Champlin, R.E., Feig, S.A., Sparkers, R.S. and Gale, R.P. (1984) Bone marrow transplantation from identical twins in the treatment of aplastic anaemia: implications for the pathogenesis of the disease. *British Journal of Haematology*, 56, 455–463.

Deka, D., Banerjee, N., Roy, K.K., Choudhary, V.P., Kashyap, R. and Takkar, D. (2004) Aplastic anaemia during pregnancy: variable clinical course and outcome. *European Journal of Obstetrics & Gynaecology and Reproductive Biology*, 94, 152–154.

de Latour, R.P., Mary, J.Y., Salanoubat, C. *et al.* (2008) Paroxysmal nocturnal haemoglobinuria: natural history of disease subcategories. *Blood*, 112, 3099–3106.

Dellinger, R.P., Mitchell, M., Levy, M.M. *et al.* (2008) Surviving Sepsis Campaign: International guidelines for management of severe sepsis and septic shock 2008. *Critical Care Medicine*, 36, 296–327.

Dokal, I. and Vulliamy, T. (2008) Inherited aplastic anaemia's/bone marrow failure syndromes. *Blood Reviews*, 22, 141–153.

Du, H.-Y., Pumbo, E., Ivanovich, J. *et al.* (2009) TERC and TERT gene mutations in patients with bone marrow failure and the significance of telomere length measurements. *Blood*, 113 (2), 309–316.

Ferdman, R.M., Wakim, M., Church, J.A., Hofstra, T.C., Thomas, D. and Genyk, Y.S. (2004) Rapid intravenous desensitization to antithymcyte globulin in a patient with aplastic anemia. *Transplantation*, 77 (2), 321–323.

Focosi, D., Kast, R.E., Benedetti, E., Papineschi, F., Galimberti, S. and Petrini, M. (2008) Phenobarbital-associated bone marrow aplasia: a case report and review of the literature. *Acta Haematol*, 119, 18–21.

Greco, B., Bielory, L., Stephany, D. *et al*. (1983) Antithymocyte globulin reacts with many normal human cell types. *Blood*, 62, 1047–1054.

Gordon-Smith, E.C. (2008) Aplastic anaemia and bone marrow failure. *Medicine*, 37 (4), 179–182.

Gordon-Smith, E.C. (2009) Haemopoiesis: the formation of blood cells. *Medicine*, 37, 129–132.

Gupta, V., Gordon-Smith, E.C., Cook, G. *et al*. (2005) A third course of anti-thymocyte globulin in aplastic anaemia is only beneficial in previous responders. *British Journal of Haematology*, 129, 100–117.

Hinterberger, W., Rowlings, P.A., Hintenberger-Fisher, M. *et al*. (1997) Results of transplanting bone marrow from genetically identical twins into patients with aplastic anaemia. *Annals of Internal Medicine*, 126, 116–122.

Jeannet, M., Rubinstein, A., Pelet, B. and Kummer, H. (1974) Prolonged remission of severe aplastic anaemia after ALG pre-treatment and HGA-semi-incompatible bone marrow cell transfusion. *Transplantation Proceedings*, 6, 359–363.

Kaufman, D.W., Kelly, J.P., Jurgelon, J.M. *et al*. (1996) Drugs in the aetiology of agranulocytosis and aplastic anaemia. *European Journal of Haematology*, 57 (suppl), 23–30.

Kwon, J.Y., Lee, Y., Shin, J.C., Lee, J.W., Rha, J.G. and Kim, S.P. (2006) Supportive management of pregnancy-associated aplastic anemia. *International Journal of Gynaecology and Obstetrics*, 95, 115–120.

Lam, R.F., Lai, J.S.M., Ng, J.S.K., Rao, S.K., Law, R.W.K. and Lam, D.S.C. (2002) Topical chloramphenicol for eye infections. *Hong Kong Medical Journal*, 8 (1), 44–47.

Lawley, T.J., Bielory, L., Gascon, P., Yancey, K.B., Young, N.S. and Frank, M.M. (1985) A study of human serum sickness. *The Journal of Investigative Dermatology*, 85, 129s–132s.

Maciejewski, J.P., Folmann, D. and Rivera, C.E. (2001) Increased frequency of HLA-DR2 in patients with paroxysmal nocturnal haemoglobinurea and PNH/aplastic anemia syndrome. *Blood*, 98, 3513–3519.

Maciejewski, J.P. and Risitano, A. (2003) Hematopoietic stem cells in a plastic anemia. *Archives of Medical Research*, 34, 520–527.

Maciejewski, J.P., Selleri, C., Sato, T., Anderson, S. and Young, N.S. (1996) A severe and consistent deficit in marrow and circulating primitive hematopoietic cells long-term culture initiating cells in acquired aplastic anemia. *Blood*, 88, 1983–1991.

Marsh, J.C.W. (1996) Long- term bone marrow cultures in aplastic anemia. *European Journal of Haematology*, 57 (suppl), 75–79.

Marsh, J. (2006) Making therapeutic decisions in adults with aplastic anemia. *Hematology*, 78–85.

Marsh, J.C.W., Ball, S.E., Cavenagh, J. *et al*. (2009) *Guidelines for the diagnosis and management of aplastic anaemia*. British Committee for Standards in Haematology, London.

McCarthy, D. (1985) Fibrosis of the bone marrow: content and causes. *British Journal of Haematology*, 59, 1–7.

Millar, M.M. and Grammer, M.D. (2000) Case reports of evaluation and desensitization for antithymocyte globulin hypersensitivity. *Annals of Allergy Asthma and Immunology*, 85, 311–316.

Montane, E., Ibanez, L., Vidal, X. *et al*. and the Catalan Group of Agranulocytosis and Aplastic Anaemia (2008) Epidemiology of aplastic anemia: a prospective multicenter study. *Hematologica*, 93 (4), 518–523.

Mohty, M. (2007) Mechanisms of action of antithymocyte globulin: T cell depletion and beyond. *Leukemia*, 21, 1387–1394.

Muir, K.R., Chilvers, C.E.D., Harriss, C. *et al.* (2003) The role of occupational and environmental exposures in the aetiology of acquired severe aplastic anaemia: a case control investigation. *British Journal of Haematology*, 123, 906–914.

Novitzky, N. and Jacob, P. (2000) In aplastic anemia progenitor cells have a reduced sensitivity to the effects of growth factors. *European Journal of Haematology*, 63, 141–148.

Passweg, J., Nissen, C., Bargetzi, M. *et al.* (1998) Repeated treatment with horse antilymphocyte globulin for severe aplastic anaemia *British Journal of Haematology*, 100, 393–400.

Polychronopoulou, S. and Koutroumba, P. (2004) Telomere length variation and telomerase activity expression in patients with congenital and acquired aplastic anemia. *Acta Haematologica*, 111, 125–131.

Rezzani, R. (2004) Cyclosporine A and adverse effects on organs: histochemical studies. *Progress in Histochemistry and Cytochemistry*, 39, 85–128.

Richman, J. and Ferber, A. (2008) Severe aplastic anemia with hot pockets following daily ecstasy ingestion. *American Journal of Hematology*, 83, 321–322.

Risitano, A.M., Maciejewski, J.P., Selleri, C. and Rotoli, B. (2007) Function and malfunction of hematopoietic stem cells in primary bone marrow failure syndromes. *Current Stem Cell Research & Therapy*, 2, 39–52.

Solomou, E.E., Rezvani, K., Mielke, S. *et al.* (2007) Deficient CD4$^+$ CD25$^+$ FOXP3$^+$ T regulatory cells in acquired aplastic anemia. *Blood*, 110 (5), 1603–1606.

Territo, M.C. (1977) Autologous bone marrow repopulation following high dose cyclophosphamide and allogeneic marrow transplantation in aplastic anaemia. *British Journal of Haematology*, 36, 305–312.

Tichelli, A., Passweg, J., Nissen, C. *et al.* (1998) Repeated treatment with horse antilymphocyte globulin for severe aplastic anaemia. *British Journal of Haematology*, 100, 393–400.

Tores, H.A., Bodey, G.P., Rolston, K.V., Kantarjian, H., Raad, I. and Kontoyiannis, D.P. (2003) Infections in patients with aplastic anemia experience at a tertiary care cancer centre. *Cancer*, 98 (1), 86–93.

Valdez, J.M., Scheinberg, P., Young, N.S. and Walsh, T.J. (2009) Infections in patients with aplastic anemia. *Seminars in Haematology*, 46, 269–276.

Wolf, H.H., Leithäuser, M., Maschmeyer, G. *et al.* (2008) Central venous catheter related infections in haematology and oncology: guidelines of the Infectious Diseases Working Party (AGIHO) of the German Society of Hematology and Oncology (DGHO). *Annals of Hematology*, 87, 863–876.

Young, N.S. (2006) Pathophysiologic mechanisms in acquired aplastic anaemia. *Hematology*, 72–76.

Young, N.S., Calado, R.T. and Schienberg, P. (2006) Current concepts in the pathophysiology and treatment of aplastic anemia. *Blood*, 108 (8), 2509–2519.

Young, N.S. and Kaufman, D.W. (2008) The epidemiology of acquired aplastic anemia. *Haematologica*, 93 (4), 489–492.

Young, N.S., Scheinberg, P. and Calado, R.T. (2008) Aplastic anemia. *Current Opinion in Hematology*, 15, 162–168.

Zand, M. (2006) B cell activity of antithymocyte globulins. *Transplantation*, 82, 1387–1395.

Chapter 6

Nutritional anaemia: pathophysiology, care and management

Marvelle Brown

By the end of reading this chapter you will:
- Have a good understanding of the causes of anaemia
- Be familiar with investigations to diagnose causes of anaemia
- Understand how iron is regulated
- Have an understanding of the importance of nutritional assessment
- Be aware of the advice required to support patients with IDA and PA

Introduction

This chapter will highlight the pathophysiology related to nutritional anaemias, with particular reference to iron deficiency anaemia, pernicious anaemia and folate deficiency anaemia. The aetiology, epidemiology and investigations undertaken and treatment, will be addressed. Nursing management will be discussed towards the end of the chapter. To put nutritional anaemias in context, a general overview of anaemia will first be reviewed.

Aetiology and epidemiology

Anaemia can be described as a reduction in the oxygen carrying capacity of red blood cells caused either by a reduction in the number of circulating erythrocytes or reduction in haemoglobin concentration. Defining the level at which anaemia is identified is not universal as factors such as age, gender and ethnicity need to be taken into consideration. UNICEF (2001) suggests that anaemia should be considered when the haemoglobin is below 13 g/dL for men and a level below 10 g/dL for women. In the UK, due to differences between populations, it has been suggested that the lower range of normal haemoglobin values should be used as a benchmark for anaemia (Goddard *et al.* 2005).

Anaemia is very common and the WHO (2008) estimated that 1.62 billion people globally have anaemia; the highest prevalence being found in pre-school children, but the

---

Haematology Nursing, First Edition. Marvelle Brown and Tracey J. Cutler.
© 2012 Blackwell Publishing Ltd. Published 2012 by Blackwell Publishing Ltd.

population group most affected by anaemia were non-pregnant women. Anaemia is not itself an illness but a symptom which warrants investigations to identify the cause. The symptoms of anaemia can range from being mild to severe. However, even if the symptoms are mild it can be an early warning sign of a serious illness such as cancer and therefore should not be ignored and identifying the cause is important.

Classifying anaemia

Anaemia can be classified by the cause of the anaemia, the morphology of red blood cells, as well as the amount of haemoglobin (Table 6.1).

With regards to the morphology of red blood cells they can be:

- Hypochromic microcytic – smaller in size than normal, with reduced haemoglobin, suggests, for example, iron deficiency, beta thalassaemia trait.
- Hyperchromic macrocytic – larger than normal in size with increased haemoglobin, suggests megablastic anaemias, for example pernicious anaemia, folate deficiency, liver disease.
- Normochromic, normocytic – normal size and colour, suggests, for example, aplastic anaemia, acute and chronic bleeding, anaemia of chronic disease, such as renal disease, haemato-oncological disease (Bain 2002).

Both the variation in size (known as anisocytosis), and variation in shape (known as poikilocytosis) are also evident in anaemia.

Table 6.1   Classification of anaemias with examples of causes.

Anaemia due to reduced erythropoiesis	Anaemia due to excessive haemolysis	Anaemia due to blood loss
Aplastic anaemia	Sickle cell disease	Gastric bleeding
Myelofibrosis	Thalassaemia syndromes	Menorrhagia
Vitamin B_{12} deficiency	Hereditary spherocytosis	Oesophageal varices
Folate deficiency	Hereditary elliptocytosis	Inflammatory bowel disease
Iron deficiency	Glucose-6-phosphate-Dehydrogenase (G6PD)	Gastric/duodenal ulceration
Crohn's disease	Pyruvate kinase (PK)	Angiodysplasia
Anaemia of chronic renal failure	Paroxysmal nocturnal haemoglobinuria (PNH)	Carcinoma of the stomach
Endocrine disorder, e.g. lack of thyroxine	Microangiopathic haemolytic anaemia	Haemorrhoids
Sideroblastic anaemia	Malaria	Uterine fibroids
Anaemia of chronic disease		
Myelodysplastic syndrome		
Lead poisoning		

Adapted from: Bain 2006; Campbell 2004; Hoffbrand *et al*. 2004.

Signs and symptoms of anaemia

Reduction in the oxygen-carrying capacity of red blood cells can have a significant negative effect on health as well as social and economic consequences, both in developed and developing countries (WHO 2001). Table 6.2 lists the general signs and symptoms of anaemia.

Table 6.2 Signs and symptoms of anaemia.

Fatigue
Pallor
Angina pectoris
Dyspnoea
Palpitations
Tachycardia
Dizziness
Insomnia
Ankle oedema
Decreased attention span
Irregular menstruation
Anorexia
Flatulence
Increased sensitivity to cold
Increased susceptibility to infection

Investigations

To determine the type of anaemia a patient has requires a number of blood investigations as listed in Tables 6.3 and 6.4 and depending on the findings or lack of a conclusive cause, further investigations maybe required.

Nutritional anaemia

Deficiencies of a number of haematinics such as iron, vitamins, including folic acid, vitamin B_{12}, B6 and vitamin A, can give rise to nutritional anaemias. The most common nutrient deficiency worldwide is iron deficiency anaemia (WHO 2001). In adults in the UK, iron deficiency anaemia (IDA), pernicious anaemia (PA), are the most common nutritional anaemias seen in adults (Campbell 2003; Hurley 2007).

Iron deficiency anaemia

Aetiology and epidemiology

Worldwide, it is estimated there are two billion people globally, with IDA (Zimmerman and Hurrell 2007). From a study undertaken by Heath and Fairweather-Tait (2002) in the UK, 21% of female teenagers aged 11–18 years and 18% of women aged 16–64 are iron deficient.

Table 6.3   Common investigations to diagnose anaemia.

Full blood count (FBC)	Normal values (indices)
RBC	Men – 4.5–5.5 x 10^{12}/L
	Women – 3.8–4.8 x 10^{12}/L
WCC	4–11 x 10^9/L
Platelets	150–400 x 10^9/L
Haemoglobin	Men – 13.5–17.5 g/dL
	Women – 11.5–15.5 g/dL
Reticulocyte	0.5–3.5%
Differential WCC	
Neutrophils	2.0–7.0 x 10^9/L
	(1.5–7.5 x 10^9/L – in blacks)
Basophils	0.05–0.1 x 10^9/L
Eosinophils	0.02–0.5 x 10^9/L
Lymphocytes	1.0–3.0 x 10^9/l
Monocytes	0.2–1.0 x 10^9/l
Mean cell volume	83–101 fl
Packed cell volume (PCV)	Men – 40–50%
	Women – 36–46%
Haematocrit	
Mean cell haemoglobin Concentration (MCHC)	32–36 g/dL
Mean cell haemoglobin (MCH)	27–32 pg*

Adapted from, MacKinney (2002), Mehta and Hoffbrand (2009).
*=picograms.

Table 6.4   Other possible investigations to establish the cause of anaemia.

Urinalysis
Screening for coeliac disease – (anti-endomysial antibody) or tissue transglutaminase
Stool examination for occult blood, parasites
Upper and lower GI investigations
Bone marrow aspiration/bone marrow trephine
Haematinics

Iron metabolism

Iron is an essential element required by nearly all cells for metabolic activity and is key to the function of red blood cells. There is a close regulatory system for controlling iron which is through a process of re-absorption and reutilisation. This is critical for two main reasons:

- Humans have no physiological route to excrete excess iron.
- Iron is a toxic substance and if not controlled could cause significant damage to cells because of its ability to convert hydrogen peroxide into oxygen free radicals which are highly acidic and toxic.

To prevent iron becoming toxic, it is bound to proteins such as haemoglobin apoferritin and ferroportin I. Iron is metabolised through processes in the gastrointestinal tract and the actions of the reticulo-endothelial system (RES) when destroying senescent red blood cells.

In the GI tract, iron is absorbed in the duodenum by enterocytes of the duodenal lining. Food can contain haem iron and non-haem iron (inorganic) compounds. The bioavailability of iron is much more readily available and easily absorbed when it is in the haem iron form, which is found in red meat, liver, fish and eggs (Gizzard 2006). Non-haem iron is primarily found in vegetables, especially green leafy vegetables, nuts, legumes, dried fruits, fortified white bread and breakfast cereals in the UK. The absorption of non-haem iron can be affected by factors as polyphenols found in nuts, tea, coffee, chocolate, pomegranates, berries and some vegetables (Barasi 2007). Both haem iron and non-haem iron have their own special molecules which act as transporters to carry the iron from the enterocytes into circulation. Brush border ferric reductase duodenal cytochrome B (DCYTB) and divalent metal ion transporter 1 (DMT1) (Gunshin *et al.* 1997) are the transporters for non-haem iron.

Prior to non-haem iron being transported it must be converted (reduced) from ferric iron to ferrous iron, which is undertaken by a number of chemicals, including ascorbic acid (Zimmerman and Hurrell 2007). Haem iron is transported by haem carrier protein (HCP1). Depending on demand some of the iron will be taken from the enterocytes into circulation by the protein, ferroportin 1. Iron that is not used is stored in the enterocytes as ferritin and if not used, is lost through intestinal sloughing. Apoferritin, a protein found in the intestinal mucosa, binds and stores iron by combining with a ferric hydroxide-phosphate compound to form ferritin which enables the liver to store iron as ferritin (De Domenico *et al.* 2008).

Macrophages in the spleen and liver are two key organs of the RES responsible for the destruction of senescent red blood cells. The normal lifespan for red blood cells is 120 days and when they reach the end of their life (as discussed in Chapter 1), the iron is separated from the 'haem'. Transferrin is a plasma protein which transports iron to the liver, spleen and the bone marrow where erythroid precursors have transferrin binding receptors sites (TfRs). This allows transferrin to be attached enabling the iron to be used in the production of new red blood cells.

The absorption and release of iron for macrophages and other cells is controlled by a hormone produced by the liver known as hepcidin (Hillman *et al.* 2005; Rossi 2005). Hepcidin (a protein) binds to ferropotin 1, decreasing the amount of iron being absorbed. In IDA and hypoxia, there is an upregulation of HCP1, DMT1, DCYTB, ferroportin 1, and a decrease in production of hepcidin, thereby increasing iron absorption.

Copper is an important element which acts as a catalyst to ensure the iron is taken up by the haemoglobin. Circulating haemoglobin contains 75% of the body's iron requirements (3–4 g). The rest of the iron is found bound to transferrin (3–4 mg) and approximately 400 mg is used for cellular activities by cytochromes found in cells and myoglobin, a pigment in muscle which has a high affinity for oxygen (Barasi 2007). The daily requirement of iron is 1 mg for men, 2–3 mg for women (childbearing women) and adolescents, which is necessary for the incidental loss of iron through sweat, intestinal loss, skin epithelial loss and urine; 20 mg can be lost monthly through menstrual loss (Cook 2005).

Iron deficiency anaemia occurs when the demand for iron is outweighed by its supply. Initially, in IDA, the iron stores are utilised so immediate effects of the lack of supply of iron do not cause symptoms. Generally symptoms occur when the stores of iron are depleted and this leads to a reduction in haemoglobin production, with the consequent result of a reduction in the oxygen carrying capacity of red blood cells.

Causes of iron deficiency anaemia

In the developing world the causes tend to be multiparity, vegetarian diet, intestinal parasites such as hook worms (*Necator americanus*), schistosomiasis and lack of copper (Leestral *et al*. 2004; WHO 2001).

In the developed world the most common causes of IDA are chronic GI bleeds, menhorrhagia and adolescent growth spurts. Other possible causes can be renal disease, small bowel disease, for example Crohn's disease, gastric cancers, hiatus hernia, oesophageal varices, uterine fibroids, increased demands in pregnancy, vegan diet and intrauterine contraceptive devices (Looker *et al*. 2007). In patients with coeliac disease malabsorption is a common cause of IDA in the UK (Goddard 2005). Nutritional insufficiency of iron intake is not generally a major cause of IDA in the developed world; however, there are potential concerns in change of dietary patterns of fast foods and less time spent cooking using fresh products, which could increase the incidence of IDA. The elderly are also at risk of IDA mainly due to an insufficient dietary intake (Allen 2009). Infective organisms such as *Helicobacter pylori*, has been associated with IDA and drug-related causes, for example NSAIDS, diclofenac. Additionally, drugs like tetracyclines, chelate with iron, thereby compromising both the functions of the antibiotic and absorption of iron.

Signs and symptoms

The general signs and symptoms of anaemia have been indicated in Table 6.2 and Table 6.5 gives signs and symptoms related to IDA.

Investigations

Obtaining a medical history, with particular attention to factors such as age, gender and diet should be considered. Information regarding previous GI surgery is important as is obtaining a dietary history to ascertain any evidence of nutritional deficiencies. A physical examination would be undertaken to identify any of the signs and symptoms outlined in Table 6.5.

Blood investigations will involve those indicated in Table 6.3 and Table 6.6. Patients with a low haemoglobin, low mean cell volume, low mean cell haemoglobin concentration, increased red blood cell distribution width (RDW) and increased red cell protoporhyrin would be suspicious of IDA. Iron studies are clearly important as low serum ferritin level, elevated TIBC and increased transferrin binding capacity receptors (STFR), are major indicators to diagnosing IDA (Goddard 2005).

On examination typical morphology of red blood cells in IDA are hypochromic (pale in colour), microcytic (small in size) and anicocytois (abnormal varying sizes) cells (Bain and Gupta 2003). Beta thalassaemia trait can mimic IDA and therefore haemoglobin electrophoresis maybe undertaken to exclude it, particularly if the patient is from the Indian sub-continent, the Mediterranean, the Middle East, Africa or the Caribbean. Differential causes such as inflammatory diseases and cancer would also be investigated.

Gastrointestinal investigations involving sygmoidoscopy, colonoscopy and stool examination for occult blood maybe considered if the cause of chronic blood loss is undetermined.

Table 6.5 Signs and symptoms of iron deficiency anaemia.

Tiredness
Weakness, fatigue
SOB
Irritability
Pallor
Tinnitus
Koilonychia (spoon shaped finger nails)
Angular stomatitis
Paterson-Kelly syndrome (oesophageal webs)
Pagophagia (pica) – craving for ice, soap
Increased susceptibility to infections
Reduced work performance abilities
Atrophic glossitis
Angular cheilitis (ulceration at the corner of the mouth)
Alopecia/hair thinning
Pruritis
Disturbance in menstrual cycle
Poor appetite

Adapted from Killip *et al.* (2007), Ramakrishnan (2000).

Table 6.6 An outline of the blood investigations which might be undertaken in addition to those in Table 6.3.

	Normal indices	Suggestive of IDA
Serum iron	50–160 µg/dL	<40 µg/L
TIBC	250–400 µg/dL	>410 µg/L
RBC protoporphyrin	30	>200 µg/L
Haemoglobin	14–18 g/dL men	<13.5 g/dL
	12–14 g/dL w4Women	<11.5 g/dL
MCH	27–32 pg	<29.5 pg
MCHC	315–345 g/L	<315 g/dL
Serum ferritin	Men 15–400 ng/mL	<10 µg/L
	Women 10–200 ng/mL	<10 µg/L
Zinc protoporphyrin (ZPP)	30–80 umol	
MCV	76–95 fL	<76 fl

Adapted from Bridges and Pearson (2008); MacKinney (2002); Mehta and Hoffbrand (2005).

Severe IDA can compromise oxygen carrying capacity and may predispose to ischaemic organ damage, for example myocardial infarction or CVA and Ioannou *et al.* (2002) highlighted that there is a significant risk of gastrointestinal cancer in patients over the age of 50.

Treatment

Identifying the cause is critical in ensuring the appropriate treatment is provided. Blood transfusion is rarely used for treating IDA, but may be considered for patients with a risk of cardiovascular complication. Oral iron administration can be in tablet or liquid suspension.

Ferrous sulphate 200 mg three times daily, is the usual ferrous compound administered. Ferrous fumarate (300 mg twice daily) or ferrous gluconate (300 mg three times a day) are other options. Oral suspension comes in the form of ferrous fumerate or ferrous glycine sulphate. The side effects of all three are nausea, diarrhoea and constipation. Vitamin C 250–500 mg may be prescribed twice daily with iron to increase its absorption.

The choice of iron preparation can depend on:

- Patient tolerance of the drug
- Any existence of gastrointestinal absorption problems
- The dosage required based on haemoglobin estimations

Rarely is parenteral iron required. This is usually necessary for one of the following reasons:

- The patient is unable to tolerate iron oral preparations.
- The patient has a severe gastrointestinal disorder.
- The patient continues to have a negative iron balance even when prescribed the maximum oral dose of iron.

The parenteral administration can be given intravenously or intramuscularly. Iron dextran (CosmoFer) and iron hydroxide sucrose (Venofer) are the two intravenous preparations and they are not without their risks. Both can cause anaphylactic reactions and adrenaline should be readily available to counter these reactions (Barberio and Gomella 2007). Hypotension, leg cramps, headaches, nausea and diarrhoea are side effects of iron sucrose (Venofer).

Sorbitol is the intramuscular preparation, but due to severe reactions it is rarely used in the United Kingdom. Iron dextran can be administered intramuscularly and the side effects are serum sickness, malaise skin rash and lymphadenopathy. Intramuscular injections of iron can be a very painful and can stain the skin, hence the Z-track technique should be used. This will be discussed in the care and management section.

Vitamin B$_{12}$ (cobalamin) deficiency

Vitamin B$_{12}$ (cobalamin) is essential for good nerve function and critical for the early development of red blood cells where it is required for DNA synthesis of methionine and for the conversion of methylmalonic acid to succinic acid (Hoffbrand *et al.* 2004). It is found primarily in meat, but also in fish, eggs poultry and dairy products, but not in any vegetables. The daily intake of cobalamin is 1–5 µg daily (Provan 2005).

Vitamin B$_{12}$ is absorbed in the presence of the intrinsic factor (IF), which is a glycoprotein found in hydrochloric acid, made from the parietal cells in the gastric mucosa. It is transported in the blood by the plasma protein transcobalamin II and stored in the liver (Hamilton and Blackmore 2006).

Aetiology and epidemiology

Vitamin B$_{12}$ deficiency can be caused by partial/total gastrectomy, coeliac disease, chronic pancreatic disease drugs like ascorbic acid, cimetidine and hormonal contraceptives can interfere with vitamin B$_{12}$ absorption.

However, the main cause of vitamin B_{12} deficiency is pernicious anaemia (PA). Although PA occurs in those of African, Asian and Chinese descent, the vast majority of cases are found in those of Northern European descent. Pernicious anaemia accounts for 80% of all megaloblastic cases (Provan 2007) and primarily occurs in those of Northern European descent, with an approximate incidence of 1:10,000.

Pernicious anaemia is a megaloblastic anaemia which occurs when vitamin B_{12} (extrinsic factor) is unable to be absorbed due to the lack of the intrinsic factor (IF), which as indicated above is normally produced by the parietal cells in the stomach. It has been suggested that PA is an autoimmune disease since many patients appear to have developed parietal cell auto-antibodies, the culprit antibody being IgA. IgA type 1 attaches itself to the IF, thereby preventing it from binding to vitamin B_{12}. The result is lack of vitamin B_{12} absorption (Leslie *et al.* 2001). As a compensatory measure, stored resources of vitamin B_{12}, mainly in the liver, become depleted and the patient exhibits signs of anaemia (Allen 2009).

Pernicious anaemia appears to be more common in people with blood group A, those who have a low level of IgA, hypoparathyroidism, carcinoma of the stomach, Crohn's disease and premature greying. Women are at a higher risk of developing PA and it tends to occur in people who are over 40 years old, increasing in incidence with age (Dignum 2009; Hughes-Jones *et al.* 2008). Interestingly, the presentation of PA in those of African descent appears to occur in a younger age group.

Symptoms of pernicious anaemia

Patients may have symptoms due to anaemia, such as pallor, dyspnoea, (orthopnoea, which relates to the urge the patient has to sit up to breathe), angina pectoria and ankle oedema. Symptoms can be gradual, with some patients presenting with congestive cardiac failure or infections. A lack of vitamin B_{12} or folic acid (folate) can place extra strain on the heart, because it raises the level of a chemical called homocysteine. High levels of homocysteine add to the build-up of fatty deposits in blood vessels, which in turn can lead to cardiovascular complications and strokes (Bønaa *et al.* 2006).

Effects on the GI tract can be glossitis, poor appetite, upper epigastric discomfort, recurring diarrhoea or constipation and potential weight loss. Major symptoms of PA are the neurological complications which have the potential to cause death. Vitamin B_{12} deficiency causes demyelination of the nerve, disrupting synaptic activity. Patients may complain of parasthesia of the fingers and toes, paranoia, delirium, depression and ataxia. Visual disturbances, such as blurred vision, are due to the degeneration of the optic nerve. Cognitive impairment has also been associated with vitamin B_{12} deficiency (Clarke *et al.* 2007) and due to some of the psychological symptoms such as depression, misdiagnosis can occur leading to delay in treatment, which is critical in preventing long-term neurological complications and death.

Investigations

As mentioned earlier, most of the investigations highlighted in Table 6.3 form the basis of tests. The lack of vitamin B_{12} leads to a disruption in the cytoplasmic and intracellular maturation, resulting in larger (hence the term megablastic), but fewer red blood cells being produced (hence the anaemia), and giant metamyelocytes (granulocytes). The red blood cell count, reticulocye count and haemoglobin level will be low. The level of vitamin B_{12} in serum will be measured, which would be expected to be reduced in PA. Folate (folic acid) is usually low when vitamin B_{12} is low. When both these vitamins are low, it is quite common to have homocysteine and methylmalonic acid in high levels. Intrinsic factor antibodies and parietal cell antibodies will also be investigated. Their presence may suggest they are destroying the intrinsic factor or parietal cells (Mehta and Hoffbrand 2009). Bone marrow aspiration and trephine might be undertaken by some clinicians and in PA the bone marrow would be hyperplasic, demonstrating excessive work.

In addition to blood investigation, a definitive diagnosis of PA is achieved from results of the Schillings test. Part 1 of this test involves the patient fasting over night or for at least eight hours, and being given radioactive cobalt 57 (cobalamin) orally and 2–3 hours later an intramuscular injection of normal cobalamin is administered. Urine is then collected over 24 hours. If there is normal gastric function producing IF, it would be expected that the injected vitamin B_{12} will bind to the IF and be carried by transcobalamin II to the liver for storage. A normal urine result will show at least 5% of the radioactive cobalt 57 being detected. A diagnosis of PA would be suggestive if the result is less than 5%. If this occurs part 2 of the test may be undertaken, which involves repeating the process of part 1, but the patient is given an oral dose of IF. If the result is normal it indicates there is a problem with the gastric sections of the IF and is usually conclusive of PA (Lewis *et al.* 2006).

Folic acid deficiency

Aetiology and epidemiology

Folate (folic acid) is a very important vitamin in helping red blood cells to mature. It is part of the B-group of vitamins, found in many foods such as, broccoli, brussels sprouts, asparagus, peas, chickpeas and brown rice. Other useful sources include fortified breakfast cereals and bread, fruits (such as oranges and bananas). Folate is absorbed at the small intestine and a small reserve is stored in the liver. The required daily intake of folic acid is 100–200 µg. Folate deficiency is most common in people over 75 years of age; however, pre-menopausal women can develop folate deficiency and are encouraged to take folic acid at time of pregnancy to reduce the risk of neural tubal defects occurring in the foetus.

Causes of folate deficiency

Primary cause is lack of dietary intake of folic acid. Alcoholism is also associated with folate deficiency due to hepatic damage, which compromises its ability to store folic acid. Alcoholism can lead to a poor appetite, adding to the reduced intake of folate. Malabsorption conditions such as coeliac disease and other bowel inflammatory disease, poor appetite, older age group and poverty are other causative factors. Drugs such as methotrexate, cholestyramine and some anticonvulsants, for example phenytoin can lead to folate deficiency. Excessive haemolysis of red blood cells in conditions such as sickle cell disease and thalassaemia can lead to folate deficiency. In addition, folate deficiency has been associated with the potential development of cancer (Duthie, 1999).

Symptoms

Most patients with folate deficiency are generally asymptomatic and tend to have incidental diagnosis. Symptoms may be present once the stores of folate have been depleted, which usually takes 3–4 months and are similar to PA, except it is rare for patients to have the neurological problems.

Investigations

Folate deficiency is a megaloblastic anaemia, therefore the red blood cells are macrocytic, the MCV maybe be high, the haemoglobin level, mean cell volume and reticulocyte will be low. Serum folate lower than 5 nmol/L is suggestive of folate deficiency. Levels of vitamin B_{12} will also be investigated and anti-endomysial and antitransglutaminase antibodies, endoscopy and duodenal biopsy, may be done to exclude or confirm coeliac disease (Mehta and Hoffbrand 2005). Liver function tests may be undertaken if liver disease is suspected and investigations for other haemanetics such as vitamin B6, vitamin A, as well as iron, maybe undertaken to establish nutritional status.

Treatment

Straightforward folate deficiency anaemia is treated with oral folic acid, 5 mg daily for four months to replenish stock. It is important that serum B_{12} levels are normal as treatment with folic acid can precipitate subacute combined degeneration of the cord. Patients may develop potassium or iron deficiency once folate treatment is started. These should be monitored and supplements provided as required.

Care and management

Iron deficiency anaemia and PA are the most common nutritional anaemias in the United Kingdom and it is important that nurses are confident and knowledgeable to provide patient education and nutritional advice, to prevent re-occurrence. Nutrition advice and provision of meals should be seen as fundamental key roles in nursing practice and are clearly indicated in the NICE guidance (2006). Care must be adapted to suit individual patients needs, with the aim being to alleviate any symptoms the patient may have, increase oxygen carrying capacity of erythrocytes and to prevent complications.

Assessment and effective care planning is important in addressing and identifying the advice needed by patients. Whether the patient is being managed as an in-patient, outpatients or in day care, a nutritional assessment should be undertaken to establish and identify any deficiencies in the patient's diet and the impact the nutritional deficiency is causing (Coxall *et al.* 2008; Hand 2001). The outcome of the nutritional assessment will determine if the patient requires referral to a dietician.

The British Association for Parenteral and Enteral Nutrition (BAPEN 2007), have developed a screening tool called Malnutrition Universal Screening Tool (MUST) and NHS Scotland, 'Nutrition – assessment and referral in the care of adults in hospital: best statement' document (2002) provides an excellent clear illustration of the role of nurses in meeting the nutritional needs of patients. Involving the patient and working in partnership is critical in gaining their compliance and ensuring their concerns are being addressed (Beckford-Ball 2006).

Managing the patient with iron deficiency anaemia

Nursing assessment is important to identify dietary patterns, ascertain whether the patient has a past history of gastrointestinal surgery, whether the patient has been experiencing any overt bleeding such as epistaxis, rectal bleeding (Gizzard 2006). In the case of pre-menopausal women questions should be asked about the regularity of her menstrual cycle and whether there have been changes such as menhorrhagia. Identifying any medication the patient may have taken is important, as drugs such as corticosteroids can impair iron absorption. Ascertain whether the patient has travelled abroad recently, particularly to developing countries were gastrointestinal parasites such as *Trichuris trichiura* (whipworm) *Necator americanus* (hookworm) are prevalent (Laroque *et al.* 2005; Zimmerman and Hurrell 2007).

Observations of pulse, blood pressure and respirations are important to gain a baseline to detect signs for tachycardia, pallor or dyspnoea. In severe cases palpitations, angina, dizziness and shortness of breath can be symptoms experienced by patients (Brooker and Nicol 2003).

The baseline findings will determine how regular the recording of those observations needs to be. It is important not only to carry out the above observations, but also to establish whether the anaemia is aeffecting the patient's ability to carry out activities of living. Ineffective tissue perfusion related to low oxygen carrying capacity can lead to increased fatigue, which can impact negatively on the patient's quality of life. Brownlie *et al.* (2002) highlighted in their study that being iron deficient even in the absence of anaemia, affects physical activities and compromises an individual's health. Assessment should be made of the level of fatigue the patient is experiencing and whether normal sleep patterns have altered and identify activities which may cause tiredness. In older patients having IDA has been shown to have a negative impact on physical activities (Phenninx *et al.* 2003). Working with the patient, the nurse can assist in developing a schedule of activities, rest periods and sleep, and encourage exercises to help increase endurance and strength.

In patients with IDA, the heart will have been beating faster to compensate for reduced oxygen levels; hence cardiac assessment should also be undertaken. Hepatomegaly, cardiomegaly and peripheral oedema are signs of cardiac failure. In such cases, where these signs are confirmed, the head of the bed should be elevated, oxygen should be provided, vital signs monitored and fluid intake and urine output recorded.

Providing advice on foods which are a rich sources of iron is essential and examples of some food high in iron can be found in Table 6.7. Encourage the patient to drink citrus fruit drinks such as orange juice with meals to increase the absorption of iron. Polyphenols

Table 6.7 Examples of food rich in iron.

Fish (mackerel)
Seafood (mussels, clams, oysters)
Red meat (especially liver)
Poultry
Dark green leafy vegetables, prunes, raisins apricots, goats' milk as opposed to cows' milk
Eggs
Legumes
Fortified cereals
Nuts, but important to check the patient does not have a nut allergy
Asparagus
Sprouts
Broccoli
Lentils
Soya beans
Chickpeas
Wheat germ
Barley
Rice
Yeast extracts, Vecon, vegetable stock
Veggie burger mixes
Textured vegetable protein

found in tea and coffee can impair iron absorption and therefore it is worth suggesting to patients that they reduce their intake temporarily until the iron stores are increased (Heath *et al.* 2002; Killip *et al.* 2007).

Iron supplements will usually be prescribed as highlighted earlier in this chapter. It is essential that nurses stress the importance of taking the iron medication. Many patients can recover quickly once commencing their treatment. This can lead to a false sense of security in which patients will feel well enough to discontinue taking the iron supplements. It should be stressed to patients that they must continue for the prescribed period of time, which is usually 3–6 months. The rationale for this is to help replenish the iron stores and if the patient ceases taking the iron supplements before this period of time, there will be insufficient stores for erythrocyte production and the anaemia will be unresolved. If a patient is having iron in a liquid form it may stain the teeth, it is therefore advisable to suggest the patient uses a straw and drinks water afterwards. Iron supplements should not be taken on their own as it can cause gastric irritation. It should be taken with meals and a citrus drink to aid the absorption of iron. Nurses should advise patients of the side effects of iron supplements, which include nausea, black stools, dyspepsia and epigastric discomfort, discolouration of urine, constipation or diarrhoea (Gwynne and Nandi 2008).

Parenteral iron administration is rarely used and the rationale has been discussed earlier. Iron dextran can be administered intramuscularly. Nurses need to be skilled in using the Z-track technique as the injection is very painful and can stain the skin.

The Z-track involves the following:

- Allow a small amount of air in the syringe and use a one inch needle for injection to avoid tracking medication through subcutaneous tissue and resulting in painful administration.

- Choose an appropriate site and not one where the patient has nodules or lumps. The most suitable areas are: ventrogluteal muscles (in the hip) dorsogluteal muscle (upper outer quadrant of the buttocks) or vastus lateralis (upper outer thigh) site.
- Having chosen the site, clean it with alcohol, applying some friction and allow to completely dry.
- Laterally retract the skin over muscle (Z-track technique) and insert the needle at a 90° angle to prevent leakage along the track and staining of the skin. Aspirate for blood and if present withdraw the needle, start the process again with a new needle and syringe.
- Inject deeply and slowly, wait a few seconds before withdrawing the needle, (usually about ten seconds).
- Don't massage the area as this can lead to the iron dextran being directed into the needle track causing skin irritation.

(McConnell 2009; Timby 2008)

Anaphylactic reaction can occur and therefore patients must be monitored for hypertension or stridor after having the iron dextran administered (Barberio and Gomella 2007; Nettina 2006). If the patient has been administered IV iron sucrose or IV dextran for the first time, it is critical that a test dose is first administered and the patient observed for 15 minutes for anaphylactic reactions. If there are no reactions the patient is usually prescribed 200 mg in 100 ml normal saline to infuse over one hour.

Nursing and management for patients with pernicious anaemia and folate deficiency

Treatment is aimed at correcting the deficiency of vitamin B_{12}. Initially the patient is prescribed 1 mg hydroxocobalamin (vitamin B_{12}), intramuscularly every 2–3 days, for a total of six injections. Once stabilised the patient is put on three monthly lifelong injections of hydroxocobalamin 250 μg. Pernicious anaemia is a lifelong problem and will warrant lifetime hydroxocobalamin treatment. Side effects of hydroxocobalamin can be dizziness, hot flushes, fever and hypokalaemia (Turgeon 2004). As pernicious anaemia appears to increase the risk of developing carcinoma of the stomach and thyroid dysfunction, doctors may do periodic thyroid function tests and stool examination for occult blood (Brenner 2009; Kim *et al.* 2007).

Since pernicious anaemia is a chronic illness, nurses need to spend time not only advising the patient about how they have developed it, but also that the treatment is lifelong, and this can have a negative psychological impact. The main aims of nursing care are to support the patient through their acute phase of the illness, to administer vitamin B12 (hydroxocobalamin) to restore supply and to help the patient to accept the lifelong maintenance treatment (Hamilton and Blackmore 2006).

Nurses should assess for parasthesia, gait disturbances, changes in bladder or bowel function, altered thought processes and refer to the appropriate specialist if required. Lifelong three-monthly intramuscular injections of hydroxocobalamin is usually administered in primary care. If the patient is being managed in the community, it is advisable that the patient is administered the hydroxocobalamin in the general practitioner's surgery, as there is a risk of anaphylactic reactions. Generally the patient is advised to stay in the surgery for 20–30 minutes to be monitored for such reactions. Once commenced on their treatment, some symptoms may soon resolve, such as poor appetite. However, neurological symptoms such as parasthesis and numbness may take up to a year to resolve and other complications such as degeneration of the optic nerve may be irreversible (Smeltzer and Bare 2000).

Encouraging patients to attend for outpatient appointments is important as pernicious anaemia is associated with gastric cancer and thyroid dysfunction (Brenner *et al.* 2009; Kim *et al.* 2007; Leslie *et al.* 2001). Therefore periodic stool examination for occult blood and thyroid function tests may be undertaken for early diagnosis.

Most patients with folate deficiency tend to be managed in the community, unless it is secondary to an illness that the patient is being treated for in hospital. Folic acid is found in meat, green leafy vegetables, whole grain and fortified cereal products. It is useful to advise on cooking methods as folic acid can be rapidly destroyed with inappropriate cooking. Steaming is the best method to retain folic acid. Advising pre-menopausal women of the importance of having sufficient intake of folic acid is important to build their folic acid stores to reduce the risk of having babies with neural tubal defects. Banning (2005) in a study has suggested that consuming fish can be helpful in reducing cardiac disease in folate and pernicious anaemia deficiency.

Conclusion

Iron deficiency anaemia and PA are important nutritional anaemias for nurses to be aware of and understand how to manage. The insidious nature of these anaemias can lead to delay in diagnosis and in the case of PA, because it occurs in older people, can be misdiagnosed. The chronic nature of PA and the life changing potential of PA makes it incumbent on nurses to help support patients. Iron deficiency anaemia can occur as a consequence of particular treatments patients may be receiving; therefore nurses should be alert to its symptoms. It might be of value to advise other family members to prevent them developing the deficiencies

References

Allen, L.H. (2009) How common is vitamin B12 deficiency? *Am J Clin Nutr*, 89, 693 S–696 S.

Bain, B.J. (2006) *Blood Cells – a Practical Guide*. Blackwell Publishing Ltd, Oxford.

Bain, B.J. and Gupta, R. (2003) *A–Z of Haematology*. Blackwell Publishing Ltd, Oxford.

Banning, M. (2005) The role of Omega-3; fatty acids in the prevention of cardiac events. *BJN*, 14 (9), 503–508.

Barasi, M. (2007) *Nutrition at a Glance*. Blackwell Publishing Ltd, Oxford.

Barberio, J. and Gomella, L.G. (2007) *Nurse's Pocket Drug Guide*. McGraw-Hill, New York.

Beckford-Ball, J. (2006) Guidelines on the provision of nutritional support in adults. *Nursing Times*, 102 (10), 25–26.

Benner, H., Rothenbacher, D.M. and Arndt, V. (2009) Epidemiology of stomach cancer. In: *Methods of Molecular Biology, Cancer, Epidemiology* (ed. M. Verma) Vol. 472, pp. 467–478. Humana Press, Totowa, NJ.

Bønaa, K.H., Njølstad, I., Ueland, P.M. *et al.* (2006) Homocysteine lowering and cardiovascular events after acute myocardial infarction. *New England Journal of Medicine*, 354, 1578–1588.

Bridges, K.R. and Pearson, H.A. (2008) *Anaemias and Other Blood Disorders*. MacGraw-Hill, New York.

British Association for Parenteral and Enteral Nutrition (2007) *Malnutrition Universal Screening Tool*, www.bapen.org.uk/must_tool.html (last accessed 28 October 2011).

Brooker, C. and Nicol, M. (2003) *Nursing Adults: the Practice of Caring*. Mosby, Elsevier, London.

Brownlie, T., Utermohlen, V., Hinton, P.S. *et al.* (2002) Marginal iron deficiency without anaemia impairs aerobic adaptation among previously untrained women. *American Journal of Clinical Nutrition*, 75, 734–742.

Campbell, K. (2003) Anaemia; causes and treatment. *NursingTimes*, 99 (43), 30–33.

Campbell, K. (2004) Pathohysiology of anaemia. *Nursing Times*, 100 (47), 40–43.

Clarke, R., Birks, J. and Nexo, E. (2007) Low vitamin B-12 status and risk of cognitive decline in older adults. *American Journal of Clinical Nutrition*, 86 (5), 1384–1391, November.

Cook, J.D. (2005) Diagnosis and management of iron deficiency anaemia. *Best Practice Research Clinical Haematology*, 18 (2), 319–332.

Coxall, K., Dawes, E. and Forsythe, E. (2008) Applying the key principles of nutrition to nursing practice. *Nursing Standard*, 22 (36), 44–48.

De Domenico, I., McVey Ward, D. and Kaplan, J. (2008) Regulation of iron acquisition and storage: consequences for iron-linked disorders. *Nature Reviews Molecular Cell Biology*, 9, 72–81.

Dignum, H. (2009) Investigation of anaemia. *InnovAiT*, 2 (3), 148–157.

Duthie, S.J. (1999) Folic acid deficiency and cancer: mechanisms of DNA instability *British Medical Bulletin*, 55, 578–592.

Gizzard, D. (2006) Diagnosing and treating iron deficiency. *Nursing in Practice* (Jul/Aug), 57–61.

Goddard, A.F., James, M.W., McIntyre, A.S. and Scott, B. (2005) *Guidelines for the Management of Iron Deficiency Anaemia*. British Society of Gastronerology, London.

Gunshin, H., Mackenzie, B. and Berger, U.V. (1997) Cloning and characteristics of a mammalian proton-coupled metal-ion transporter. *Nature*, 388, 482–488.

Gwynne, M. and Nandi, A. (2008) Managing iron deficiency anaemia. *Nursing in Practice* (Mar/Apr), 44–48.

Hamilton, M. and Blackmore, S. (2006) Investigations of megaloblastic anaemia – cobalamin, folate and metabolic staus. In: *Practical Haematology* (eds S.M. Lewis, B.J. Bain and I. Bates), 10th edition. Churchill Livingston. Elsevier. Philadelphia.

Hand, H. (2001) Blood and the classification of anaemia. *Nursing Standard*, 15 (39), 45–53.

Heath, A.L. and Fairweather-Tait, S.J. (2002) Clinical implications of changes in the modern diet; iron intake, absorption and status. *Best Practice Research Clinical Haematology*, 15 (2), 225–241.

Hillman, R.S., Ault, K.A. and Rinder, H.M. (2005) *Hematology in Clinical Practice*, 4th edition. McGraw-Hill, New York.

Hoffbrand, A.V., Pettit, J.E. and Moss, P.A.H. (2004) *Essential Haematology*, 4th edition. Blackwell Publishing Ltd, Oxford.

Hughes-Jones, N.C., Wickramasinghe, S.N. and Hatton, C. (2008) *Haematology Lecture Notes*. Wiley-Blackwell, Oxford.

Hurley, G. (2007) Anaemia, overview and management. *Primary Health Care*, 17 (6) (July), 25–30.

Ioannou, G.N., Rockey, D.C., Bryson, C.L. and Weiss, N.S. (2002) Iron deficiency and gastrointestinal malignancy: a population-based cohort study. *Am J Med*, 113 (4) (Sept), 276–280.

Killip, S., Bennett, J.M. and Chambers, M.D. (2007) Iron deficiency anaemia. *Amercian Family Physician*, 1 (75) (March) (5) 671–678 (abstract).

Kim, B.S., Kim, J.W., Lee, I.K. *et al.* (2007) Gastric adenocarcinoma in patient with pernicious anemia: a case report. *J Korean Gastric Cancer Assoc*, 7 (1) (March), 38–41.

King, M. (2005) Helping to understand the pathophysiology of anaemia. *Nursing Times*, 101 (9).

Larocque, R., Casapia, M., Gottuzzo, E. and Gyorkos, T.W. (2005) Relationship between intensity of soil-transmitted helminth infections and anaemia during pregnancy. *Am J Trop Hygiene*, 73, 783–789.

Leenstra, T., Kariuki, A.K., Kurtis, J.D. *et al.* (2004) Prevalence and severity of anemia and iron deficiency: cross-sectional studies in adolescent schoolgirls in western Kenya. *European Journal of Clinical Nutrition*, 58, 681–691.

Leslie, D., Lipsky, P. and Notkins, A.L. (2001) Autoantibodies as predictors of disease. *J. Clin. Invest*, 108 (10), 1417–1422.

Lewis, S.M., Bain, B.J. and Bates, I. (2006) *Practical Haematology*, 10th edition. Churchill Livingston, Elsevier, Philadelphia.

Looker, A.C., Dallman, P.R. and Carroll, M.D. (1997) Prevalence of iron deficiency in the United States. *JAMA*, 277, 973–976.

MacKinney, A.A. (2002) *Haematology for Students*. Martin Duntiz, USA.

McConnell, E. A. (2009) Administering a Z-track IM injection. *Nursing* (20 Sept), http://findarticles.com/p/articles/mi_qa3689/is_199901/ai_n8831313/ (last accessed 28 October 2011).

Mehta, A. and Hoffbrand, V. (2009) *Haematology at a Glance*. Wiley-Blackwell, Oxford.

Nettina. S.M. (2006) *The Lippincott Manual of Nursing Practice*, 8th edition. Lippincott Williams & Wilkins, Philadelphia.

NHS Scotland (2002) *Nutrition and Referral in the Care of Adults in Hospital: Best Practice Statement*. NHS Scotland, Edinburgh.

Phenninx, B.W. (2003) Anemia and decline in physical performance in older persons. *American Journal of Medicine*, 115, 104–110.

Provan, D. (2005) Iron deficiency anaemia. *Independent Nurse* (Oct), 26.

Provan, D. (2007) *ABC of Clinical Haematology*. Blackwell Publishing Ltd, Oxford.

Ramakrishnan, U. (2000) *Nutritional Anemias*. Lewis Publishers, Boca Raton, FL.

Rossi, E. (2005) Hepcidin – the iron regulatory hormone. *Clin Biochem Rev*, 26 (3) (Aug), 47–49.

Smeltzer, S.C. and Bare, B.G. (2000) *Brunner and Suddarth's Textbook of Medical Surgical nursing*, 9th edition. Lippincott, Philadelphia.

Timby, B.K. (2008) Fundamental nursing skills and concepts. In: *Lippincott's Practical Nursing*, 9th edition. Lippincott Williams & Wilkins, Philadelphia.

Turgeon, M.L. (2004) *Clinical Hematology: Theory and Procedures*. Lippincott Williams & Wilkins, Philaldelphia.

UNICEF (2001) Iron deficiency anaemia; assessment, prevention and control. A guide for programme managers. www.who.int/nut/documents/ida (accessed 10 July 2009).

Verma, M. (ed.) (2009) *Methods of Molecular Biology, Cancer Epidemiology*, vol. 472. Humana Press, Totowa, NJ.

World Health Organisation (2001) *Iron Deficiency Anaemia: Assessment, Prevention, and Control. A Guide for Programme Managers*. Geneva, World Health Organization.

World Health Organisation (2008) *Worldwide Prevalence of Anaemia 1993–2005 WHO Global Database on Anaemia*. WHO, Geneva.

Zimmerman, H. and Hurrell, R. (2007) Nutritional iron deficiency. *Lancet*, 370 (9586), 511–520.

Chapter 7

Acquired haemolytic anaemia: pathophysiology, care and management

Marvelle Brown

By the end of the chapter you should:
- Have an awareness of the different types of acquired haemolytic anemias
- Know the common types of antibodies which cause autoimmune haemolytic anaemias
- Have an appreciation of the pathophysiology of the acquired haemolytic anaemias
- Understand the causes of non-immune haemolytic anaemias
- Be familiar with some of the treatment options for the different types of acquired haemolytic anaemias
- Know key nursing principles for patients with acquired haemolytic anaemia

Introduction

Acquired haemolytic anaemia refers to the premature destruction of red blood cells, caused by external factors, leading to a reduction in their lifespan. These factors can include immune disorders, infective organisms, mechanical trauma of red blood cells and other miscellaneous factors (Mack and Freedman 2000). Acquired haemolytic anaemia can be classified as immune and non-immune. Table 7.1 provides a list of some of the common causes of this type of anaemia.

Immune haemolytic anaemia

Immune haemolytic anaemias refer to the way red blood cells react to antibodies or the complement cascade system. Haemolysis can occur in circulation and this is known as 'intravascular haemolysis'. In this case, the activation of the complement system causes red blood cell lysis and its destruction. 'Extravascular haemolysis' occurs within organs which make up the reticulo endothelial system (RES), where macrophages detect antibody-coated red blood cells, and instigate phagocytosis, leading to red blood cell destruction (Gehrs and Friedberg 2002).

Haematology Nursing, First Edition. Marvelle Brown and Tracey J. Cutler.

Table 7.1   Common causes of acquired haemolytic anaemias.

Causes	Examples
Immune	Alloimmune
	Autoimmune
	Drug induced*
Infectious	Malaria
	Clostridium perfringens
	Bartonellosis
Chemical	Lead
Venom/poison	Snake venom
	Snake venom
Severe burns	
Hypersplenism	
Mechanical damage to RBC	Trauma caused following cardiac surgery; aortic valve replacement, heart valve repair
	Haemolytic ureamic syndrome
	Disseminated intravascular coagulation
	Thrombotic thrombocytopenia purpura
	March haemoglobinuria
	Metastatic malignancy

Adapted from Hughes-Jones *et al*. (2008), Kelton *et al*. (2002).
*Drugs can either cause haemolysis by directly attacking the red blood cells or acting as an antigen, trigger antibody reactions to cause the haemolysis.

Immune reactions can occur due to:

- Alloantibodies – the individual produces antibodies against antigens received from another individual (see Chapter 17 for more on haemolytic reactions).
- Auto-antibodies – the individual is producing antibodies against their own red blood cells.

Autoimmune haemolytic anaemia

Autoimmune haemolytic anaemia (AIHA) refers to a group of disorders in which the individual produces autoantibodies against their own red blood cells, which leads to symptoms of anaemia. These anaemias can be classified as either 'warm' or 'cold' AIHA. In the warm antibody type, the autoantibodies attach to and destroy red blood cells at temperatures equal to or in excess of normal body temperature of 37°C. In the cold antibody type, the autoantibodies become most active and attack red blood cells at temperatures below 32°C (Gehrs and Friedberg 2002; Hughes-Jones *et al*. 2008).

Warm autoimmune haemolytic anaemia

Warm AIHA is the most common of the two autoimmune haemolytic anaemias. It occurs across all races, gender and ages, although it is most commonly seen in individuals over 50 years of age, with a higher incidence in women. Generally for half of the patients, the cause is idiopathic; for other patients it is an underlying illness such as systemic lupus erythematosis (SLE), viral infections, immunodeficiency, chronic lymphocytic leukaemia (CLL) or lymphoma. Evans syndrome is the name given to the association between AIHA and autoimmune idopathatic thrombocytopenic purpura (ITP) (Michel *et al.* 2009).

IgG is the prime polyclonal antibody associated with causing this type of autoimmune haemolytic anaemia. IgM coated red blood cells can also cause warm AIHA, but this is much less common. Approximately 50% of warm autoantobodies have specificity for the Rh antigen system, which comprise antigens Cc, Dd and Ee (Hoffbrand *et al.* 2004). Coated red blood cells with IgG are taken up by macrophages in the RES. These macrophages have receptor sites for IgG and when presented with red blood cells, the macrophage will cause haemolysis through the process of phagocytosis. This process is enhanced by opsonisation, a function of the complement proteins which increases destruction. IgG has the ability to activate the complement cascade and red blood cells coated with C3d and C4d attract macrophages. Furthermore, these proteins make the red blood cell less deformable than normal red blood cells and these activities together may increase IgG-mediated phagocytosis. As a result, the extravascular haemolytic process may be enhanced by the presence of complement on the cell, facilitating the phagocytic process (Kelton *et al.* 2002).

Signs and symptoms

These can vary from mild to life threatening and are outlined in Table 7.2. In patients where the cause is identified as an autoimmune disorder such as SLE, the remission and relapsing of the AIHA appear to parallel that of the disorder.

Table 7.2   Signs and symptoms of warm AIHA.

Fatigue
Pallor
Shortness of breath following exercises
Tiredness
Dizziness
Haemoglobinuria
Irritability
Tachycardia
Increased heart murmur
Hypotension
Headaches
Jaundice
Splenomegaly
Hepatomegaly
Concentration/attention difficulties
Difficulty in sleeping

Adapted from (King and Ness 2005, Tefferi 2000).

Investigations

A number of haematological and biochemistry tests are undertaken to establish the diagnosis of warm AIHA. Generally patients will have a reduced red cell count and both the haemoglobin and haematocrit will be low. Reticulocytosis, erythroblastaemia and neutrophilia, can be present.

Red cell morphology is usually altered, with the red blood cell becoming spherical and larger in size. The spherical shape is due to the partial loss of the coated membrane when attached to the antibody. The change in shape aims to try and maintain volume, but the abnormal shape (for example spherical) leads to premature destruction of the red blood cell. The enzyme lactate dehydrogenase (LDH) will be raised due to the increased destruction of red blood cells, and the plasma protein haptoglobulin is usually decreased. A positive DAT (direct-globulin test) also known as a Coombs test, confirms IgG with or without complement antibodies causing the anemia (Adamson and Longo 2001).

Management

Initial treatment for warm AIHA is generally high dose prednisolone with a gradual reduction as the symptoms of the anaemia are addressed. The dosage of 60–100 mg per day for 1–3 weeks is a usual starting dose (King and Ness 2005). The rationale for prednisolone includes aiming to suppress autoantibody production, inhibit lysozomal enzymes by macrophages and suppression of red blood cell clearance by the RES (Kelton *et al.* 2002). If prednisolone is not effective, splenectomy maybe done but 50% of patients tend to relapse. As the spleen is the main site of extravascular haemolysis, splenectomy aims to reduce red cell destruction. The spleen has a significant role in immunity, thus the loss can compromise the patient's immune system. Therefore vaccination against *Haemophilus. influenzae, pneumococcus* and *meningococcus* prior to surgery and lifetime penicillin post-surgery is essential. If the patient is not responding positively to either prednisolone or splenectomy, immunosuppressive medication such as azathioprine or cyclophosphamide maybe prescribed (Tefferi 2001). Generally, regardless of the type of treatment, folate supplementation of 1 mg/day is commonly part of the patient's regime. If the patient has an underlying illness, treating that condition most often leads to remission of the AIHA.

Cold autoimmune haemolytic anaemia

Like warm AIHA, this is a chronic haemolytic anaemia and the cause can be idopathic, secondary to lymphoma, or infection with *Mycoplasma* (pneumonia), Epstein Barr virus (EBV) (infectious mononucleosis), or *Treponema pallidum* (syphilis). Cold AIHA can be divided into cold agglutination syndrome and paroxysmal cold haemoglobinuria (Petz 2008).

Cold agglutination syndrome is generally seen in older people in the sixth or seventh decade of life. The main antibody culprit is IgM. Haemolytic anaemia caused by IgM antibodies can be polyclonal or monoclonal. Polyclonal IgM is associated with EBV, cytomegalovirus (CMV), *Mycoplasma pneumoniae*; monoclonal IgM are associated with CLL, Waldenström's macroglobulinemia (Gertz 2006).

IgM binds to the red blood cell at temperatures below 32°C and causes agglutination. Capillary blood flow can be at 25°C, allowing for cold-reactive agglutination, triggering the complement cascade, leading to intravascular and extravascular haemolysis, obstruction of blood flow and potentially causing haemoglobinuria and haemoglobin anaemia. Capillary obstruction is reversible but overtime necrotic damage can occur, potentially leading to gangrene.

Signs and symptoms

Intravascular and extravascualr haemolysis occurs with varying degrees of severity. The severity of the anaemia depends on the antibody titre in serum, the antibody's ability to bind to complement proteins and affinity with red blood cells (Rodak *et al.* 2007). Because the haemolysis occurs in peripheral circulation this can lead to significant circulatory problems as mentioned above and can lead to Raynaud's phenomenon, depicted by blue discoloration of extremities, for example fingers, toes, nose and ears, in cold conditions. Mild jaundice may be present and some degree of splenomegaly.

Investigations

The investigations are similar to warm AIHA. There is less spherocytosis occurring, but the red blood cells will agglutinate at cold temperature. A positive DAT may demonstrate complement C3d on red cells and a there is a high IgM antibody titre. Reticulocytosis and neutrophil leucocytosis can be evident and LDH will tend to be high. In addition, serum haptoglobulin is decreased and urinary urobilinogen is raised (Lichtman *et al.* 2003).

Treatment

If the RBC destruction is mild, generally no treatment is required except to advise the patient to keep warm. If there is an underlying illness, treating it can ameliorate the symptoms. In some cases corticosteroids (prednisolone) may be prescribed. Plasmapheresis may be undertaken to lower antibody titre and if blood transfusion is necessary, cold AIHA is one of the few conditions in which a blood warmer might be used (Gertz 2006).

Paroxysmal cold haemoglobinuria

Paroxysmal cold haemoglobinuria (PCH) is very rare in adults, more commonly seen in children and mainly associated with viral infections such as measles, mumps, adenovirus and syphilis. The cause of PCH is a polyclonal IgG autoantibody, known as the Donath-Landsteiner (DL). The antibody has an affinity for P antigens on the red cell surface and binds to the red blood cell when exposed to cold (Dacie 1992). Paroxysmal cold haemoglobinuria is biphasic, requiring both cold and warmth to agglutinate. The DL-antibody, when exposed to cold, coats red blood cells causing them to become sensitised. This occurs around 15°C. Once warming has occurred, the sensitised red blood cells instigate complement cascade leading to rapid intravascular haemolysis.

Signs and symptoms

These are similar to those of cold agglutination syndrome. The symptoms are sometimes preceded by, but not always, respiratory or other acute viral/bacterial infection or following vaccination. Symptoms may occur within minutes or hours, following exposure to cold. Acrocyanosis can occur due to agglutination of red blood cells in the blood vessels. The nose, ear lobes, fingers and toes are particular areas which are affected. Other signs and symptoms of PCH are listed in Table 7.3.

Table 7.3 Additional signs and symptoms of paroxysmal cold haemoglobinuria.

Jaundice
Fever
Rigors
Headaches
Paraesthaesia of the hands and feet
Nausea
Affected adult males may suffer with impotence due to microvascular occlusion
Oliguria or anuria
Urticarial rash
Hepatosplenomegally
Haemoglobinuria

Adapted from Gertz (2006); Thomas (2004).

Investigations are similar to those mentioned earlier, with the addition of undertaking the Donath-Landsteiner test. This demonstrates that antibody binds to the red blood cell at low temperature (4°C) but causes red blood cell lyis when warmed at 37°C. Treatment of PCH is primarily to advise the patient to keep warm and treat any underlying cause. Prednisolone may also be prescribed to alleviate symptoms (Hoffbrand *et al*. 2006).

Drug induced haemolysis

Haemolysis induced by drugs may be immune or non-immune mediated. Drug-induced immune haemolysis is idiosyncratic (an unusual) reaction, while non-immune mediated haemolysis results from exposure to oxidative factors (for example oxygen free radicals which are toxic interact with other molecules in a cell causing damage to membranes and proteins) (Sinxadi and Maartens 2007).

Drug induced non-immune haemolytic anaemia tends to occur due to oxidative processes which cause the denaturing of haemoglobin to methahaemoglobin. This tends to occur when the red blood cell lacks defensive oxidant properties such as the enzyme glucose-6-phosphate dehydrogenase (G6PD). This is essential in enabling enzymes nicotinamide adenine dinucleotide phosphate-oxidase (NADPH) and glutathione (GSH) to carry out their function, which is to remove toxic substances such as oxygen free radicals from the red blood cells. The lack of G6PD means they are unable to carry out their functions effectively, rendering the red blood cells susceptible to oxidant drugs. Drugs such as primaquine, chloroquine, co-trimoxazole, dapsone and chloramphenicol are examples of drugs which cause haemolysis in G6PD deficiency (Frank 2005). See Chapter 8 for more information on G6PD.

Drug induced immune haemolytic anaemia

The main antibodies involved in drug induced immune haemolytic anaemia are IgG and IgM. This is usually confirmed by a positive Coombs (DAT) test. The haemolysis can occur through one of three mechanisms:

- *Antibody directed against a drug red blood cell membrane complex*   The drug binds to the red blood cell membrane, and acts as a hapten, stimulating IgG antibody production. Haptens are small molecules which can cause an antigenic stimulation but cannot do this alone. However, when attached to larger carrier molecules such as a protein, that attachment then stimulates an immune response. Penicillins and cephalosporins are examples of haptens which can cause drug induced haemolytic anaemia (Gehrs and Friedberg 2002).
- *The drug causes a drug antigen-antibody complex*   Usually this involves the antibody IgM and the drug anti-body immune complex, which is formed, binds to the red blood cell, initiating the complement cascade. This results in intravascular haemolysis and can be severe. Examples of drugs which cause drug antigen antibody complex are quinine, rifampicin, paracetamol, sulphonamides, streptomycin, tetracycline and fludarabine. Since the red blood cell is not generally the target, this type of haemolysis is sometimes known as 'innocent bystander' immune haemolysis (Ammus and Yunis 1989).
- *The drug induces the formation of autoimmune antierythrocyte IgG antibodies*   The role of the drug is not clear in this mechanism, but the behaviour of this type of drug induced haemolysis is very similar to warm autoimmune and tends to be mild in its effect. Methyldopa, diclofenac and ibuprofen are examples (Sinxadi and Maartens 2007).

Treatment is the discontinuation of the drug, which resolves the haemolysis (see Figure 7.1).

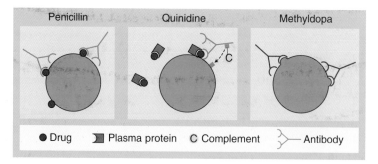

Figure 7.1   Three different mechanisms of drug-induced immune haemolytic anaemia. In each case the coated (opsonised) cells are destroyed in the reticuloendothelial system (from Hoffbrand *et al*. 2006). Reprinted with permission of John Wiley & Sons, Inc.

Paroxysmal nocturnal haemoglobinuria

Paroxysmal nocturnal haemoglobinuria (PNH) is an acquired haemolytic anaemia, depicted by a somatic clonal mutation of haemopoietic stem cells, leading to complement-mediated haemolysis. The mutation results in defective membranes found on red blood cells, leukocytes and platelets. Glycosyl-phosphatildylinositol (GPI) is an important anchor glycolipid, which binds a number of membrane proteins to the cell membrane. In PNH these membrane proteins are either missing or defective because of a fault in the synthesis of a GPI anchor. The defective synthesis is caused by a deficiency of phosphatidylinositol glucosyltransferase (PIG) because of a mutation of the X-linked PIG-A gene.

Some of the membrane proteins which are affected include: decay accelerating factor (DAF), also known as CD55, which normally binds to C3b and C4 on the membrane surface, thus inhibiting C3 activity. In doing so it protects the cells from haemolysis. Membrane inhibitor of reactive lysis (MIRL) also known as CD59, normally protects red blood cells from complement mediated lysis by inhibiting the development of complement membrane attack complex C5b-9 (Pallister 1997). Homologous restriction factor (HRF) binds to C8 preventing complement cascading. Other membrane proteins which are affected by the fault in GPI anchorage include CD14, CD16, CD24, CD55 and CD56 (Parker *et al.* 2005). The lack of these proteins prevents any protection of the cell against complement mediated lysis and as a consequence the marrow cells are destroyed.

Signs and symptoms

The patient may have intravascular haemolysis, recurrent thrombosis especially in unusual veins such as the hepatic, mesenteric and portal veins and severe abdominal pain may occur because of the mesenteric thrombosis. The haemolysis is chronic, with nocturnal haemaglobinuria, hence the name of the condition, and the haemolysis may be mild but exacerbated, for example by infections. Pancytopenia may occur, leading to aplastic crisis (Young *et al.* 2006) and other signs and symptoms can be iron deficiency and there is a risk of PNH transforming into acute leukaemia (Luzzato 2000).

Investigations

As well as the haematological investigations mentioned in earlier sections, Ham test maybe be undertaken, but more definitive tests for PNH are flow cytometry to detect the presence or absence of these GPI-linked proteins and fluorescently labelled inactive toxin aerolysin (FLAER). In PNH there is an absence of all the GPI-linked antigens. Although flow cytometry confirms the diagnosis of PNH, further studies are required to determine whether the patient has PNH type 1, 2 or 3. The type relates to how sensitive the red blood cells are to complement activation. In type 1, the red blood cells have a normal response to complemented activation; in type 2, cells have some moderate degree of increased sensitivity to complement lysis and type 3 shows a significant increase in sensitivity (Nishimura *et al.* 2004).

Management

The symptoms determine treatment options. A number of drugs might be considered, either on their own or in combination. Patients may lose iron through haemoglobinuria and therefore iron supplements such as ferrous sulphate would be prescribed. Corticosteroids are thought to be useful in limiting haemolytic crisis and may have positive effects in reducing blood transfusion requirements. Immunosuppressive regimens such as antithymocyte globulin and cyclosporine have also been used to manage PNH (Risitano and Rotoli 2008; Young 2005). Androgenic medication such as oxymetholone may be prescribed to increase erythropoiesis or recombinant erythropoietin therapy would be an alternative.

Anticoagulants such as heparin might be used following thrombotic episodes. However, heparin can exacerbate the thrombosis and therefore aspirin or ibuprofen might be used to prevent heparin activating the complement cascade. Prophylactic use of the anticoagulant warfarin has been suggested for some patients, although there is some debate about the use (Hall *et al.* 2003). Blood transfusion may be required to increase haemoglobin and to reduce the haemolysis by suppressing erythropoiesis. Immunosuppressives such as antithymocyte globulin might be used as part of a treatment regime if the patient develops aplastic anaemia.

Recently, a biological agent which acts as a complement inhibitor named eculizumab has been undergoing trials to treat PNH. Eculizumab is a monoclonal antibody that binds and prevents activation of complement C5, interrupting the complement cascade. It appears to modify the symptoms, the biology and the natural history of PNH, improving the quality of life of patients (Hillmen *et al.* 2006; Risitano and Rotoli 2008). Parker (2009) also alludes to the positive benefits of eculizumab, being the inhibition of the intravascular haemolysis, reduction in transfusion requirements and stabilisation of haemoglobin concentration. The main adverse effect of treatment is an increased susceptibility to infections with *Neisseria meningitides*, causing meningococcal meningitis; therefore it is standard practice to vaccinate patients before treatment. However, eculizumab is not widely available in the UK, partly because it is still on trial but also because it is an expensive drug (Parker 2009) and it is not a curative treatment, which potentially means long-term usage. In addition, the variation in PNH means that not all patients will be suitable for treatment.

Paroxysmal nocturnal haemoglobinuria is a long-term condition, with a medial survivorship of 10–15 years. Rarely is there spontaneous recovery as the clonal mutation is permanent, therefore the only curative treatment is allogenic stem cell transplantation.

Key principles of nursing for a patient with acquired haemolytic anaemia

Managing the patient with anaemia is addressed in several chapters and the reader is guided to those for additional reading. Nursing assessment should be able to determine what impact the anaemia is having on the patient's quality of life and how it is affecting the patient's ability to carry out activities of living (Lemone and Burke 2004). In knowing that some of these anaemias can be secondary to other illness, nurses should be familiar with haematological and biochemistry investigations in order to understand treatment options. The patient may be prescribed or need advice for example, if the patient is on iron medication, it is important to advise the patient of the appropriate timing of taking the iron medication with food and to be aware of side effects such constipation, dyspepsia and black stools. Further details on iron medication management can be found in Chapter 6.

Being cognisant of the different types of acquired anaemia is useful to understand what symptoms to anticipate and therefore know what kind of monitoring will be necessary (Jones 2004; Smeltzer *et al.* 2008). The patient should be observed for symptoms of anaemia, such as fatigue, breathlessness, lethargy, increased tiredness and jaundice. If the patient is having an acute episode of haemolysis the nurse should monitor oxygen saturations, undertake vital signs monitoring, record fluid intake and output and cardiovascular activity. A reduction in haemoglobin leads to increased workload on the heart and the patient will shows signs of this by having tachycardia, palpitations and dyspnoea. If the patient requires blood transfusion, safe administration is essential and this is addressed in detail in Chapter 17.

Conclusion

Acquired haemolytic anaemias are varied in their cause, presentation and treatments. Understanding of the disease process of the anaemia and assisting the patient in managing their symptoms are significant aspects of the nurse's role to enable the patient to improve their welfare.

References

Adamson, J.W. and Longo, D.L. (2001) Hematologic alterations. In: *Harrison's Principles of Internal Medicine* (eds E. Braumwald, A.S. Fauci, D.L. Kasper, S.L. Hauser, D.L. Longo and J.L. Jameson). pp. 348–365. McGraw Hill, New York.

Ammus, S. and Yunis, A.A. (1989) Drug-induced red cell dyscrasias. *Blood Rev*, 3, 71–82.

Dacie, J.V. (1992) *The haemolytic anaemias*. 3rd edition. Vol. 3: *The Auto-Immune Haemolytic Anaemias*. Churchill Livingstone, Edinburgh.

Frank, J.E. (2005) Diagnosis and management of G6PD deficiency. *Am Fam Physician*, 72, 1277–1282.

Gehrs, B.C. and Friedberg, R.C. (2002) Autoimmune haemolytic anaemia. *Am J Hematol*, 69, 258–271.

Gertz, M.A. (2006) *Cold hemolytic syndrome. Hematology*. American Soc. Hematology, (Jan), 19–23.

Hall, C., Richards, S. and Hillmen, P. (2003) Primary prophylaxis with warfarin prevents thrombosis in paroxysmal nocturnal hemoglobinuria (PNH). *Blood*, 102 (10), 3587–3591.

Hillmen, P., Young, N., Schubert, J. *et al.* (2006) The complement inhibitor eculizumab in paroxysmal nocturnal hemoglobinuria. *N. Engl. J Med*, 355 (12), 1233–1243.

Hoffbrand, A.V., Moss, P.A.H. and Pettit, J.E. (2006) *Essential Haematology*, 5th edition. Blackwell Publishing Ltd, Oxford.

Hughes-Jones, N.C., Wickramasinghe, S.N. and Hatton, C.S.R. (2008) *Lecture Notes: Haematology*. Blackwell Publishing Ltd, Oxford.

Jones, K.J. (2004) Nursing management hematologic problems. In: *Medical-surgical Nursing: Assessment and Management of Clinical Problems* (eds S.M. Lewis, M.M. Heitkemper and S.R. Dirksen). pp. 705–755. Mosby, St Louis.

Kelton, J.G., Chan, H., Heddle, N. and Whittaker, S. (2002) Acquired hemolytic anaemia. In: *Blood and Bone Marrow Pathology* (eds S.N. Wickramasinghe and J. McCullough). pp. 185–202. Churchill Livingstone, New York.

King, K.E. and Ness, P.M. (2005) The appropriate therapy of autoimmune hemolytic anemia (AIHA) is dependent. *Semin Hematol*, 42, 131–136.

Lemone, R. and Burke, K. (2004). Nursing care of clients with hematologic disorders. In: *Medical Surgical Nursing: Critical Thinking in Client Care*. pp. 931–979. Prentice Hall, New Jersey.

Lichtman, M., Beutler, E.M., Kipps, T.J. and Williams, W.J. (2003) *Williams Manual of Hematology*, 6th edition. Chapter 28, pp.133–137. McGraw-Hill, New York.

Luzzatto L. (2000) *Paroxysmal nocturnal hemoglobinuria. Hematology*, 28–38. American Society of Hematology Education Program.

Mack, P. and Freedman, J. (2000) Autoimmune haemolytic anaemia: a history. *Transfusion Medicine Reviews*, 14 (3), 223–223

Michel, M., Chanet, V., Dechartres, A. *et al.* (2009) The spectrum of Evans syndrome in adults: new insight into the disease based on the analysis of 68 cases. *Blood*, 114 (15), 3167–3172.

Nishimura, J.I., Kanakura, Y., Ware, R.E. *et al.* (2004) Clinical course and flow cytometric analysis of paroxysmal nocturnal hemoglobinuria in the United States and Japan. *Medicine (Baltimore)*, 83 (3), 193–207.

Pallister, C. (1997) *Blood-Physiology and Pathophysiology*. Butterworth-Heinemann, Oxford.

Parker C., Omine M., Richards S. *et al.* and International PNH Interest Group (2005) Diagnosis and management of paroxysmal nocturnal haemoglobinuria. *Blood*, 106, 3699–3709.

Parker, C. (2009) Eculizumab for paroxysmal nocturnal haemoglobinuria. *Lancet*, 373 (9665), 759–767.

Petz, L. (2008) Cold antibody autoimmune hemolytic anemias. *Blood Rev*, 22 (1), 1–15.

Rodak, B.F., Fritsma, G.A.M. and Doig, K. (2007) *Hematology; Clinical Principles and Applications*. Chapter 25, pp. 325–332. Saunders-Elsevier, St Louis, Missouri.

Risitano, A.M. and Rotolu, B. (2008) Paroxysmal nocturnal hemoglobinuria: pathophysiology, natural history and treatment options in the era of biological agents. *Biologics : Targets and Therapy*, 2, 205–222.

Sinxadi, P. and Maartens, G. (2007) Clinical pharmacology: drug-induced haemolytic anaemia. *CME*, 25 (6), 286–288.

Smeltzer, S.C., Bare, B.G., Hinkle, J.L. and Cheever, K.H. (2008) Assessment and management of patients with hematologic disorders. In: *Brunner and Suddarth's Textbook of Medical Surgical Nursing*. pp. 1035–1117. Lippincott Williams & Wilkins, Philadelphia.

Teffery, A. (2000) *Primary Hematology*. Humana Press, Totowa, New Jersey.

Thomas, L. (2004) Anaemia of chronic disease – pathophysiology and laboratory diagnosis. *Laboratory Hematology*, 10 (3), 163–165.

Young, N.S. (2005) Paroxysmal nocturnal hemoglobinuria: current issues in pathophysiology and treatment. *Current Hematology Reports*, 4 (2), 103–109.

Young, N.S., Calado, T.C. and Scheinberg, P. (2006) Current concepts in the pathophysiology and treatment of aplastic anemia. *Blood*, 108, 2509–2519.

Chapter 8

Inherited haemolytic anaemia: pathophysiology, care and management

Marvelle Brown

By the end of the chapter you will:

- Have an understanding of hereditary spherocytosis (HS) and glucose-6-phosphate-dehydrigenase deficiency (G6PD)
- Know the mode of inheritance for HS and G6PD deficiency
- Be familiar with the signs, symptoms and investigations to diagnose HS and G6PD deficiency
- Be aware of treatment options
- Understand key nursing principles in managing patients with HS and G6PD deficiency

---

Introduction

Inherited haemolytic anaemias can either affect red cell membrane proteins, enzymes necessary for glycolysis or haemoglobin. This chapter will discuss the more common membrane protein disorder, hereditary spherocytosis (HS), and the most common enzyme defect, glucose-6-phosphate dehydrogenase (G6PD). Chapter 9 will review inherited haemolytic anaemias caused by haemoglobin dysfunction.

Hereditary spherocytosis

To understand the effect of red blood cell membrane disorders, an overview of the red blood cell membrane will be discussed.

Red blood cell membrane

The red blood cell membrane is a bilipid layer composed of phospholipids and cholesterol. α-spectrin, β-spectrin, actin, ankyrin and protein 4.1 are membrane proteins which interweave and interact with the bilipid layer and make up the cytoskeleton of the red blood cell (Perrotta *et al.* 2008). These contractual and structural proteins are essential in

---

Haematology Nursing, First Edition. Marvelle Brown and Tracey J. Cutler.

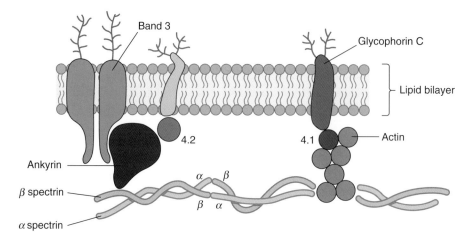

Figure 8.1   Schematic diagram of the red cell membrane cytoskeleton.

enabling the red blood cell to deform and retain cellular morphology (for example the biconcave shape), maintain elasticity (for example the ability to contract in size to pass through microcirculation) and have the capability to withstand the stress of arterial circulation (Van Dort *et al.* 2001).

Spectrin proteins are located on the cytoplasmic side of the lipid bilayer with α and β spectrin amino acids at one end of the spectrin protein and protein 4.1 and actin located at the other end. The vertical attachment of spectrin is enabled by proteins band 3 and glycophorin C. Band 3 interacts with ankyrin which binds to β spectrin. This protein and band 3 interacts with protein 4.2 to provide stability. Glycophorin C interacts with protein 55 and protein 4.1 which also binds to β spectrin. It is evident that any defect of membrane proteins will disrupt the stability of the cytoskeleton, resulting in morphological changes (Bolton-Maggs 2004; Perrotta *et al.* 2008). Figure 8.1 provides a schematic diagram of the red blood cell membrane cytoskeleton.

Hereditary spherocytosis (HS) occurs due to genetic mutations of the genes which encode for the membrane proteins, spectrin (α and β), actin, protein 4.1 and ankyrin. The mutation leads to either a defect or dysfunction of one or more of these membrane proteins (Delaunay 2007). Hereditary spherocytosis is inherited in an autosomal dominate mode, causing either deletions or translocation of the chromosomes 1, 8 and 14. Chromosome 1 encodes for α-spectrin and protein 4.1, chromosome 8 encodes for ankyrin and chromosome 14 encodes for β-spectrin (Eber and Lux 2004; Eber *et al.* 1996; Gallagher 2004). An example of the mode of the inheritance can be seen in Table 8.1. This illustration gives an example of the inheritance of HS. The mother has HS and the father has normal genes. In this scenario, there is a 50% chance of having an affected child with HS and a 50% chance the child will be unaffected.

The pathophysiology of HS is underpinned by two factors, namely: loss of membrane stability due to defective membrane protein and the effect of an efficient functioning spleen destroying red blood cells (Gallagher and Jarolim 2005). The defect of the membrane proteins leads to a loss of cohesion between the lipid layer and membrane skeleton, thus causing destabilisation of the lipids, which are released. The end result is a reduction

Table 8.1   Modes of inheritance.

Mother	Father	
	a	a
A_{hs} a	A_{hs} a	A_{hs} a
	aa	aa

Key: A_{hs} = HS
Designed by Marvelle Brown.

in surface area volume. The lack of proteins leads to an increased intake of sodium ions, which attracts increased water into the red blood cell. This places increased pressure on the cation 'pump' (an active transport mechanism) which is responsible for removing sodium from the cell. The cation pump is unable to keep up with increased workload, resulting in excess water entering the cell, eventually altering its shape from biconcave to spherical. Haemolysis is a significant feature of HS and the spleen is the major site where the haemolysis takes place. The abnormal shape of the red cells leads to their entrapment in the spleen, causing intrasplenic haemolysis. Hereditary spherocytosis is highly prevalent in Caucasian Northern European populations (1 in 5000), North Americans (1 in 2000) and appears to be significantly common in Japan (Bolton-Maggs *et al.* 2004; Pallister 2005).

Signs and symptoms

The severity of HS is very varied. In some adults diagnosis can occur following a secondary illness such as aplasia or severe infection. Infections can exacerbate the anaemia and jaundice. For some patients aplastic crisis caused by parvovirus B19 can also occur. The virus infects erythroblastic cells, inhibiting their growth, leading to anaemia. Aplastic crisis is rare, but can lead to major haemolytic crisis, severe anaemia and significant complications such as congestive cardiac failure.

Anaemia, pallor and jaundice are common presenting symptoms due to haemolysis. Pigment gallstones (cholelitiasis), can also be present and associated with right upper abdominal pain. The cholelitiasis can be severe if the individual has co-inheritance of Gilbert syndrome. This is a condition which causes hyperbilirubinaemia due to reduced activity of the enzyme glucuronyltransferase, which conjugates bilirubin, (Beutler *et al.* 2002; Bolton-Maggs 2004). Hereditary spherocytosis can co-exist with other haematological conditions such as beta thalassaemia major, sickle cell disease, iron deficiency, vitamin B_{12} deficiency, which can worsen or ameliorate the condition (Ustun *et al.* 2003). The severity of HS is classified as mild, moderate or severe, and is based on haemoglobin, bilirubin levels and reticulocyte count.

Investigations

Diagnosis involves family history, haematological investigations and presenting symptoms mentioned earlier. Mild HS can be difficult to diagnose as bilirubin and haemoglobin levels can be normal, and iron, folate and vitamin B_{12} deficiencies, can mask diagnosis. Laboratory investigations would find spherocytes, increased levels of mean cell haemoglobin concentration (MCHC), red cell distribution width (RDW) and reticulocyte count. Haemoglobin will be low and the direct anti-globulin test (DAT) will be negative. The DAT is done to exclude an autoimmune cause of the haemolysis. Ultrasonography may be undertaken to detect gall stones.

Clinical and nursing management

In mild to moderate cases of HS, there is increased erythropoiesis which occurs due to the haemolysis; this can be a compensatory response to the reduced lifespan of red blood cells and the haemoglobin concentration may be normal. However, the increased erythropoiesis may lead to folate deficiency and hence folate supplements maybe necessary. The dosage is variable and nurses should be aware of advising patients of food which is rich in folate and the reader is directed to Chapter 6 on nutritional anaemias, for further information. Cholecystectomy may be undertaken in those with mild haemolysis who have troublesome cholestasis.

Splenectomy may be considered. This can be very successful in controlling the haemolysis, effectively 'curing' the patient. Splenectomy can eradicate the anaemia and hyperbilirubinaemia and the reticulocyte count returns to normal. Spherocyte shaped red blood cells will still persist but the haemolysis is generally no longer problematic following the splenectomy. However, splenectomy is not undertaken lightly because of the spleen's importance in immunity. There are significant risks of infections caused by encapsulated bacterial organisms, such as *Streptococcus* pneumonia, *Neisseria meningitides*, meningococcal organisms and *Haemophilus influenza*.

Nursing management for splenectomy

Pre-operative preparation should involve history taking, checking blood and biochemistry results and ensuring baseline observations of vital signs are recorded on the observation chart. If the operation is elective, it is important as part of the assessment process that the nurse checks the patient has had a pre-operative pneumococcal and meningococcal vaccination, at least two weeks prior to surgery as indicated by Davies *et al.* (2002). Blood should have been cross-matched and grouped. The nurse should confirm with the patient their understanding of the procedure they are having and ascertain any anxieties the patient may have. The consent form should be checked and signed by the patient.

Post-surgical management

Significant risks are bacterial infections and therefore penicillin V, amoxicillin or erythromycin will be prescribed. Diligence in infection control practice is essential, particularly when handling intravenous lines and wound management. Blood transfusion might be required and the safe administration by following local policy and guidelines are important. Appropriate analgesia should be prescribed and administered. Chest physiotherapy to prevent chest infections would be beneficial and administering analgesia prior to chest physiotherapy would be good practice to aid the patient's comfort. Thrombocytosis may occur, which may warrant prophylactic aspirin if the platelet count is very high.

Of fundamental importance is the discharge advice regarding the patient's vulnerability to infections and the lifelong risk of sepsis. Written information should be provided regarding vaccinations required and what actions to take if they become febrile, feel lethargic or experience shivering. The patient will also be advised of the need to have annual influenza vaccination. Lifelong antibiotic prophylaxis of either of the penicillin V (250–500 mg bd), or amoxicillin (250–500 mg daily), or erythromycin (250–500 mg daily) orally, is usually prescribed. Patients should be advised to wear an alert bracelet or pendant.

Glucose-6-phosphate dehydrogenase deficiency

Glucose-6-phosphate dehydrogenase (G6PD) deficiency is known to be one of the commonest enzymopathies worldwide (Scriver *et al.* 1995). The G6PD gene is located on the X chromosome, resulting in the vast majority of people with G6PD deficiency being male and females being carriers. Nurses should be aware of G6PD deficiency in adult patients as it can co-exist with other haematological conditions such as sickle cell disease.

Functions of glucose-6-phosphate dehydrogenase

Red blood cells gain their energy through a sequence of enzymatic reactions which ultimately lead to the conversion of glucose to lactic acid. This occurs along two metabolic pathways: the Embden-Meyerhof pathway (EMP) and the other alternate pathway is the pentose phosphate shunt (PPS). It is along the PPS pathway that the enzyme G6PD is active (Mehta *et al.* 2000) There is a close working relationship between the enzymes, enabling the red blood cell to function and to produce energy. G6PD is essential for a number of reasons: namely, it is one of many enzymes the body requires to convert carbohydrates into energy and in relation to its role in red blood cells, it protects them from oxidation. Oxidant substances can be drugs, infective organisms, chemicals or toxins. G6PD carries out its protective function of the red blood cell by:

- Converting glucose-6-phosphate into 6-phosphogluconate, which ensures that there are appropriate levels of the co-enzyme nicotinamide adenine dinucleotide phosphate (NADPH).
- NADPH is necessary for keeping glutathione (GSH), a tri-peptide, in its reduced form to enable it to function.
- The role of GSH is to clear the red cell of oxygen free radicals which produces hydrogen peroxide, a toxic substance to red blood cells. Glutathione converts hydrogen peroxide to water with the help of the enzyme, glutathione peroxidise.

(Cappellini and Fiorelli 2008; Zanella 2000)

Unlike other cells which have a number of enzymes to help generate NADPH, the red blood cell only has G6PD and therefore a fault of G6PD compromises the functions of NAPDH and GSH.

There are over 400 variants of G6PD, and they all result from a single point mutation on the X chromosome. The coding region for G6PD gene is Xq28 (see Chapter 3 Genetics

Table 8.2   Example of the inheritance of G6PD.

	Father	
Mother	X	Y
X	XX	XY
Xg	XgX	XgY

Key: Xg = G6PD mutated gene
Designed by Marvelle Brown.

for more detail on chromosome structure and terms). Table 8.2 provides a schematic example of the inheritance of G6PD. In this example there is carrier mother for G6PD deficiency and her partner has a normal X chromosome. This can result in a 25% chance a daughter will have 2 normal X chromosomes, a 25% a daughter will be a carrier for G6PD deficiency. In the case of son's there is a 25% chance there will be an unaffected male and a 25% of a son with G6PD deficiency.

The extent of the impact of a variant of G6PD can range between mild to severe deficiency. The lack of G6PD results in compromising the functions of haemoglobin and the enzymes NADPH and GSH. Due to insufficient levels of G6PD, these enzymes are unable to be in sufficient concentration to protect the red blood cells from oxidant drugs or infective organisms which can cause oxidation. The deficiency of these enzymes allows oxidant substances to attach to haemoglobin, causing it to denature (change the nature/ feature of the haemoglobin molecule, stopping it from functioning). This results in forming black mass compounds known as Heinz bodies. In addition, the build up of oxygen free radicals due to the lack of GSH increases the acidity of the red blood cells and therefore when these red cells travel through the spleen, splenic macrophages recognise them as being abnormal and destroy them, leading to haemolytic anaemia.

Although there are 400 variants of G6PD deficiency, 95% of all cases come under two types; the African (A) and the Mediterranean (B) type (Gregg and Prcha 2000). The African (A) type is the most common and is less severe than the Mediterranean (B) type. The difference in effects between the two is that the African (A) type tends to affect the older red blood cells and therefore the haemolysis is self-limiting and mild. Whereas in the Mediterranean (B) type, the deficiency of G6PD affects all ages of the red blood cells and therefore the haemolysis can be potentially more severe (Beutler 2008).

An evolutionary benefit of G6PD deficiency is that it offers protection against the most fatal malarial infection, *Plasmodium falciparum*. This provides some explanation as to why G6PD deficiency is prevalent in countries where malaria is endemic. It is believed that the rapid destruction of G6PD deficient red blood cells, possibly reduces the severity of malarial infections caused by *P. falciparum* (Scriver *et al.* 1995; Tripathy and Reddy 2007). Glucose-6-phosphate dehydrogenase deficiency is categorised by the World Health Organisation (WHO) into five classes, based on enzyme activity. Classes 1–3 are considered the more clinically significant (WHO 1989).

1 Severe deficiency (<10% activity), with chronic (non-spherocytic) haemolytic anaemia
2 Severe deficiency (<10% activity), with intermittent haemolysis

3   Mild deficiency (10–60% activity), haemolysis with stressors only
4   Non-deficient variant, no clinical sequalae
5   Increased enzyme activity, no clinical sequalae

Glucose-6-phosphate dehydrogenase deficiency is most common among people of Mediterranean, African, Asian and Middle Eastern decent and in Kurdish and Sephardic Jews (Kaplan *et al*. 1996; Oppenheim *et al*. 1993; Tripathy and Reddy 2007). Table 8.3 provides a breakdown in prevalence.

Table 8.3   Prevalence of G6PD deficiency across the world.

Approximately:
• 1 in every 12 Greek Cypriots are G6PD deficient
• 1 in every 5 Africans are G6PD deficient
• 1 in every 10 African-Caribbeans are G6PD deficient
• 1 in every 5 Indians are G6PD deficient
• 1 in every 30 Chinese are G6PD deficient
• 1 in every 5 Thais are G6PD deficient

Signs and symptoms

Most patients are generally well, but if they ingest oxidant drugs or develop an infection, acute haemolysis can occur and this tends to be the main issue in adults. *Salmonella, Escherichia coli*, beta-haemolytic streptococci, rickettsial infections, viral hepatitis, and influenza A tend to be common culprits in causing haemolysis (Frank 2005). Patients may become pale and this can be seen in black and other dark-skinned patients by looking at the lips or tongue. The haemolysis may lead to splenomegaly, tachycardia and dyspnoea. Signs of anaemia such as tiredness, fatigue and lethargy are possible. Jaundice occurs due to haemoglobin being metabolised and therefore excessive bile is produced and haemoglobinuria causes the urine to be dark in colour. Abdominal pain and back pain can also be symptoms patients complain of, particularly if they have acute renal failure.

Favism can cause haemolysis in the presence of G6PD deficiency. Favism is a haemolytic response to eating broad beans and its name is derived from the Italian name of the broad bean (fava) Legumes, particularly but not exclusively the fava bean, contain proteins vicine, convicine and isouramil, which generate oxygen free radicals, causing haemolysis (Beutler 1994). The haemolytic reaction is varied and does not always require hospitalisation. However, frequent mild episodes of haemolysis can, over time, lead to more serious complications, particularly ocular damage. Table 8.4 provides examples of food and drugs patients with G6PD should be advised to avoid.

Investigations

Full blood count is undertaken, which would demonstrate a reduced haemoglobin level, the enzyme lactate dehydrogenase (LDH) will be high due to the excessive haemolysis.

Table 8.4 Examples of food and drugs patients with G6PD should be advised to avoid.

Food	Drugs

Beans
  Fava beans
  Broad bean
  Butter bean
  Red kidney bean
	Antibiotics
	  Sulphanamides
	  Chloramphenicol
	  Co-trimoxazole

Other legumes
  Alfalfa sprouts
  Astragalus (herbal medicine)
  Carob (chocolate substitute)
  Fenugreek
  Liquorice
	Analgesia
	  Paracetamol
	  Aspirin
	  Phenazopyridine
	  Acetanilide

Tamarind
Other chemicals
  Mothballs
  Methylene and toluidine blue
  Vitamin K (water soluble)
  Red wine
	Suphonmides
	  Primaquine
	  Pentaquine
	  Sulfanilamide
	  Sulfamethoxazole
	  Mafenide
	Anti-malarial
	  Primaquine
	  Pentaquine
	  Mepacrine (quinacrine)
	  Chloroquine

This is not an exhaustive list.

The plasma protein haptoglobin will be low and a Coombs test may be done to exclude an autoimmune cause. The Beutler test, also known as the fluorescent spot test is a test undertaken to identify enzyme defects under ultraviolet light in the presence of G6PD deficiency. The test is positive if the blood spot fails to fluoresce under ultraviolet light, meaning that there is a reduction in NADPH levels (Frank 2005). Additionally, other confirmatory investigations would be the presence of Heinz bodies. Liver enzymnes, such as gamma-glutamyl transferase (GGT); alanine aminotransferase (ALT or SGPT); aspartate aminotransferase (AST or SGOT); and alkaline phosphatase (ALP) may be measured to exclude other causes of jaundice.

Clinical and nursing management

The severity of the anaemia would determine treatment options. Identifying the trigger of the haemolyisis is the main feature and once identified and addressed the haemolysis generally tends to resolve. Hospital admission may occur when the patient has acute haemolysis and is symptomatic. In the acute phase of haemolysis, blood transfusions might be necessary, or even dialysis in acute renal failure. Monitoring fluid intake and urine output is important to detect early signs of deterioration of renal function. Blood transfusion could be useful in having a positive symptomatic role, as the transfused red cells are not G6PD deficient and will live a normal lifespan in the recipient's circulation. Nursing care for managing blood transfusion is addressed in Chapter 17. If the haemolysis is causing significant clinical concerns, splenectomy may be undertaken since this organ is the major site of haemolysis. Managing a patient who has a splenectomy is outlined earlier in this chapter. Some clinicians may vaccinate against some common pathogens, for example hepatitis B, which may prevent this organism causing haemolysis (Monga *et al.* 2003).

Nurses must be able to reinforce the importance of advising patients on avoiding drugs and foods known to cause oxidation. A patient information sheet of the known drugs and foods which can cause haemolysis, would be of benefit for patients to have as an aide-memoire.

Conclusion

Hereditary spherocytosis and G6PD deficiencies are two commonly inherited haemolytic anaemias. Understanding their inheritance patterns, the investigations to ascertain a diagnosis and treatments have been reviewed. Nurses should have a good understanding of the genetics to help advise patients regarding the potential for effects on any children the individual may have or may intend to have in the future. It is essential to be familiar with the nursing care required for a splenectomised patient and know the advice required for patients with G6PD deficiency. Education is an important part of helping the patient to maintain their health and activities.

References

Beutler, E. (2008) Glucose-6-phosphate dehydrogenase deficiency: a historical perspective. *Blood*, 111 (1), 16–24.

Beutler, E., Gelbart, T. and Miller, W. (2002) Severe jaundice in a patient with a previously undescribed glucose-6-phosphate dehydrogenase (G6PD) mutation and Gilbert syndrome. *Blood Cells Mol Dis*, 28 (2), 104–107.

Bolton-Maggs, P.H.B. (2004) New guidelines hereditary spherocytosis. *Arch Dis Child*, 89, 809–812.

Bolton-Maggs, P.H., Stevens, R.F. Dodd, N.J., Lamont, G., Tittensor, P. and King, M.J. (2004) Guidelines for the diagnosis and management of hereditary spherocytosis. *Br. J. Haematol*, 126 (4), 455–474.

Cappellini, M.D. and Fiorelli, G. (2008) Glucose-6-phosphate dehydrogenase deficiency. *Lancet*, 371 (9606), 64–74.

Davies, J.M., Barnes, R. and Milligan, D. (2002) Update of guidelines for the prevention and treatment of infection in patients with an absent or dysfunctional spleen. *Clinical Medicine: Journal of the Royal College of Physicians of London*, 2, 440–443.

Delaunay, J. (2007) The molecular basis of hereditary red cell membrane disorders. *Blood Rev*, 21, 1–20.

Eber, S. and Lux, S.E. (2004) Hereditary spherocytosis-defects in proteins that connect the membrane skeleton to the lipid bilayer. *Semin Hematol*, 41, 118–141.

Eber, S.W., Gonzalez, J.M., Lux, M.L. *et al.* (1996) Ankyrin-1 mutations are a major cause of dominant and recessive hereditary spherocytosis. *Nature Genetics*, 13, 214–218.

Frank, J. (2005) Diagnosis and management of G6PD deficiency. *Am Fam Physician*, 72, 1277–1282.

Gallagher, P.G. (2004) Update on the clinical spectrum and genetics of red blood cell membrane disorders. *Curr Hematol Rep*, 3, 85–91.

Gallagher, P.G. and Jarolim, P. (2005) Red cell membrane disorders. In: *Hematology: Basic Principles and Practice* (eds R. Hoffman, E.J. Benz, JR., Shattil *et al.*), 3rd edition. pp. 576–610. WB Saunders, Philadephia.

Gregg, X.T. and Prchal, J.T. (2000) Red cell enzymopathies. In: *Hematology: Basic Principles and Practice* (ed. R. Hoffman), 4th edition. pp. 657–660.Churchill Livingstone, Philadelphia.

Kaplan, M., Vreman, H.J., Hammerman, C., Leiter, C., Abramov, A. and Stevenson, D.K. (1996) Contribution of haemolysis to jaundice in Sephardic Jewish glucose-6-phosphate dehydrogenase deficient neonates. *Br J Haematology*, 93, 822–827.

Mehta, A., Mason, P.J. and Vulliamy, T.J. (2000) Glucose-6-phosphate dehydrohenase, deficiency. *Baillière's Best Practice and Research in Clinical Haematology*, 13, 21–38.

Monga, A., Makkar, R.P., Arora, A., Mukhopadhyay, S. and Gupta, A.K. (2003) Case report: Acute hepatitis E infection with coexistent glucose-6-phosphate dehydrogenase deficiency. *Can J Infect Dis*, 14 (4), 230–231.

Oppenheim, A., Jury C.L., Rund, D., Vulliamy, T.J. and Luzzatto, L. (1993) G6PD Mediterranean accounts for the high prevalence of G6PD deficiency in Kurdish Jews. *Human Genetics*, 91 (3), 293–294.

Pallister, C.J. (2005) *Haematology*, 2nd edition. Edward Arnold, London.

Perrotta, S., Gallagher, P.G. and Mohandas, N. (2008) Hereditary spherocytosis. *Lancet*, 372 (9647), 1411–1426.

Scriver, C.R., Beaudet, A.L., Sly, W.S. and Valle, D. (1995) *The Metabolic and Molecular Basis of Inherited Disease*. McGraw-Hill, New York.

Tripathy, V. and Reddy. B.M. (2007) Present status of understanding on the G6PD deficiency and natural selection. *J Postgrad Med*, 53, 193–202.

Ustun, C., Kutlar, F., Holley, L., Seigler, M., Burgess, R. and Kutlar, A. (2003) Interaction of sickle cell trait with hereditary spherocytosis: splenic infarcts and sequestration. *Acta Haematol*, 109, 46–49.

Van Dort, H.M., Knowles, D.W., Chasis, J.A., Lee, G., Mohandas, N. and Low, P.S. (2001) Analysis of integral membrane protein contributions to the deformability and stability of the human erythrocyte membrane. *J Biol Chem*, 276, 46968–46974.

World Health Organisation Working Group (1989) Glucose-6-phosphate dehydrogenase deficiency. *WHO Working Group. Bull World Health Organ*, 67, 601–611.

Zanella, A. (2000) Inherited disorders of red blood cell metabolism. *Clin. Haematology*, 13, 1–150.

Chapter 9

Sickle cell disease and thalassaemia: pathophysiology, care and management

Marvelle Brown

After reading this chapter you should be able to:

- Know the difference between being a 'carrier' and having SCD or thalassaemia
- Understand the mode of inheritance for SCD and thalassaemia
- Be aware of the investigations necessary to diagnose SCD and thalassaemia
- Be cognisant of the potential complications that SCD and thalassaemia can cause
- Understand the key principles of managing a patient with SCD or thalassaemia

Introduction

Sickle cell disease (SCD) and thalassaemia are recessively inherited genetic conditions, which affect the haemoglobin molecule. Haemoglobinopathy is the generic term to describe genetic faults of the haemoglobin. The fault can either be structural such as SCD, or relate to an absence or reduction in globin chain synthesis, namely the thalassaemia syndromes (Weatherall and Clegg 2001). Both these pathologies are very complex and although they adversely affect the haemoglobin, they do so in very different ways, which will be discussed later in this chapter. An overview of the potential complications of these conditions as well as investigations to diagnose SCD and thalassaemia will be outlined. The clinical and nursing management will be addressed in the section on nursing care.

Haemoglobin is composed of a 'haem' component in which ferritin is attached and where oxygen reversibly combines. Each 'haem' is attached to a 'globin' group formed from four polypeptide chains (protein), which are two alpha chains and two non- α chains (Bain 2005) (Figure 9.1). The globin molecular structure, genetically determines an individual's haemoglobin type. The genes which code for the alpha chains are located on the short arm of chromosome 16 and the genes which code for beta, delta and gamma chains are located on the short arm of chromosome 11 (Pallister 2005).

Haematology Nursing, First Edition. Marvelle Brown and Tracey J. Cutler.
© 2012 Blackwell Publishing Ltd. Published 2012 by Blackwell Publishing Ltd.

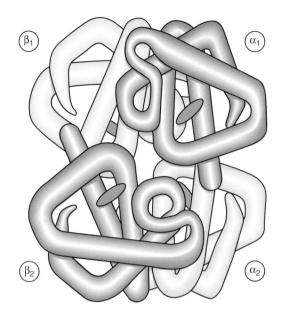

Figure 9.1   Composition of haemoglobin.

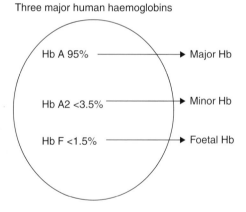

Figure 9.2   Types of haemoglobin. Designed by Marvelle Brown.

In adult humans, there are three types of normal haemoglobin found in each red blood cell:

Hb A = major haemoglobin
Hb A^2 = minor haemoglobin
Hb F = foetal haemoglobin

The globin molecular structure of haemoglobin A is composed of (α2 β2). Hb A^2 is comprised of two alpha chains and two delta chains (α2, δ2) and Hb F is formed from two alpha and two gamma chains (α2, γ2).

As illustrated in Figure 9.2, Hb A forms the vast majority of the haemoglobin in red blood cells.

The clinical manifestations and management for SCD and thalassaemia are distinctly different and will be addressed separately. Prior to discussing the pathologies of these conditions we will first address what the terms 'trait', 'carrier' and 'minor' mean.

Sickle cell trait and thalassaemia trait

As with any genetically determined characteristic such as eye or hair colour, there are variations and in relation to haemoglobin, there are over 1000 haemoglobin variants (NHS Antenatal and Neonatal Screening Programme 2006). However, the most common and clinically significant haemoglobin variants are S, C, D, E and thalassaemia. The words 'trait' and 'carrier' are sometimes used interchangeably in relation to sickle cell and can be confusing. Similarly, thalassaemia trait can also be known as thalassaemia 'minor'. All these terms have the same meaning, that is, the individual is asymptomatic and for consistency the term 'trait', will be used in this chapter. An individual who has sickle cell trait, means they have inherited Hb A (the normal/usual haemoglobin) from one parent and a haemoglobin variant from the other. Using the example of a sickle cell trait as illustrated in Figure 9.3, it demonstrates that the person inherits Hb A from one parent and HbS from the other, giving the genotype Hb AS.

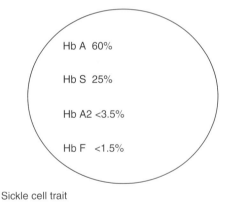

Hb A 60%

Hb S 25%

Hb A2 <3.5%

Hb F <1.5%

Sickle cell trait

Figure 9.3   An example of a haemoglobin variant. Designed by Marvelle Brown.

Having a haemoglobin variant generally does not cause any haematological concerns and daily life is unaffected. Sickle cell trait has been linked to haematuria, particularly during pregnancy and in the case of extreme exercise as seen, for example, in intense, extreme army training, sudden deaths have occurred (Hughes-Jones *et al.* 2009; Williams 1996). It is well known that sickle cell trait offers some innate protection against *Plasmodium falciparum* malarial infections.

Incidence and prevalence

The incidence of the most common types of haemoglobin variants can be seen in Table 9.1. Approximately 300 million people worldwide have sickle cell trait (Tsaras

Table 9.1 Carrier frequency of haemoglobin genes in selected ethnic groups.

Haemoglobin variant	Ethnic group	Population frequency
Beta thalassaemia	Mediterranean	1 in 7–20
	Asians – Bangladesh	1 in 10–30
	Pakistani, Chinese, Indian	
	African-Caribbean	
	West Africans	1 in 30–100
	White British	1 in 1000
Sickle cell trait	West African	1 in 5
	African-Caribbean	1 in 8–10
	Middle East/Mediterranean	1 in 100
C trait	Ghana	1 in 30
	African-Caribbean	1 in 30–50
D trait	Indians	1 in 50–100
	Also found in Pakistani,	
	Caribbean and White British	
E trait	Bangladesh	1 in 25–30
	Also occurs in Pakistani,	
	African-Caribbean, Chinese	
	and Indian population	
Alpha zero thalassaemia trait	Chinese, Far Eastern	1 in 20
	Mediterranean	1 in 30–100
Alpha plus thalassaemia trait	Occurs frequently in populations around the world	

Adapted from SMAC Report 1994.

et al. 2009). The sickle gene is predominately found in Africa, the Caribbean, the Middle East, the Mediterranean and India. West Africa has the highest incidence of sickle cell trait, with almost 24% of Nigerians having sickle cell trait (WHO 2006). In the UK, 1 in 10 of the black population have sickle cell trait and in India, the Orissa state has the highest concentration of Indians with sickle cell trait (Patel *et al.* 2009). In the United States, 7–9% of the African American population, and 1 in 100 American Hispanics have sickle cell trait (Derebail *et al.* 2010; NHGRI 2011; NHLBI 2011). The World Health Organisation in 2006 recognised SCD as a global health issue, encouraging countries to provide effective health promotion interventions and an integrated health care system to manage SCD.

Since sickle cell screening has been added to the national neonatal screening programme in England via the blood spot test (formerly known as the Guthrie test), it has been confirmed that sickle cell trait is also found in the indigenous population, children from mixed race parentage, in addition to those communities identified in Table 9.1 (Streetly *et al.* 2008).

Sickle cell disease

Sickle haemoglobin was first discovered by Dr Herrick in 1910 (Herrick 1910). Sickle cell disease (SCD) is a complex condition, with long-term chronicity, exacerbated by episodes of acute vaso-occulsive painful crisis, which at times for some patients can

	Mother	
	A	S
Father A	AA	AS
S	AS	SS

Figure 9.4 Inheritance of sickle cell anaemia (HbSS). Designed by Marvelle Brown.

be life threatening and life shortening. The severity, frequency and the intensity of sickling crisis varies from one individual to the next and varies with each crisis for the patient.

Sickle cell disease is a qualitative problem of haemoglobin production because there is a structural fault with the beta chain. This fault relates to a DNA point mutation in which adenine is replaced by thymine on the sixth position of the beta chain. This substitution leads to the production of the protein valine which produces Hb S (sickle) haemoglobin, instead of the protein glutamic acid, which normally produces Hb A (Hoffbrand and Moss 2011).

Sickle cell disease encompasses a number of heterogeneous combinations of haemoglobin variants, which can be inherited along with the sickle gene. The commonest type of sickle cell disease is sickle cell anaemia (HbSS). Here, if both parents have sickle cell trait (HbAS), the potential genotype for their offspring can be seen in Figure 9.4.

Figure 9.4 illustrates that there is a 1 in 4 (25%) chance the parents will have an off-spring with normal Hb AA, a 1 in 2 (50%) chance the parents will have an offspring with sickle cell trait (HbAS) and a 1 in 4 (25%) chance the parents will have a child with sickle cell anaemia (HbSS). These statistics will always been the same for every conception that occurs. If one parent has sickle cell trait (HbAS) and the other has sickle cell anaemia (HbSS), there is a 1 in 2 chance (50%) that the child will inherit sickle cell trait or a 1 in 2 chance (50%) the child will have sickle cell anaemia.

Haemoglobin SC disease, is the second commonest form of sickle cell disease. Haemoglobin C is one of the haemoglobin variants mentioned earlier and like Hb S, it is a structural fault. In this case, the DNA base substitution at the sixth position of the beta chain results in the protein lysine which produces Hb C. Illustrated in Figure 9.5 is the potential inheritance pattern. Here there is a 1 in 4 (25%) chance of an infant inheriting Hb AA, 1 in 4 (25%) chance of having sickle cell trait, 1 in 4 (25%) chance of having haemoglobin C trait and a 1 in 4 (25%) chance of having Hb SC disease.

The third commonest form of sickle cell disease is sickle betathalassaemia and Figure 9.6 below illustrates the potential inheritance pattern for the offspring. Again here, there is a 1 in 4 (25%) chance of an infant inheriting Hb AA, 1 in 4 (25%) chance of having sickle cell trait, 1 in 4 (25%) chance of having haemoglobin β thalassaemia trait and a 1 in 4 (25%) chance of having Hb S/beta thalassaemia. It is estimated that there are approximately 12,500 people living with sickle cell disease in the United Kingdom, making it more common than cystic fibrosis and the equivalent of haemophilia (Streetly *et al.* 1997).

Mother

	A	S
Father A	AA	AS
C	AC	SC

Figure 9.5   Inheritance of haemoglobin sickle cell disease. Designed by Marvelle Brown.

Mother

	A	S
Father A	AA	AS
β	Aβ	Sβ

Figure 9.6   Inheritance of sickle/beta thalassaemia. Designed by Marvelle Brown.

Diagnosis of sickle cell disease

The solubility test (sickle test) uses a reducing agent sodium dithionite. If there is sickle haemoglobin present this agent will cause the blood to become turbid in appearance because of precipitation (oxidation) of the haemoglobin (Stuart and Nagel 2004). However, the solubility test cannot distinguish between sickle cell trait and sickle cell disease and therefore haemoglobin electrophoresis is undertaken to determine the haemoglobin genotype. Each globin chain has its own electronic charge based on the composition of its amino acids. The haemoglobin electrophoresis is able to identify those charges, thereby establishing the haemoglobin genotype. High performance liquid chromatography (HPLC) is another diagnostic tool which can be used to determine haemoglobin genotype.

In the case of SCD, no Hb A would be present and the Hb F can vary from 0.1% to 9%. The higher the Hb F, the greater the oxygen carrying capacity of the red blood cell and the potential for fewer and less severe vaso-occulusive crises. Some patients can inherit a mutation of Hb F, which is called persistent hereditary foetal haemoglobin (PHFH). This is not common, but if it occurs has a positive effect on the function of the haemoglobin by enabling it to increase its oxygen carrying capacity. By doing so it has the potential to reduce the severity and frequency of vaso-occulusive crises.

Other investigations include full blood count; reticulocyte count, bilirubin and lactate dehydrogenase (LDH), would be undertaken (Sickle Cell Society 2008; Wethers 2000). Haemoglobin is usually 9 g/dL or lower, the reticulocyte count, bilirubin and LDH will all be high. Due to excessive haemolysis of sickle red blood cells, the bone marrow shunts out more reticulocytes into circulation, thereby increasing their number. High levels of the enzyme LDH, are associated with sickle red blood cell breakdown and can be a marker for complications such as pulmonary hypertension, leg ulcers, priapism and increased risk of mortality. Lactate dehydrogenase is also a useful marker for chemical reactions occurring in the bloodstream that deplete the patient of nitric oxide, which normally works to dilate blood vessels. A deficiency of nitric oxide causes the endothelium of the blood vessels to thicken, causing narrowing and leading to nitric oxide resistance (Kato *et al.* 2006).

Signs and symptoms of sickle cell disease

Signs and symptoms do not manifest until after the age of 3–6 months because foetal hae-moglobin has a high affinity for oxygen and enables the infant to have successful gaseous exchange. After the period of 3–6 months, molecular changes occur in the haemoglobin and the haemoglobin genotype inherited from the parents will gradually manifest itself.

In sickle cell disease, when the red blood cells are oxygenated, they retain their normal biconcave shape. However, when sickle haemoglobin releases its oxygen into tissues, and becomes deoxygenated, the sickle haemoglobin forms crystals and polymerisation occurs. This leads to a distortion in the shape of red blood cells into a sickle shape (depranocyte – is the name for sickle shaped red blood cell). These abnormally shaped red blood cells revert back to their normal shape when oxygenated. However, the constant changing of shape eventually leads to the red blood cells becoming irreversibly sickle-shaped and they are then destroyed by macrophages in the reticulo-endothelial system. The lifespan of red blood cells in sickle cell disease is 10–20 days in comparison with 120 days of a normal red blood cell. This excessive breakdown of red blood cells leads to chronic haemolytic anaemia (Buchanan *et al.* 2004).

Painful vaso-occulsive crisis is the most common presenting symptom of sickle cell disease and Ballas (1995) identified four phases of painful crisis: prodromal, initial, established and resolving. Other types of crisis can be found in Table 9.2. Vaso-occlusive crises cause pain when the sickle-shaped red blood cells clump and stick together, causing occlusion and preventing oxygen and nutrients from being supplied to the tissues. This will ultimately lead to tissue hypoxia and tissue necrosis. In addition, by sticking to the endothelial lining of blood vessels the sickle-shaped red blood cells trigger the release of inflammatory mediators, such as histamine and tumour necrosis factor-α (TNF-α), which exacerbate the pain. These inflammatory mediators instigate pain impulses across the alpha and C nerve fibres towards the dorsal horn of the spinal cord. Impulses are then sent up to the spinothalamic tract to the brain stem, hypothalamus and thalamus. The thalamus also interconnects with the limbic system which is responsible for mood and emotion. The pain stimulus continues onto the parietal lobe where the pain sensation is perceived. The role the limbic system plays in the pain phenonomen, demonstrates the added socio-logical, psychological and emotional factors that make the pain experience subjective and a real challenge for health care professionals. The complexity of sickling pain is further

Table 9.2   Other types of crisis.

Sequestration crisis	This relates to pooling of blood in organs, particularly the lungs, spleen and liver.
Haemolytic crisis	Occurs due to excessive haemolysis, leading to a fall in haemoglobin and haematocrit, causing fatigue, lethargy, headaches and cardiac failure. Jaundice is a result of haemolysis, leading to excessive production of bilirubin formed from the metabolised haem part of the haemoglobin. This type of crisis occurs more commonly inpatients who also have glucose-6-phosphate-dehydrogenase deficiency (G6PD).
Aplastic crisis	This crisis can be caused by folate deficiency or infection and the culprit virus, parvovirus B19. This virus directly disrupts the production of RBC by invading red cell precursors. The result is a drop in haemoglobin, patients complaining of tiredness, and having signs of tachycardia and appearing pale.

compounded by such as factors as: previous experiences of pain management, anxiety, fear of dying, stress and mood (Ress *et al.* 2003; Stuart and Nagel 2004).

Some of the inflammatory mediators are also procoagulant, increasing the adherence ability of the sickle red blood cells to the endothelium. The release of adhesive molecules such as vascular cell adhesion molecule-1 (VCAM-1), and intracellular adhesion molecule-1(ICAM-1) from damaged endothelial tissue, increases the adherence of the sickle red cells to the wall of the blood vessel (Telen 2007). The combination of the activated mediators coupled with the sticky, rigidity of the red blood cells, bind to the von Williebrand factor and thrombospondin, a substance secreted by activated platelets. The end result is vascular stasis, haemolysis and vaso-occlusion of capillary vessels, ultimately causing tissue necrosis (Phillipots and Doung 2005).

Acute painful vaso-occulsive crisis can occur in any part of the body, but typically in adults the femur, humerus, vertebrae, ribs and abdomen are common sites. Ischaemia and infarction are the main cause of bone pain. Chronic pain usually occurs due to chronic arthritis, vertebral collapse and avascular necrosis. Avascular necrosis is the main cause of joint pain. Organ dysfunction, referred pain from the ribs and bowel dysfunction can be the cause of abdominal pain (Firth 2005). Frequency of painful crisis has been suggested as a gauge of the severity of the condition. However, Van Beers *et al.* (2008) suggest that significant organ damage such as pulmonary hypertension and microalbumuria, occur in patients without painful crisis, causing significant organ dysfunction.

Acute chest sequestration occurs in both adults and children and is a life-threatening complication caused by sickle cells blocking the alveoli. Hepatic sequestration occurs in adults; patients will complain of right upper quadrant abdominal pain and hepatomegaly will be present. Splenic sequestration only occurs in childhood. Jaundice is a consequence of excessive haemolysis and the excessive bilirubin produced can lead to gallstones.

Potential predisposing factors of sickling crisis

Dehydration is a significant cause of sickling crisis as it leads to increased plasma viscosity, which slows the movement of red blood cells, increasing the opportunity for sickle-shaped red blood cells to stick together. Alcohol consumption can also be a cause of dehydration.

Smoking can potentially increase the anaemia since the carbon monoxide requires the same position as the oxygen molecule on the haemoglobin. The end result is a lower level of circulating oxygen and increased risk of increasing the severity of the anaemia.

Infections are a significant problem in sickle cell disease, due to chronic anaemia, functional asplenia, hepatic dysfunction and defective opsonisation of the alternative complement pathway and a deficiency of circulating antibodies (Allen 2005). *Streptococcus pneumonia, Haemophilus influenzae* type B and *Salmonella* osteomyelitis are main culprits. Parvovirus B19 is a common infective organism in patients on hypertransfusion programme.

Changes in environmental temperature can cause sickling crisis. This is particularly the case during the winter months. During cold weather the blood vessels vasoconstrict, making it difficult for sickle-shaped red blood cells to flow through micro-blood vessels. In hot weather, the blood vessels dilate which enables a smoother flow of red blood cells in circulation. Excessive exercise can lead to dehydration and cell lysis, causing a crisis. Stress is known to be associated with sickling crisis, both physical and mental stress. Gill *et al.* (2004) reported that daily mood and stress can be a predictor of painful crisis. Pregnancy is an additional strain on the body of the woman which is compromised by chronic anaemia. During pregnancy, there are increased risks, including infection, particularly respiratory and urinary tract infections, cholecystitis and cardiomegally due to anaemia. Potential obstetric complications are: pre-eclampsia, miscarriage and premature labour. Cerebrovascular accidents are also a risk during pregnancy. Complications for the foetus can include intrauterine growth retardation (poor foetal growth), intrauterine death, preterm birth (before 37 weeks of pregnancy), low birth weight (less than 5.5 pounds (2.4 kg) and stillbirth. Women with sickle cell disease who become pregnant are always managed by a consultant haematologist and consultant obstetrician.

Complications of sickling crisis

Any organ can be affected in a sickling crisis, which makes management very challenging and for patients it poses significant emotional and psychological challenges. As patients are living longer, dysfunction of major organs is not uncommon.

Dactycitis (swelling of the fingers, hands and feet) are indicative signs of sickling crisis in children.

Cerebrovascular accidents (CVAs) are a major complication of sickling crisis. The sticky adhesive nature of sickle red blood cells can cause occlusion in the cerebral arteries, leading to cerebrovascular accidents. Cerebral haemorrhage may also occur secondary to berry aneurysms and moyamoya vascular abnormalities (Adams *et al.* 2001).

Priapism is painful involuntary erection of the penis. Blood becomes trapped in the blood vessels and the stagnant blood causes an erection that can last from hours to days. There are two types of priapism in sickle cell disease: stuttering priapism which can last 30–60 minutes; it resolves but occurs again sometimes several times in a day, but clears up without medical treatment. Acute priapism can last hours or days, potentially causing permanent blood vessel damage (Clare *et al* 2002; Nolan *et al.* 2005). Both stuttering and acute priapism can cause impotence. Delayed puberty and problems with fertility can occur for both sexes.

Retinopathy is most commonly seen in patients with Hb SC disease. Vascular occlusion causes retinal hypoxia, ischemia and in some cases neovascularisation. Retinal damage in sickle cell disease is classified as non-proliferative sickle retinopathy (NPSR) or proliferative sickle retinopathy (PSR). This involves neovascularisation which occurs from repeated ishaemic episodes related to peripheral arterial occlusion (Phillpots and Doung 2008).

As adults with sickle cell disease get older, through improved management and increasing understanding about the condition, pulmonary, renal, cardiac and hepatic function poses significant challenges. Pulmonary artery hypertension (PAH) is strongly associated with early death in adults with SCD. Secondary PAH related to SCD leads to the potential problem of reduced oxygen for prolonged periods through the lungs (Castro *et al.* 2003; Hayes Jr and Pack-Mabien 2007). Cardiac impairment occurs due to a number of factors, including hypoxic stress on endothelia tissues, reduced elasticity of the myocardium, PAH and cor pulmonae, exacerbated by hepatic and renal dysfunction (Aessopas 2006). Renal dysfunction can be caused by damage to the distal renal tubules, producing type IV renal acidosis and haematuria secondary to necrosis (Abbot *et al.* 2002).

Leg ulcers are a debilitating complication of sickle cell disease. Occlusion of blood vessels, poor circulation, reduced oxygenation, all lead to difficulty with leg ulcers healing. Kato *et al.* (2006) highlighted in their study that patients with leg ulcers had lower haemoglobin levels, high levels of lactate dehydrogenase, bilrubin, aspartate aminotransferase and high reticulocyte count, which could be factors potentially causing difficulties with the healing process. Skeletal damage caused by sickling can lead to significant problems with mobility, chronic pain and reduced quality of life.

Pathology of thalassaemia

Thalassaemia syndromes can be broadly divided into two groups: alpha thalassaemia and beta thalassaemia. There are many mutations and gene deletions in thalassaemia, which occur in different populations globally. Both alpha and beta thalassaemia cause quantitative problems with haemoglobin production (Thein 2005).

Incidence and prevalence

Thalassaemia trait, like sickle cell trait, offers some protection against plamasmodium falciparum malaria infections (Danquah and Mochenhaupot 2008; Weatherall 1997). The prevalence of alpha thalassaemia is approximately 0.01% in the United Kingdom. This is in distinct contrast to other parts of the world, such as Thailand, India, Saudia Arabia and Papua New Guinea, where the prevalence is 60–80% and in West Africa it is approximately 20–30% (Casas-Castenda 1998). The prevalence of beta thalassaemia trait is found in individuals who originate from the Mediterranean, the Middle East, Indian subcontinent, Pakistan and Eastern Europe, and can be found in Table 9.1.

Alpha thalassaemia

Alpha thalassaemia relates to the number of α (alpha) globin chains that are deleted. Normally, an individual inherits 2 α genes on each of chromosome 16; the more α chains missing, the greater the clinical severity (see Tables 9.3 and 9.4). To identify which type of alpha deletion an individual has, DNA analysis using polymerase chain reaction (PCR) is usually required (Liu *et al.* 2009).

Table 9.3   Alpha thalassaemia trait.

αα/-α	One α globin chain deletion is not problematic and is sometimes called a silent carrier.
αα/-	Two α globin chain deletion (also known as α thalassaemia trait) generally does not cause the individual any problems. Laboratory investigations may identify the red blood cells as being microcytic and hypochromic. However, individuals do not require any treatment.

Table 9.4   Alpha thalassaemia deletions of clinical significance.

-/-α	Three α globin chain deletion causes a clinical condition known as haemoglobin H disease and is a chronic haemolytic illness.
-/- no alpha chains	Alpha thalassaemia major

Haemoglobin H disease

The signs and symptoms are very varied, including anaemia, jaundice, fatigue, spleno-megaly and it has been recognised that osteoporosis is a significant problem in adults with haemoglobin H disease (Chui *et al.* 2003). Pyrexia, infections, pregnancy, inhalation of the fumes of moth balls (naphthalene) and eating fava beans, can worsen the anaemia. In addition, the red blood cells of individuals with haemoglobin H disease are susceptible to oxidant drugs which also cause haemolysis, leading to increased anaemia. Table 9.5 lists the drugs known to oxidise red blood cells in haemoglobin H disease.

Investigations to diagnose haemoglobin H disease will identify red blood cells as being microcytic, abnormally shaped, and hypochromic. Haemoglobin can be between 7–10 g/dL and the mean cell volume (MCV), mean cell haemoglobin (MCH) and mean cell haemoglo-bin concentration (MCHC) will be reduced. The reticulocyte count will be high >4–10% and the higher the reticulocyte the more severe the anaemia. Haemoglobin electrophoresis will identify haemoglobin A, A_2, Hb F and the high level of haemoglobin Barts, which is indicative of haemoglobin H disease (Williams 1996).

Patients with haemoglobin H disease are regularly reviewed to detect any changes in haemolytic status. Management is primarily supportive care, which includes, prescribing vitamin D to minimise osteoporotic problems and folic acid to help with red blood cell matu-rity. Periodic blood transfusion for severe anaemia maybe required. Splenectomy may be done if the patient has severe hypersplenism which is causing leucopenia, thrombocytopenia or anaemia is worsening. Haemoglobin H disease is associated with myeloproliferative or myel-odysplastic conditions and in some rare cases can cause mental retardation (Turgeon 2005).

Alpha thalassaemia major

In alpha thalassaemia major, all four α globin chains are deleted and this leads to Barts hydrops foetalis, causing the foetus to either die *in utero* or within hours of birth. The neonate is very oedematous with very little circulating haemoglobin, all of which contains

Table 9.5   Drugs and food known to oxidise red blood cells in haemoglobin H disease.

Sulpha drugs Sulphacetamide (eye drops) Sulphapyridine Sulphasalazine (salicylazosulphapyridine) Sulphanilamide Dapsone	**Other antibacterials** Nalidixic acid (negram) Nitrofurantonin Furazolidone Chloramphenicol Beta-aminosalicylic acid Ciprofloxacin Doxycycline
Antimalarials Primaquine Chloroquine Hydrozychloroquine sulphate	**Analgesics** Aspirin Phenacetin Acetanilide
Other items Iron supplements Vitamin K analogues Quinidine gluconate Phenazopyridine (pyridium) Toluidine blue (a dye) Methylene blue (a dye) Naphthalene (mothballs) Fava beans	**Tuberculosis drugs** Isoniazid Rifampicin Folic acid antagonists Pyrimethamine

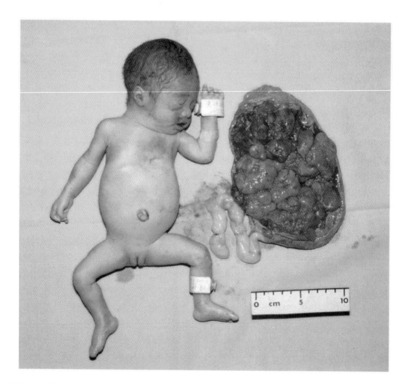

Figure 9.7   α- Thalassaemia: hydrops foetalis, the result of deletion of all four α- globin genes (homozygous α°-thalassaemia). The main haemoglobin present is Hb Barts (γ4). The condition is incompatible with life beyond the foetal stage (courtesy of Professor D. Todd, from Hoffbrand and Moss 2011). Reprinted with permission of John Wiley & Sons, Inc.

Mother

		A	β
Father	A	AA	Aβ
	β	Aβ	ββ

Figure 9.8   The potential haemoglobin genotype of offspring of parents who have beta thalassaemia trait. Designed by Marvelle Brown.

haemoglobin Barts. Investigations to identify couples who are at risk of having a child with alpha thalassaemia major would include haemoglobin electrophoresis and DNA analysis.

Beta thalassaemia

There are approximately 200 mutations of the β (beta) chain, which results in a fault with synthesis, causing either a reduction in the β chain production (β thalassaemia plus), or total absence of β chain production (β thalassaemia zero) (Higgs *et al*. 2001).

Beta thalassaemia trait

This occurs when the individual has inherited one normal β globin gene and one affected β (thalassaemia) gene, and results in a raised level of Hb A^2 (Bain 2005). People with beta thalassaemia trait typically have red blood cells which are microcytic, hypochromic, with a low mean cell volume (MCV). Such a picture mimics iron deficiency anaemia and therefore it is important that beta thalassaemia trait is confirmed or excluded prior to a patient commencing iron medication, as this could cause problems of increased iron absorption. Individuals with beta thalassaemia trait are asymptomatic and do not require any treatment.

Beta thalassaemia major

Beta thalassaemia major (BTM) is also known as Cooley's anaemia, named after Professor Cooley, a paediatrician who first identified the condition (Steensman *et al*. 2001). Beta thalassaemia major can be defined as beta thalassaemia major zero (B^0B^0), which is total absence of beta chain production or beta thalassaemia major plus (B^+B^+) where there is limited β chain synthesis. Normal α globin chain production is unaffected in beta thalassaemia major, but due to the lack of or reduction in the amount of beta chains being produced, the alpha chains are in excess in red blood cells. This results in a compensatory rise in α chains, leading to an increase in the Hb A^2. However, this has no positive effect on the haemoglobin function but instead increases haemolysis. The excess α chains also accelerates apoptosis in red blood cells (Rund 2005), resulting in excessive haemolysis. The haemolysis triggers increased production of erythropoietin as an attempt to stimulate red blood cell production in the bone marrow. However, this is to no avail since haemoglobin synthesis is lacking due to insufficient beta chains to make haemoglobin (Schrier 2002). The incidence of beta thalassaemia major is a mixed picture globally. B°B° predominates in India, Pakistan; B+B+ predominates in Sardinia and Cyprus, and both are found in Greece, the Middle East and Thailand.

Blood investigations will identify severe anaemia; haemoglobin can be 3–4 g/dL, the red blood cells will be hypochromic microcytic, evidence of reticulocytosis and haemoglobin electrophoresis will show no haemoglobin A and a very high A^2. The bone marrow will show extensive erythroid hyperplasmia, abnormal erythroblastic cells and iron studies tend to demonstrate high serum iron.

Figure 9.7 illustrates the potential haemoglobin genotype of offspring of parents who have beta thalassaemia trait. There is a 1 in 4 (25%) of having a child with normal haemoglobin genotype Hb AA), a 1 in 2 (50%) chance of having a child with beta thalassaemia trait and a 1 in 4 (25%) chance of having a child with beta thalassaemia major.

Symptoms of beta thalassaemia major

Unlike alpha thalassaemia major, beta thalassaemia major is compatible with life, but is associated with significant morbidities and mortality, due to iron overload toxicity (Cunningham *et al.* 2004; Model *et al.* 2000). Anaemia in beta thalassaemia major occurs because of three interrelated factors: ineffective erythropoiesis, excess alpha chain production and reduced haemoglobin synthesis (Schrier 2002). As a result, tiredness, lethargy and fatigue can occur. Like SCD, jaundice is a consequence of the excessive haemolysis, and hepatomegaly and splenomegaly occurs, partly in response to the increase workload of destroying red blood cells and as a result of increased iron load in the liver (Telfer *et al.* 2000).

Cardiomegaly may occur because of the increased workload, due to the reduction in circulating red blood cells. Hyperplasia is a compensatory mechanism to try and encourage increased bone marrow production of red blood cells. The bone expansion causes pain as well as thinning of the bone, making fractures an increased risk. Hyperplasia can also cause thrombocytopenia and neutropenia. In addition, patients who may have been diagnosed late in childhood or had ineffective transfusion regime or who are non-complaint with iron chelation therapy can develop significant bone abnormalities. These can include frontal and parietal bossing of the cranium, enlarged maxillary bones which can lead to dental deformities, malocclusion of the teeth and depression of the bridge of the nose (Hoffbrand and Moss 2011) (see Figures 9.8 and 9.9).

Complications of beta thalassaemia major

Management will be discussed in detail the next section. However, to understand the cause of complications associated with BTM, it is important to note that many of the

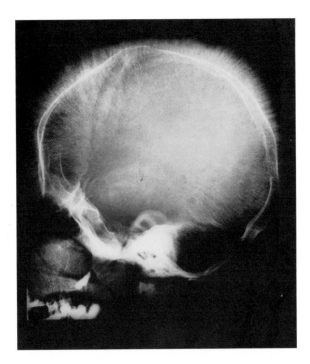

Figure 9.9   The skull X-ray in β-thalassaemia major. There is a 'hair-on-end' appearance as a result of expansion of the bone marrow into cortical bone (from Hoffbrand and Moss 2011). Reprinted with permission of John Wiley & Sons, Inc.

complications stem from the management, which is blood transfusion and iron chelation therapy. As indicated in Chapter 6 (Nutritional anaemia), iron is controlled through a closed loop system. Humans do not have a normal excretory route for excess iron and because of this the management of BTM is very challenging (Fleming and Bacon 2005). In BTM, the main treatment is lifelong monthly blood transfusion and each unit of packed red blood cells contains 250 mg of iron. In addition, Gantz (2003) and Papanikolaou *et al.* (2005) highlighted the problem of the peptide hepcidin in patients with BTM. Hepcidin inhibits iron absorption from the small intestine. When there are high iron levels, there is an increase in hepicidin; however, in patients with BTM, hepcidin levels are very low. This gives some explanation as to why gastrointestinal absorption of iron is high in BTM.

High iron absorption from the gut coupled with transfusional iron, illustrates the problem of excess iron in BTM. Ultimately the excess iron overwhelms the body and without iron chelation therapy, iron deposits will be deposited into major organs. The heart, liver and endocrine glands are significant targets for excess iron deposits and, unfortunately, iron targets the parenchymal cells (the functional tissue or cells of an organ or gland), causing organ dysfunction.

Multi-endocrinological dysfunctions are common in beta thalassaemia major, potentially resulting in diabetes mellitus, hypoparathyroidism, hypothyroidism, and hypogonadotrophic hypogonadism (Malik *et al.* 2009). The anterior pituitary gland is particularly sensitive to iron disrupting hormonal secretion, leading to its dysfunction. The anterior pituitary produces follicle-stimulating hormone (FSH), luteinising hormone (LH), adrenocorticotropic hormone (ACTH), thyroid-stimulating hormone (TSH), prolactin (PRL) and growth hormone (GH).

An understanding of the impact of iron on the function of the anterior pituitary, indicates why it is not surprising that patients with beta thalassaemia have delayed puberty, stunted growth, secondary amenorrhea, menstrual irregularities and fertility challenges (De Sanctis *et al.* 1988; Toumba *et al.* 2007). In addition to endocrinological challenges, chronic anaemia, infections, poor nutrition malabsorption of vitamin D, deficiencies of calcium, zinc copper, and lower serum levels of insulin-like growth factor-1 (IGF-1) and IGF-binding protein-3 (IGFBP-3), have also been linked to poor pubescent growth, causing short stature in adults (Malik *et al.* 2009). Deficiency of trace elements such as zinc is considered to be one of the main factors contributing to growth and puberty disorders in thalassaemic patients.

Cardiac dysfunction, especially, left-sided heart failure is responsible for more than half of the deaths in patients with beta thalassaemia major (Hahalis *et al.* 2005). Signs of cardiac disease can manifest as arrhythmias, systolic/diastolic dysfunction, pericardial effusion, myocarditis or pericarditis, heart failure, pulmonary hypertension and cardiomopyapthy due to haemosiderosis (Borgna-Pignatti 2007). MRI investigations (cardiac T2* MRI and either R2 or T2* of liver) for monitoring myocardial and liver iron, is undertaken at specialist centres (St Pierre *et al.* 2005). Low bone mass prevalent in patients with beta thalassaemia major, which tends to manifest as osteoporosis or osteopenia, is caused by a number of factors: lack of spontaneous puberty, malnutrition, multi-endocrine dysfunction and deficiencies of vitamin D, calcium and zinc (Voskaridou *et al.* 2001). The high risk of liver failure and potential hepatocellular carcinoma in a liver already damaged by iron toxicity and frequent blood transfusions can be manifested by hepatomegaly, high liver enzyme levels (aspartate and alanine transaminase) as well as hepatitis B and C.

Other infective organisms such as *Yersinia entercolitica* occur in an iron-rich environment, which is produced by the blood transfusion regime and the use of desferal (an iron chelator) aids their growth. *Yersinia entercolitica* causes abdominal pain, diarrhoea, skin rashes, vomiting and can mimic appendicitis. Neurological symptoms can be another complication of beta thalassaemia major, which include visual, auditory, and somatosensory problems that are mainly attributed to desferal neurotoxicity.

Beta thalassaemia intermedia (BTI)

This type of beta thalassaemia relates to clinical symptoms which cross between being mild, such as beta thalassaemia trait to being clinically severe, such as beta thalassaemia major. The diagnosis is more often a clinical one based on the patient being able to maintain haemoglobin of 6–8 g/dL without requiring blood transfusion. The differences in the complexity of the clinical severity of BTI is based on a number of factors, including the genetic globin mutation combinations the patient has and whether there is an increased production of Hb F which would help to improve the oxygen carrying capacity of red blood cells.

Ineffective erythropoiesis is the main cause of the symptoms seen in BTI, leading to chronic anaemia and extramedullary haemopoiesis. In addition, excess iron absorption from the gut due to increased demand for RBC development can lead to iron overload. There is a down-regulation of hepcidin which controls iron haemostasis in the gut, leading to excess iron and as a consequence after some years the iron overload may necessitate chelation therapy.

Particular complications in BTI are skeletal and growth problems, vertebral disc disease, splenomegally, tumour masses in the spine, pressing on nerves causing severe back pain. Due to the skeletal problems and chronic anaemia, adults may have a small stature. Cappellini *et al.* (2005) indicated in their study complications of hypercoagulability and pulmonary hypertension in patients with thalassaemia intermedia, especially after having a splenectomy. Penicillin maybe prescribed for those patients who have had a splenectomy to reduce the risk of bacterial infections and aspirin to prevent thrombotic complications. Blood transfusion maybe required if the person develops a severe infection or during pregnancy (Aessopas *et al.* 2007).

Patients with BTI are closely monitored and have frequent outpatient appointments as the clinical status can transform from being intermedia to major. Patients are sometimes advised to reduce vitamin C intake as this increases iron absorption and to increase drinking tea with meals as it helps to inhibit iron absorption. Vitamin E may also be advised as it helps to minimise some of the toxic effects of the free oxygen radicals and other iron-related toxicity. For those patients whose condition transforms to beta thalassaemia major, their management follows that of beta thalassaemia major.

Nursing care of patients with sickle cell disease and thalassaemia

This section is divided into two, to review the nursing issues for patients with SCD and thalassaemia. Both SCD and thalassaemia are considered long-term conditions and the majority of care is undertaken in the community. In SCD hospitalisation primarily relates to acute painful sickling crisis and for thalassaemia, hospitalisation is necessary for their blood transfusion regime. Readers are guided to read the *British Standards for Clinical Haematology* – guidelines for managing acute sickling crisis (BSCH) (2003), the *Standards for Managing Adults with SCD* (Sickle Cell Society 2008) and the *Standards for the Clinical Care of Adults and Children with Thalassaemia* in the UK (UK Thalassamia Society 2008), in conjunction with this chapter. NICE in 2012 will be publishing updated guidelines on managing patients in acute sickling crisis.

Nursing care of for acute vaso-occlusive crisis in sickle cell disease

Increasing understanding of the pathology of sickle cell disease has led to improvements in interventions, leading to an increase in the lifespan of people with SCD (Quinn *et al.* 2004), transferring SCD into a long-term chronic illness. However, as patients are living longer, there is an increase in morbidities of neurological, cardiopulmonary and renal disease, adding to the complexity in managing adults with SCD. A multidisciplinary approach is essential in providing holistic care.

Hospitals with large populations of sickle cell patients may have dedicated sickle cell day treatment clinics. In hospitals with smaller populations, sickle cell patients can be treated alongside oncology patients in chemotherapy day units. Both options for outpatient day treatment have several advantages over the use of emergency departments for a number of reasons:

- Staff are familiar with the patient, particularly those admitted on a regular basis.
- Intravenous or intramuscular pain medications are usually given quicker and more aggressively than in accident and emergency.
- Aggressive outpatient treatment of moderate to severe painful episodes and consistent, supportive care from familiar staff can often prevent the need for inpatient admissions for these same crises.

General nursing management principles include monitoring the effectiveness of analgesia, vital sign monitoring, ensuring the patient is well hydrated, fluid monitoring, monitoring major organ functioning, observing for signs of infection, encouraging a healthy diet and supporting the patient in undertaking activities of living. Ultimately, the primary aims of nursing must be to control the pain, minimising potential organ damage and provide supportive, sensitive and high quality care. Acute painful crisis should be managed and treated like cancer pain.

Pain management

Many patients who are experiencing a vaso-occulsive crisis, tend to aim to manage themselves at home, with a combination of analgesia, NSAIDS, increasing their fluid intake, resting, reducing their activities and keeping warm. The type of medication used at home is listed in Table 9.6. However, there will be times when the vaso-occlusive crises are so acutely painful that hospital admission becomes necessary. Vaso-occlusive crisis is the cause of 90% of hospital admissions for adults with SCD (Streetly *et al.* 1997). Prompt and effective pain relief should be a priority intervention for sickle cell crises. The consequences of unrelieved pain can ultimately make pain itself a disease in its own right. Detrimental effects of unrelieved pain can lead to depression, heighten anxiety levels, lead to debilitation and patients feeling dehumanised, all of which have a major negative effect on quality of life.

On admission, sensitive and empathetic questioning should ascertain when the patient last took their medication, what medication they took and the dosage. This is important to ensure the patient is not overdosed and to monitor for any side effects related to the drugs the patient may have taken. Nurses need to reassure the patient that nursing staff acknowledge and understand they are in pain and will work with them to develop an acceptable pain management programme. Patients should receive pain relief within 30 minutes of arriving at the emergency department and effective analgesia by 60 minutes (BCSH 2003).

Pain assessment tools are important in helping the patient to describe their pain and are an objective measure for practitioners to use to assess the effectiveness of pain interventions. There are a wide range of pain assessment tools; an assessment tool which uses a numerical scoring, from 0–10 (zero being least pain), combined with front and back body

Table 9.6 Selection of analgesia and NSAIDS used at home for sickle pain.

Paracetamol
Co-codamol
Sevredol
Oxycodone
Fentanyl patches
Fentanyl lozenges
Ibuprofen
Oramorph
MST
Diclofenac

On the picture below place a cross where you are feeling the pain.

Please place a circle around the number which best describes your pain now.
   0 1 2 3 4 5 6 7 8 9 10
   (no pain)   (severe pain)

Has the pain affected your daily activities (personal hygiene, cooking)?

Please circle the number
   0 1 2 3 4 5 6 7 8 9 10
   (no pain)   (severe pain)

How much has the pain affected your ability to walk?
   0 1 2 3 4 5 6 7 8 9 10
   (no effect)   (severely affects)

Is the pain making it difficult to concentrate?
   0 1 2 3 4 5 6 7 8 9 10
   (no difficulty)   (severe difficulty)

Is the pain affecting your appetite?
   0 1 2 3 4 5 6 7 8 9 10
   (no effect)   (severely affects)

Is the pain affecting your mood?
   0 1 2 3 4 5 6 7 8 9 10
   (no effect)   (severely affects)

Figure 9.10 Brief pain inventory assessment tool. Designed by Marvelle Brown.

outline charts, enables the patient to indicate both severity and position of pain, providing additional informative information. Figure 9.10 provides an example of a brief pain inventory assessment tool.

As part of assessing pain, non-verbal signs such as facial grimacing, restlessness, diaphoresis (excessive sweating) and limited activity, should also be noted as part of a pain assessment. Identify and record factors which alleviate or trigger the patient's pain. The severity of the pain determines the pharmacological approach. The World Health Organisation (WHO 1986) pain ladder has been seen to be a useful framework to base this approach on. Although first designed to manage cancer pain, its rationale and simplicity has made it a very valuable tool to manage patients in sickle pain.

Narcotic analgesic (morphine, diamorphine) infusion, either continuous or patient controlled (PCA), is preferable to IM or IV bolus dosing. PCAs not only maintain a constant blood level of analgesic (Van Beers *et al.* 2007) but allow the patient to have some sense of control and prevents the patient feeling they are a burden to nurses by frequently asking for analgesia. Intravenous infusion of morphine is typically adjusted to deliver between 2 to 12 mg per hour or 0.05–0.10 mg per kilogram/hour with the availability of 'rescue' doses as needed (Brookhoff and Polomano1992; Shapiro 1989). Evidence suggests patients will use far less of the opioid and hospital admissions have been shortened (Vichinsky *et al.* 1982). This dispels the myth that many sickle patients are 'drug addicts'. Brookoff (2009) and Solomon (2010) argue that many health professionals lack an understanding of the illness, lack pharmacological knowledge of pharmokinetics, and act as a major barrier to effective opioid management, underpinned by an unsubstantiated fear of addiction. This issue will be discussed further later in this section.

If the patient is not using PCA prescribing and administering of analgesia should be scheduled and not written as 'prn'. Routine doses of analgesics facilitate a steady state serum level of the drug, eliminating 'peaks and valleys' of analgesia and the breakthrough pain common with intermittent dosing. Opioids like morphine and diamorphine can cause constipation due to morphine receptors along the mysenteric plexus in the intestinal tract, reducing gut motility. Constipation can therefore exacerbate pain, especially if the patient is having an abdominal crisis and therefore use of laxatives such as stool softeners are often prescribed. Morphine and diamorphine can cause emesis and pruritus and therefore antiemetics such as prochlorperazine cyclizine are commonly prescribed. To manage pruritus, antihistamines such as hydroxyzine chlorpheniramine are added to the patient's drug regime. To lesson anxiety and stress, anxiolytic drugs like haloperidol may be very helpful.

In making patients aware of the rationale for the choice of morphine, the choice of diamorphine instead of pethidine is important. Many adult patients will have been used to and feel safer with pethidine, mainly because it relieves pain quicker in comparison to morphine. In addition morphine and diamorphine can also cause nausea and pruritus as mentioned earlier, necessitating additional medication to address these problems. For these reasons patients may not like using morphine or diamorphine. However, frequent administration of high doses of pethidine has been well associated with the risk of cerebrovascular seizures caused by norpethidine, the metabolite of pethidine. Hence pethidine is not viewed as the first drug of choice by clinicians. If a patient is allergic to morphine or diamorphine, oxycodone has proven to be an effective option and a useful alternative to pethidine. Along with analgesia, non-steroidal anti-inflammatory drugs may be prescribed to reduce the inflammatory damage caused by cytokines realised by damaged endothelial cells of the blood vessel.

Once the patient has been assessed and commenced on pain management, it is important to monitor the effectiveness of the analgesia frequently. It is advisable to re-assess the pain 30–40 minutes after administration to ascertain the patient's scoring of their pain. Monitoring of respiration to detect signs of respiratory depression is critical. It is recommended that vital sign monitoring oxygen saturation should be monitored every 30 minutes until pain is stable and then every two hours (BCSH 2003). Oxygen saturation should be >94% and respiration rate should be >12/minute. Humidified oxygen is preferable or continuous positive air pressure (CPAP). The mask used can be claustrophobic for the patient, making it very uncomfortable. The lips can become very dry, therefore petroleum Vaseline should be used for comfort. Naxolone should be available on the ward for quick response to treat respiratory depression. If the patient has been prescribed sedation, vital sign monitoring should be done regularly until they are able to respond satisfactorily to instructions.

Non-pharmacologic measures for pain control may include ensuring the room is warm and the patient has sufficient bedding to maintain warmth. Comfortable positioning and support of painful body areas can also be helpful. Various types of distraction therapy (television, reading) or relaxation techniques, therapeutic massage, hydrotherapy may also help, especially with mild to moderate pain (Rivers and Williamson 1990). It should not be assumed, however, that non-pharmacologic means of pain relief will replace the need for analgesics. Patients rating of their pain must be the guide to appropriate nursing interventions.

Fluid hydration

In an acute crisis patients tend to be dehydrated and may find it difficult to drink sufficient fluids and therefore intravenous hydration should commence. Three to four litres over 24 hours of normal saline should be administered. When possible, patients should be encouraged to have fluids, but vomiting, nausea, diarrhoea, tiredness and uncontrolled pain might make this initially difficult. Venous access can be extremely difficult, particularly for patients who are frequent admitters. No more than three attempts on one vein by a practitioner should be attempted. For patients with no venous access, it may be necessary to have skin tunnel catheters such as a Groshong, Hickman line, portacath or Broviac catheter.

It is essential that an accurate fluid balance chart is maintained to monitor input and output for early signs of renal failure or fluid overload. Renal complications are common in adults due to sickling damage of the distal renal tubules. Urinalysis is important to detect protein as proteinuria could be suggestive of glomerular sclerosis. Some patients may complain of polyuria or have nocturia, both symptoms potentially indicating renal dysfunction. The urine should be observed for haematuria and cloudiness, which may indicate renal damage or pyelonephritis.

Acute chest syndrome is a common cause of death. Fat emboli and infectious organisms have been associated with ACS (Claster and Vichinsky 2003). This is a medical emergency and the patient will either be managed with exchange blood transfusion and CPAP, or exchange transfusion and ventilation. It is important for nurses to undertake accurate recording of respiration, auscultation and patterns of breathing. Psychological support is essential as patients will be frightened, and constant reassurance is important. Ideally these patients should have a nurse allocated to them for close monitoring. The positioning of the patient on the ward is important and where possible the patient should be easily visible from the nurses' station.

Table 9.7 Health concerns.

Neurological	Headaches Ataxia Dizziness Visual disturbances Paraesthesia Facial numbness
Cardiopulmonary	Palpitations Angina chest pain Tachycardia Hypotension/hypertension Signs of shock (particularly hypovolaemic shock)
Respiratory	Dyspnoea on exertion or at rest Crackles, wheezes, Increased anteroposterior (AP) diameter of the chest (barrel chest)
Skin	Paleness Cyanosis – greyish/ashen appearance in black patients, observe the mucous membranes and nail beds for discolouration, and lips may have a bluish appearance
Hepatic	Right upper quadrant pain may indicate hepatomegaly Increased jaundice Gallbladder tenderness and pain
Gynaecological	The menstrual cycle is known to trigger VOC, but the cause is not well understood

The importance of accurate fluid recording and vital sign monitoring cannot be stressed enough, as illustrated in the outcomes of the NCEPOD report of unexpected deaths in the NCEPOD Enquiry (2008). Encourage the patient to eat a healthy diet, particularly high in protein to aid tissue repair; fibre to minimise the problem of constipation; and iron to reduce the effects of anaemia and support haemoglobin development.

Assessing for other symptoms

Once the pain has been controlled it is important to assess if there are other health problems that the patient may have. It should be remembered SCD patients can have co-morbidities which may also be causing clinical problems, independently of their sickling crisis. Other health concerns may include areas highlighted in Table 9.7.

Patient with SCD have a defective immune system and it is therefore important to monitor the patient for signs of sepsis and septicaemia. Antibiotics may be administered as some patients may have a low grade infection and be asymptomatic.

Blood transfusion

Advances in blood transfusion, have made the procedure much safer, but it is not without risks, hence blood transfusions are administered for specific complications in sickle cell disease, which are listed in Table 9.8. Blood groups are co-dominate, which means humans inherit more than one blood group and for haemoglobinopathy patients,

Table 9.8   Reasons for blood transfusion in SCD.

Cerebrovascular accident
Acute chest syndrome
Pre-post surgery
Frequent sickling crisis causing organ dysfunction
Aplastic crisis possible option during pregnancy

cross-matching donor blood for other minor blood groups the patient has is critical to prevent alloimmunisation. Blood groups such as C, E and Kell are commonly found in patients with sickle cell disease (Claster and Vinchinscky 2003).

Patients may either have a simple blood transfusion or exchange blood transfusion. Simple blood transfusion is the administration of blood units to the patient. An exchange blood transfusion is commonly undertaken via apheresis and involves the patient having a specific amount of blood removed and replaced with healthy blood from the donor.

For patients who have frequent sickling crisis, an alternative option to blood transfusion has been the use of hydroxycarbamide (hydroxyurea (HU)) (Charache 1997; Eckman 2010). Hydroxyurea increases foetal haemoglobin, enabling greater oxygen carrying capacity. The result of this is a reduction in frequency and severity of sickling crisis. It has also been suggested that HU aids red blood cell deformability, making it easier for red cells to pass through microvessels, reducing vaso-occlusion. Nurses should be aware of the importance of advising patients about the possible side effects, which include constipation; drowsiness; hair loss; inflammation of the mouth; loss of appetite; nausea; myelosuppression, particularly neutropenia (Liebelt *et al*. 2007).

Hydroxyurea has been used as a carcinogenic drug to treat chronic myeloid leukaemia; there have been some concerns about whether there is a risk of HU causing leukaemia in SCD patients (Platt 2008). Advice on contraception should be provided. It is suggested that a patient planning to start a family should discontinue hydroxycarbine at least 3–6 months prior to conception and the partner screened for their haemoglobin genotype. It is appropriate to offer advice on having the partner screened for their genotype.

Psychological issues

Sickle cell disease is a complex syndrome and for the patient can pose many psychological, sociological and emotional challenges. The unpredictable nature of the painful VOC disrupts family and social life as well as education and employment. When a patient is in a sickling crisis the fear of dying cannot be underestimated. Anger and frustration at the illness are not uncommon emotions and may be deflected onto nursing staff, particularly if the patient feels they are not being listened to. Creating a calming and reassuring environment along with highly skilled nursing care is paramount. Altered body image, possibly caused by leg ulcers, jaundice, impotency due to priapism and CVA, can impact on self-confidence, self-worth and self-esteem.

Many patients can be concerned about addiction because they have to use opioids to manage their acute pain and nurses may have concern about patients becoming addicts because of the regularity of opioid usage. However, most authorities stress that fear of addiction should not be a major concern with these patients (Brookoff 2009). Drug tolerance and/or physical dependence can occur with long-term narcotic use; however, addiction is rare in patients using narcotics for chronic intermittent pain. Addiction is a psychological dependence associated with behaviours marked by drug craving, efforts to secure drugs and interference with physical and/or psychosocial functioning. Tolerance refers to a decrease in the effectiveness of the drug over time, necessitating an increased dosage for pain relief. Physical dependence results in physical withdrawal symptoms when the drug is abruptly stopped.

Patients may have poor short-term memory, difficulties with concentration, recall and therefore nurses need to be aware of the need for repeating information. Depression is also not uncommon. These problems are associated both with the illness as well as with opioid management and clearly further compound the challenges faced by patients.

Cognitive behaviour therapy (CBT) is a very useful psychological management therapy to help patients manage and develop coping strategies for living with their illness (Anie 2005). Nurses should advise patients of voluntary organisations such as the Sickle Cell Society which can provide peer support and information about relevant services.

Discharge planning and long-term management of SCD

Education continues throughout a patient's life and is important to evaluate and review patients' understanding of their disease. Self-care management is critical to decrease hospital admissions, minimise organ dysfunction and improve the health status and quality of life. As part of discharge planning ensure that the patient has analgesia to take at home. Adults with sickle cell disease often experience daily, chronic pain as well as episodic, acute painful events. Anecdotally, concerns have been raised regarding the use of opioids as self-management at home and the possible link with increasing difficulty with controlling acute VOC crisis in hospital. This may possibly due to increased tolerance of the drug (Robinson 2011).

Provide the patient with their follow-up appoint and if they are managed by specialist counsellors in the community it is good practice to advise them of the discharge to enable a home visit. Remind patients of the importance of taking their medication, which is usually folic acid and some haematologists will prescribe long-term use of antibiotics for some adults.

Encourage patients to continue drinking regularly to avoid dehydration. Three litres a day should be the aim. If the patient plays any sport it is essential they remember to drink fluids, before, during and after their sporting activity. Advise the patient that if they drink alcohol they should limit consumption as this can cause dehydration. Suggest having isotonic drinks such as fruit juice with any alcohol to help limit the hydration. Advise on eating a well-balanced diet to help with tissue repair, high in fibre to prevent constipation and food rich in iron. If necessary refer the patient to a dietician to advise the patient. Keeping warm in the winter is especially important.

Finance can be an issue for some patients and referral to a benefits advisor maybe helpful. Minimising stress is a subject that should be discussed with the patient to identify any support that maybe required. A balance between rest and exercise is important in reducing fatigue but also helping to keep muscles active and reduce stiffness. Remind the patient that if they have any signs of infection to seek medical advice urgently. Occupational therapy referral may be required to assist the patient with home adaptations if they have had a stroke.

Nursing care for beta thalassaemia major

Beta thalassaemia major (BTM), like SCD, is a chronic illness, necessitating lifelong treatment and patients need to be supported in living with and managing the chronicity of this condition. A multidisciplinary approach is required, involving the haematologist, cardiologist, endocrinologist, gastroenterologist and specialist nurse, who are all key players in supporting the patient. Chronic blood transfusion and iron chelation therapy are the main features of managing beta thalassaemia major. The aims of blood transfusion are to improve the anaemia and suppress ineffective erythropoiesis (UK Thalasaemia Society 2008). The patient will require blood transfusion every three or four weeks throughout their life. Understandably, the realisation by patients that they have such a dependency on the hospital to treat them and the potential consequences of blood borne infections, can create anxiety and stress for patients. Once the patient commences their blood transfusion regime, the challenges related to transfusion of blood become of significant concern.

Blood transfusion preparation

Prior to commencement of transfusion assessing the patient for health changes since the previous transfusion period should be undertaken. If the patient is having desferal for chelation, nurses should ask the patient about any problems with hearing or vision. Discussing dental care is important, as dental and orthodontic occlusion can be a common problem with thalassaemia (Cutando *et al.* 2002). Although appropriately administered units of blood can prevent dental problems, it is important to encourage dental check-ups, at least once a year.

If a patient is complaining of increased fatigue, breathlessness and ankle oedema, these symptoms might indicate signs of heart failure, which would affect the frequency of the transfusion regime, making it more likely that the blood transfusion regime would increase. Complaints of bone pain may be due to hyperplasia, which could require an adjustment in the amount of units prescribed. Hyperplasia may suggest that the blood transfusion regime is insufficient in causing suppression of the bone marrow. Assessing the patient if they have any mobility problems or back pain is useful as a possible indicator of extramedullary haemopoiesis tumour masses in the paraspinal region, leading into spinal cord compression.

Nurses should ensure patients are up to date with their vaccinations of hepatitis B and influenza. Depending on hospital protocol, the patient may be screened annually for hepatitis A, B and C antibodies to identify any early treatment requirements. The risk of cirrhosis or renal carcinoma require regular patient monitoring. Nurses should be familiar with protocols for assessing the patient prior to administering blood and be aware of the timing for routine investigations for hepatic, cardiac, skeletal, endocrinology, virology and iron assessments. Nurses are guided to review the *Standards for Clinical Care of Children and Adults with Thalassaemia in the UK* (UK Thalassaemia Society 2008), which provides excellent guidance on investigations and should be read in conjunction with this section of the chapter on the care of patients living with thalassaemia.

Blood transfusion management in beta thalassaemia major

Patients' weight and height measurements are taken and pre-transfusion haemoglobin levels are ascertained to determine the right amount of units of blood the patient will require. Pre-transfusion haemoglobin is usually aimed to be maintained between 9.5–10 g/dL and the aim of post-transfusion haemoglobin level generally planned to be no more than 15 g/dL (Cazzola *et al.* 1995). Nurses should be aware of their trust policy of administration of blood and blood products. Generally the patients are managed in haematology day units, and may be well known to the nursing staff. However, it is important that the patient wears their identity wristband for safety checks when blood is being administered.

Checking the compatibility form information against the unit of blood should be done at the bedside with the patient being involved. Many hospitals will have a policy of two practitioners checking, one of whom should be a registered practitioner. However, following reports from the Severe Hazards of Transfusion committee which reports on near misses and actual adverse incidents with blood and blood transfusion administration, some hospitals are considering or have changed their policy to having one registered practitioner to conduct checking and administration. This has been because the SHOT reports have highlighted the greatest percentage of errors occurs at the point of the administration of the blood. Involving the patient in the process of identifying their name, date of birth and hospital number is good practice.

Pre-transfusion observations of TPR and BP should be recorded and again 15 minutes after the commencement of each unit. Hospitals will have different policy procedures regarding whether observations are then conducted hourly until completion of the unit of blood. Generally a blood unit should complete within four hours and nurses should record not only commencement but completion of each unit as this can be useful information as part of an audit trail if the patient has any adverse reactions. Each unit of blood transfused carries a small risk of an acute or late adverse effect and therefore nurses should observe the patient throughout the time the transfusion is being administered. For further information on blood transfusions see Chapter 17.

Venous access can be challenging with such regularity of blood transfusion, and skills in cannulation are essential. It is recommended that no more than three attempts should be made by any one practitioner on a patient (UK Thalassaemia Society 2008). For patients with heart failure or pulmonary hypertension, transfusion regimens will increase and diuretics should be administered with the transfusion. If the patient is on diuretics, serum electrolytes – sodium, potassium and magnesium, need to be monitored at regular intervals.

Iron chelation therapy

Since the human body has no normal excretory route for excess iron, ultimately all patients with beta thalassaemia major will commence iron chelation therapy. This is a crucial part of the patient's management since iron overload, as mentioned earlier in this chapter, can have damaging effects, on the liver, heart and endocrinology organs. Compliance with iron chelation is essential and nurses have a major role in supporting patients in understanding the importance of iron chelation and educating the patient on reporting any problems or side effects of the chelation therapy.

The main drugs used in iron chelation therapy are desferroxiamine (desferal), deferiprone, and deferasirox (Exjade) either singularly or in combination. Desferal can only be administered parenterally – subcutaneously or intravenously and works by converting iron into the compound ferroxamine which is excreted in urine. For adults, subcutaneous dosage of desferal varies between 20/40 mg/per kg. Patients usually administer desferal via a syringe pump driver over 8–12 hours a night, 5–6 nights per week. Nurses need to ensure patients are taught how to inject themselves properly, ensuring they inject through the dermis and rotate the injection sites, which are usually the abdomen and upper areas of the legs. Rotation of sites is important to avoid the development of fibrotic tissue and local reactions occurring. Injecting properly also prevents the development of painful blisters and inflammation. Side effects of desferal include, hearing loss, temporary blindness, cataracts, tinnitus, in rare cases analphylactic reaction may occur (Trachtenberg *et al*. 2011).

Not surprisingly, compliance with desferal can be problematic and nurses should work with the patient in establishing how best to rotate the administration of desferal around the patient's lifestyle. Deferiprone (Ferriprox) was the first oral iron chelator to be developed. It can be given as syrup as well as in tablet form. It is prescribed three times a day and the number of tablets the patients is prescribed is based on body weight and iron levels. There are a number of side effects with deferiprone, which include: nausea and vomiting, abdominal pain, diarrhoea, joint pain, hepatoxicity, agranulocytosis and zinc deficiency (Neufeld 2006).

Deferasirox (Exjade) is the most recent oral iron chelator, which works by combining with iron which is then excreted in faeces. Deferasirox is in tablet form and the patient takes one tablet a day. The dosage may initially commence at 10 mg/kg/day and can increase to 3 mg/kg/day to achieve serum iron levels of 500–1000 µg/L. The tablet needs to be dissolved in water or fruit juice and should be taken on an empty stomach at least 30 minutes before eating. Side effects of deferasirox are renal and hepatic impairment and gastrointestinal haemorrhage. Serum creatinine/creatinine clearance, serum transaminase and bilirubin levels are closely monitored for early signs of organ failure.

Diet advice for patients

Nutritional deficiencies are common in thalassaemia, secondary to the use of desferrioxamine, the haemolytic anaemia and iron overload that accompanies this disease. Nurses can advise on eating smaller, less spicy meals and eating or drinking ginger to help with the nausea. If nausea and vomiting is severe antiemetics maybe prescribed. For diarrhoea, patients should be encouraged to drink plenty of fluids to avoid dehydration. Drinking tea may help to reduce iron absorption through the intestinal tract and vitamin C 100–250 mg orally is often prescribed as it is improves the efficacy of desferal with iron excretion. Vitamin D and calcium 1200 mg can help with bone structure and can be offered to patients. Nurses should advise patients of foods which are rich in calcium, vitamins D and E and folic acid. Table 9.9 provides some advice on food types rich with these nutrients.

Table 9.9   Food types.

Food high in calcium	Yogurt, fruit Milk, low fat, non-fat or whole milk shakes Cheese, including American, ricotta, cheddar cheese and mozzarella cheese Okra Baked beans Peas, broccoli, sprouts, spinach
Food rich in vitamin E	Soya Corn Olive oil Nuts and seeds
Food rich in vitamin D	Oily fish, such as salmon and sardines Powdered milk Fortified fat spreads Fortified breakfast cereals Eggs
Food rich in folic acid	Spinach Asparagus Turnips Greens Legumes such as dried or fresh beans, peas, lentils Egg yolks Pasta Cereal Sunflower seeds Liver Kidney

Psychological support

Beta thalassaemia major can have a wide reaching impact on the individual and their family. Management of the illness can disrupt studying and employment. Altered body image of the skin due to jaundice, excess iron deposits in the skin which can give a greyish appearance, lack of sexual development and short stature are some issues which can affect the development of relationships. Many psychological issues have a major bearing on the patient's quality of life and with compliance of treatment. As with SCD, cultural and ethnic differences between the patient and practitioner means nurses and doctors must be aware of the cultural, social, developmental and behavioural issues that affect this patient population.

Fertility challenges may also make people feel a lack of self-confidence, lack of self-worth and have a low self-esteem. Nurses need to spend time listening to patients, gaining an understanding of the patients' issues and identifying what support interventions maybe helpful. They can also inform patients of self-help groups such as the UK Thalassaemia Society for patient information and peer support. The UK Thalassaemia Society has produced a 'patient held records' booklet, which enables the patient to be more involved with their care, be aware of what investigations are required and records their results. This can aid in empowering the patient and also provides a basis for a dialogue with the nurse and clinician. If patients are concerned about fertility and want to plan to have children, genetic counselling is important and referral to the obstetrician for assessment with the possibility of commencing IVF treatment is usually the process.

Messina *et al.* (2008), in their study, highlighted significant psychological problems which impacted on treatment compliance, challenges with self-image and that many patients used escape-avoidance as a coping strategy. Such findings illustrate the importance of having a clinical psychologist providing culturally sensitive psychological services as a major part of comprehensive care.

Conclusion

Sickle cell disease and thalassaemia are complex conditions, but there is increasing knowledge about them which has led to changes in treatment and increased longevity. The ultimate advance would be to have the availability of safe gene therapy intervention, but that remains elusive at the moment. Haemopoietic stem cell transplantation is the current curative option for some people with BTM and for some children with SCD. In the UK, stem cell transplantation is only offered for SCD up to the age of 16 years. Nurses need to have a good understanding of the pathologies and recognise the challenges patients living with a chronic illness face in order to provide effective care.

References

Abbot, K.C., Hypolite, I.O. and Agodoa, L.Y. (2002) Sickle cell nephropathy at end-stage renal disease in the United States; patient characteristics and survival. *Clinical Nephrology*, 58, 9–15.

Adams, R.J., Ohene-Frempong, K. and Wang, W. (2001) Sickle cell and the brain. *Hematology*, 1 January (1), 31–46.

Aessopas, A. (2006) The heart in sickle cell disease. In: *New Developments in Sickle cell Disease*. (ed. P.D. O'Malley). Chapter 8, pp. 211–250. Nova Science Publishers, New York.

Allen, S. (2005) Understanding sickle cell anaemia. *The Pharmaceutical Journal*. July. 275, 25–28.

Anie, K.A. (2005) Psychological complications in sickle cell disease. *British Journal of Haematology*, 129 (6), 723–729.

Bain, B. (2005) *Haemoglobinopathy Diagnosis*, 2nd edition. Blackwell Publishing Ltd, Oxford.

Ballas, S.K. (1995) The acute sickle cell painful crisis in adults: Phases and objective signs. *Hemoglobin*, 19, 323.

Borgna-Pignatti, C., Cappellini, M.D., De Stefano, P.D. and El Vecchio, G.C. (2006) Cardiac morbidity. *Blood*, 107 (9), 3733–3737.

British Committee for Standards in Haematology (2003) Guidelines for the management of acute painful crisis in sickle cell disease. *British Journal of Haematology*, 120 (5), 744–752.

Brookoff, D. (2009) Pain in sickle cell disease. In: *Current Therapies in Pain* (ed. H.S. Smith). Chapter 46. Saunders.Elsevier, Philadelphia.

Brookoff, D.S. and Polomano, R. (1992) Treating sickle cell pain like cancer pain. *Annals of Internal Medicine*, 116 (5), 364–368.

Buchanan, G.R., Debaun, M.R., Quinn, C.T. and Steunberg, M.H. (2004) Sickle cell disease. *Am. Soc Hematology Education Progra*, 35–47.

Cappellini, M.D., Grespi, E., Cassinerio, E., Bignamini D. and Fiorelli, G. (2005) Coagulation and splenectomy: an overview. *Ann N Y Acad Sci*, 1054, 317–324.

Casas-Castaneda, M., Hernandez-Lugo, I., Torres O. *et al.* (1998) Alpha-thalassaemia in a selected population of Mexico. *Rev Invest Clin, Sep-Oct*, 50 (5), 395–398.

Castro, O., Hoque, M. and Brown, B.D. (2003) Pulmonary hypertension in sickle cell disease: cardiac catheterization results and survival. *Blood*, 101, 1257–1261.

Cazzola, M., DeStafano P., Ponschio, L. *et al.* (1995) Relationship between transfusion regimen and suppression of erythropoiesis in beta thalassaemia major. *British Journal Haematology*, 118, 1, 330–336.

Charache, S. (1997) Mechanism of action of hydroxyurea in the management of sickle cell anaemia in adults. *Semin Hematol*, July, 34 (3 Suppl 3), 15–21. Review.

Chui, D.H.K., Fucharoen, S. and Chan, V. (2003) Hemoglobin H disease: not necessarily a benign disorder. *Blood*, 1 February, 101 (3), 791–800.

Clare, A., Fitzhenley Harris, J.M., Hambleton, I. and Sargeant, G.R. (2002) Chronic leg ulceration in homozygous sickle cell disease; the role of venous incompetence. *Br. J. Haematology*, 119, 576–571.

Claster, S. and Vichinsky, E.P. (2003) Managing sickle cell disease. *BMJ*, 327, 1151–1155.

Cunningham, M.J., Macklim, E.A., Neufield, E.J. *et al.* (2004) Complications of beta-thalassaemia major in North America. *Blood*, 104 (1), 34–39.

Cutando Soriano, A., Gil Montoya, J.A. and López-González Garrido, D. (2002) Thalassemias and their dental implications. *Med Oral*, Jan-Feb, 7 (1), 36–40, 41–45.

Danquah, I. and Mockenhaupt, F.P. (2008) Alpha(+)-thalassaemia and malarial anaemia. *Trends Parasitol*, 24 (11), 479–481.

Derebail, V.K., Nachman, P.H., Key, N.S., Ansede, H., Falk, R.J. and Kshiragar, A.V. (2010) High prevalence of sickle cell trait in African Americans with ESRD. *J Am Soc Nephrol*, 21 (3), 413–417.

De Sanctis, V., Vullo, C., Katz, M., Wonke, B., Tanas, R. and Bangi, B. (1988) Gonadal function in patients with beta thalassaemia major. *J Clin Pathol*, 41, 133–137.

Eckman, J.R. (2010) Hydroxyurea enhances sickle survival. *Blood.* 115 (12), 2331–2332.

Fleming, R.E. and Bacon, B.R. (2005) Orchestration of iron homeostasis. *New England Journal of Medicine*, 352 (17), 1741–1744.

Firth, P.D. (2005) Anaesthesia for peculiar cells – a century of sickle cell disease. *British Journal of Anaesthesia*, April, 1–13.

Gantz, T. (2003) Hepcidin, a key regulator of iron metabolism and mediator of anaemia of inflammation. *Blood*, 102, 783–788.

Gill, K.M., Carson, J.W., Porter, L.S., Scipio, C., Bediako, S.M. and Orringer, E. (2004) Daily mood and stress predict pain, health care use and work activity in African-American adults with sickle cell disease. *Health Psychology*, 23, 267–274.

Hahalis, G., Alexopoulos, D., Kremastinos, D.T. and Zoumbos, N.C. (2005) Heart failure in beta thalassaemia syndromes: a decade of progress. *Am J Med*, 118, 957–967.

Hayes, J.R. and Pack-Mabien, A. (2007) Sickle cell disease in adults. In: *Renaissance of Sickle Cell Disease Research in the Genome Era* Pace (ed. B.S. Pace). Imperial College Press, London.

Herrick, J.B. (1910) Peculiar elongated and sickle cell shaped red blood corpuscles in a case of severe anaemia. *Arch Intern Med*, 6, 517–521.

Higgs, D.R., Thein, S.L. and Woods, W.G. (2001) In: *The Thalassaemia Syndromes* (eds D.J. Weatherall and B. Clegg), 4th edition. pp. 133–191. Blackwell Publishing Ltd, Oxford.

Hoffbrand, A.V. and Moss P.A.H. (2011) *Essential Haematology*, 6th edition. Wiley-Blackwell, Oxford.

Hughes- Jones, N.C., Wickramasinghe, S.N. and Hatton, C.S.R. (2009) *Lecture Notes in Haematology*, 8th edition. Wiley-Blackwell, Oxford.

Kato, G.J., McGowan, V., Machado, R.F. *et al.* (2006) Lactate dehydrogenase as a biomarker of hemolysis-associated nitric oxide resistance, priapism, leg ulceration, pulmonary hypertension, and death in patients with sickle cell disease. *Blood*, 107 (6), 2279–2285.

Liebelt, E., Balk, S., Faber, W. *et al.* (2007) NTP-CERHR expert panel report on the reproductive and developmental toxicity of hydroxyurea. *Birth Defects Research. Part B, Developmental and Reproductive Toxicology*, 80 (4), 259–366.

Liu J., Tang, N., Liu, Q. *et al.* (2009) Improvement in the detection of alpha0- and Deletional alpha-thalassemia by real-time PCR combined with dissociation curve analysis. *Acta Haemato*, 15 Aug, 122 (1), 17–22.

Malik, S., Syed, S. and Ahmed, N. (2009) Complications in transfusion-dependent patients of ß-thalassaemia major: a review. *Pak J Med Sci*, 25 (4), 678–682.

Messina, G., Colombo, E., Cassinerio, E. *et al.* (2008) Psychosocial aspects and psychiatric disorders in young adult with thalassaemia major. *Internal and Emergency Medicine*, 3 (4), 339–343.

Model, B., Khan, M. and Darlington, M. (2000) Survival in beta-thalassaemia major in the UK; data from the UK Thalassaemia Register. *Lancet*, 355, 2051–2052.

National Confidential Enquiry into Patient Outcome and Death (NCEPOD) (2008) *A Sickle Cell Crisis?* NCEPOD, London.

National Heart, Lung, and Blood Institute (NHLBI) NIH. Sickle cell anemia. Available at: www.nhlbi.nih.gov/health/dci/Diseases/Sca/SCA_All.html. Accessed 18 May 2011.

National Human Genome Research Institute (NHGRI) NIH (2011) Learning about sickle cell disease. Available at: www.genome.gov/10001219. Accessed 20 May 2011.

NHS Antenatal and Neonatal Screening Programmes (2006) *Sickle Cell and Thalassaemia: Handbook for Laboratories*. NHS Antenatal and Newborn Screening Programmess, London.

Neufeld, E.J. (2006) Oral chelators deferasirox and deferiprone for transfusional iron overload in thalassaemia major: new data, new questions. *Blood*, 107, 3436–3441.

Nolan, V.G., Wyszynski, D.F., Farrer, L.A. and Steinberg, M.H. (2005) Hemolysis associated priapism in sickle cell disease. *Blood*, 106, 3264–3267.

Pallister, C.J. (2005) *Haematology*, 2nd edition. Hodder Arnold, London.

Papanikolaou, G., Tzilianos, M., Christakis, J.L. *et al.* (2005) Hepcidin in iron overload disorders. *Blood*, 105, 4103–4105.

Patel, J., Patel, A., Patel, J., Kaur, K. and Patel V. (2009) Prevalence of haemoglobinopathies in Gujarat, India: a cross-sectional study. *The Internet Journal of Hematology*, 5 (1).

Phillipots, B.A. and Duong, H.Q. (2008) Retinopathy, Hemoglobinopathies. http://emedicine. medscape.com/article/1225300-overview. Accessed 14 December 2010.

Platt, O.S. (2008) Hydroxyurea for the treatment of sickle cell anemia. *N. Engl. J. Med.* 358 (13), 1362–1369.

Quinn, C.T., Rogers, Z.R. and Buchanan, G.R. (2004) Survival of children with sickle cell disease. *Blood*, 1 June, 103 (11), 4023–4027.

Ress, D.C., Lujohungbe, A.D., Parker, N.E., Stephens, A.D., Telfer, P. and Wright, J. (2003) Guidelines for the management of acute painful crisis in sickle cell disease. *Br. J Haematology*, 120, 744–752.

Rivers, R.V. and Williamson, N. (1990) Sickle cell anaemia: complex disease, nursing challenge. *RN*, 24–28.

Robinson, S. (2011) *Pain Management at Home*. Telconference, London.

Rund, D. and Rachmilewitz, E. (2005) β-Thalassaemia. *New England Journal Medicine*, 353, 1135–1146.

Schrier, S.L. (2002) Pathophysiology of thalassaemia. *Current Opinion in Hematology. March*, 9, 123–126.

Shapiro, B. (1989)The management of pain in sickle cell disease. *Pediatric Clinics of North America*, 36 (4), 1029–1041.

Sickle Cell Society (2008) *Standards for Managing the Adult with Sickle Cell Disease*. Sickle Cell Society, London.

Solomon, L.R. (2010) Pain management in adults with sickle cell disease in a medical center emergency department. *Journal of the National Medical Association*, 102 (11), 1025–1032.

Standing Medical Advisory Committee (1994) *Report of a Working Party of the Standing Medical Advisory Committee on Sickle Cell, Thalassaemia and Other Haemoglobinopathies*. HMSO, London.

Steensman, D.P., Hoyer, J.D. and Fairbanks, V.F (2001) Hereditary red blood cell disorders in Middle East patients. *Mayo Clinic Proceedings*, 76, 285–293.

St Pierre, T.G., Clarke, P.R., Chua-Anusoem, W. *et al*. (2005) Non-invasive measurement and imaging of liver iron concentration using proton magnetic resonance. *Blood*, 105 (2), 855–681.

Streetly, A., Clarke, M., Downing, M. *et al*. (2008) Implementation of the newborn screening programme for sickle cell disease in England: results for 2003–2005. *Journal of Medical Screening*, 15, 9–13.

Streetly, A., Maxwell, K. and Mejia, A. (1997) *Sickle Cell Disorder in Greater London: a Needs Assessment of Screening and Care Services*. Fair shares for London, United Medical and Dental Schools, Department of Public Health Medicine, London.

Stuart, M.J. and Nagel, R.L. (2004) Sickle cell disease. *Lancet*, 364 (9442), 1343–1360.

Telen, M. (2007) Role of adhesion molecules and vascular endothelium in the pathogenesis of sickle cell disease. *Hematology*, 1, 84–90.

Telfer, P.T., Prescott, E., Holder, S., Walker, M.M., Hoffbrand, A.V. and Wonke, E. (2000) Hepatic iron concentration combined with long-term monitoring of serum ferritin to predict complications of iron overload in thalassaemia major. *British Journal of Haematology*, 110 (4), 971–977.

Thein, S.L. (2005) Pathophysiology of β thalassaemia – a guide to molecular therapies. *Am Soci Hematology*, 32–37.

Toumba, M., Sergis, A., Kanaris, C. and Skordis, N. (2007) Endocrine complications in patients with thalassaemia major. *Pediatric Endocrinol Rev*, 5 (2), 642–648.

Trachtenberg, F., Vichinsky, E., Haines, M.D. *et al*. (2011) Iron chelation adherence to deferoxamine and deferasirox in thalassaemia. *American Journal of Hematology*, 85, (5), 433–436.

Tsaras, G., Owusu-Ansah, A., Owusu-Boateng, F. and Amoateng-Adiepong, Y. (2010) Complications associated with sickle cell trait: a brief narrative review. National Human Genome Research Institute, NIH. Learning about sickle cell disease. Available at: http://www.genome.gov/10001219. Accessed 20 March 2010.

Turgeon, M. (2005) *Clinical Hematology: Theory and Procedures*. Lippincott Williams & Wilkins, Philadelphia.

UK Thalasaemia Society (2008) *Standards for the Clinical Care of Children and Adults with Thalassaemia in the UK*. UK Thalasaemia Society, London.

Van Beers, E.J., van Tulin, C.F., Nieuwkerk, P.T., Friederich, P.W., Vranken, J.H. and Biemond, B.J. (2007) Patient- controlled analgesia versus continuous infusion of morphine during vaso-occulsive crisis in sickle cell disease, a randomized controlled trial. *American Journal Hematology*, 82 (11), 955–960.

Van Beers, E.J., Van Tuiju, C.F.J., MacGillavry, M.R., Van der Giessen, A., Schnog, J.J.B. and Biemond, B.J. (2008) Sickle cell disease-related organ damage occurs irrespective of pain rate; implications for clinical practice. *Haematologica*, 93 (5), 757–760.

Vichinsky, E., Johnson, R. and Lubin, B. (1982). Multidisciplinary approach to pain management in sickle cell disease. *American Journal of Pediatric Hematology & Oncology*, 4 (3), 328–333.

Voskaridou, E., Kyrtsonis, M.C., Terpos, E. *et al.* (2001) Bone resorption is increased in young adults with thalassaemia major. *Br J Haematol*, 112 (1), 36–41.

Weatherall, D.J. (1997) Fortnightly review: the thalassaemias. *BMJ*, 314, 1675–1677.

Weatherall, D.J. and Clegg, J.B. (2001) *The Thalassaemia Syndromes*. 4th edition. Blackwell Publishing Ltd, Oxford.

Wethers, D. (2000) Sickle cell disease in childhood; part 1.Laboratory diagnosis, pathophysiology and health maintenance. http://www.aafp.org/afp/200000901/1013.html. Accessed 14 December 2008.

Williams, W.J (1996) *Williams Hematology*, 5th edition. McGraw-Hill, New York.

World Health Organisation (WHO) (1986) *Cancer Pain Relief*. World Health Organisation, 51, Geneva.

World Health Organisation (2006) *Sickle cell anaemia. 59th World Health Assembly A59/9. Provisional agenda item 11.4*. 24 April 2006, Geneva.

Chapter 10

Haemochromatosis: pathophysiology, care and management

Jan Green

By the end of this chapter readers should have a working knowledge of:

- Genetic haemochromatosis (GH) and its prevalence in society
- The effect on the family and an understanding of how it is inherited
- Diagnostic testing and screening
- Organs affected by GH
- The signs and symptoms of GH
- Disease monitoring
- Treatment and nursing care of the patient
- Blood donation for people with haemochromatosis

Introduction

Haemochromatosis, also known as iron overload disease or iron storage disease (BCSH 2000) is a genetic disorder, which interferes with the body's ability to maintain an effective biofeedback system to sustain iron regulation and balance. This means the body is unable to excrete surplus iron, beyond daily requirements, absorbing all iron ingested. As a result of this, excess iron accumulates in the heart, liver, pancreas, endocrine glands and joints, causing multiple pathologies. Treatment is simple and effective, but if the condition is not identified and treated early enough the outcome can be severe and sometimes fatal (Warrell *et al.* 2005).

Haemochromatosis (or GH – genetic haemochromatosis) is one of the most common genetic disorders. Recent surveys of people of northern European origin have shown a prevalence of 1 in 400 likely to be at risk of developing iron overload (BCSH 2000). In the UK the Haemochromatosis Society (2008) estimates that there are approximately 5000–6000 diagnosed patients with the disorder but there is evidence that several times that number have tissue damage and disease caused by iron overload. In the UK, about 250,000 people have a genetic predisposition to haemochromatosis (GH). It occurs twice as commonly as sickle cell anaemia and ten times more frequently than cystic fibrosis, yet was once thought to be rare. It is now realised that it was the diagnosis that is rare, not the disease, because until recently most diagnoses were either missed, or made at an advanced

Haematology Nursing, First Edition. Marvelle Brown and Tracey J. Cutler.
© 2012 Blackwell Publishing Ltd. Published 2012 by Blackwell Publishing Ltd.

stage, as the symptoms may mimic many other diseases. Routine screenings performed by doctors do not include tests for GH.

Genetic information

In 1996 the major gene involved with iron regulation in haemochromatosis, the HFE gene, was identified (Haemochromatosis Society 2008; Phatak, Bonkovsky and Kowdley 2008). It is an autosomal recessive condition. Over 90% of those diagnosed with GH are homozygous for the HFE C282Y gene mutation and another 4% are affected by compound heterozygotes for the C282Y/H63D mutation (BCSH 2000). In the general population 1 in 200 people have this genotype. Of these, most accumulate iron but only a minority will go on to develop clinical symptoms, which rarely appear before adulthood. To develop GH you have to inherit a defective gene from both parents. This can happen in three ways, see Table 10.1 and Figure 10.1.

Table 10.1 Illustration of inheritance with a defective gene from both parents (with permission from the Haemochromatosis Society).

1. If both parents are carriers (most common – about 10% of the population are carriers, so 1% of partnerships will be between carriers). On average a quarter of the children will develop GH, half will be carriers, and a quarter will be normal. See Figure 10.1.
2. If one parent has GH and the other is a carrier (about 1 in 2000 partnerships). On average half the children will develop GH, the other half will be carriers.
3. If both parents suffer from GH (a rare event, occurring in about 1 in 100,000 partnerships) all the children will inherit two defective genes, and will have GH.

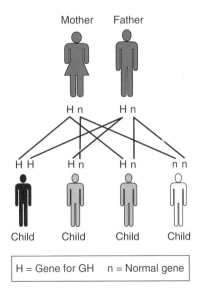

Figure 10.1 How recessive inheritance works when both parents are carriers. (with permission from the Haemochromatosis Society).

Who does it affect?

Genetic haemochromatosis affects those of European ancestry, particularly those of Nordic and Celtic ancestry (BCSH 2000; Warrell *et al.* 2005); it affects men and women equally, but women often develop symptoms later as they are protected by menstruation and pregnancy. Being a regular blood donor is thought to have the same protective qualities, delaying the build up and accumulation of iron in the organs.

Clinical symptoms

Iron overload disease can give rise to a wide range of non-specific symptoms and clinical findings, leading to potential misdiagnosis. This is linked to where iron accumulates and how much has accumulated.

Symptoms include (BCSH 2000, p. 11):

- Unexplained weakness, fatigue or lethargy
- Abdominal pain; sometimes in the stomach region or the upper right hand side, sometimes diffuse
- Bronze skin pigmentation or a permanent tan
- Liver disorders, abnormal liver function tests, enlarged liver or cirrhosis
- Arthralgia or arthritis may affect any joint, but is particularly common in the knuckle and first joint of the first two fingers
- Diminished sex drive or impotence
- Diabetes (late onset type)
- Abnormal heart rhythms
- Sexual disorders; loss of sex drive, impotence in men, absent or scanty menstrual periods and early menopause in women, and/or decrease in body hair
- Cardiomyopathy, disease of the heart muscle (not to be confused with disease of the arteries of the heart)
- Neurological/psychiatric disorders, impaired memory, mood swings, irritability, and / or depression

Most of these symptoms are often found in other disorders, explaining the difficulties with early diagnosis. Chronic fatigue may be ascribed to after-effects of a viral infection or to psychological causes, and abdominal pain to irritable bowel syndrome. Similarly, liver disorders may be put down to excessive alcohol intake, even in someone who is only a moderate drinker. However, patients presenting with any of these symptoms and clinical findings, particularly a combination of two or more, should be considered for investigation for possible iron overload (particularly for individuals aged under 50). Arthritis, particularly if it occurs initially in the first and second knuckles, is highly suggestive of GH (Haemochromatosis Society 2009).

Organs affected and disease monitoring

As previously discussed, iron overload can cause many things, but equally, many of the organs concerned may have become diseased without the patient ever developing haemochromatosis.

Thus, awareness of haemochromatosis, genetic heritage, symptomology and the fact that it affects so many different organs, producing the symptoms listed, is essential.

The liver and biliary system

The liver is a complex organ performing a number of functions, for example it:

- Processes:
  - carbohydrates
  - proteins
  - fats
- Produces:
  - most of the cholesterol in the body
  - bile acids
  - urea
  - proteins and amino acids
- Stores:
  - glucose
  - vitamins

To determine if the liver is working effectively some tests can be performed.
These are:

- Blood tests
- Liver biopsy
- Imaging, usually MRI scanning

See under 'Diagnostic testing' for further information.

While these do not measure system function they can indicate the presence of abnormality such as damage or inflammation and consequently are useful indicators of malfunction, especially in the context of the patient's full medical history, along with physical examination.

Liver cirrhosis means liver scarring. Scarring can occur as a result of many different liver diseases, including iron overload and can lead to primary liver cancer (hepatoma) (Cancer Backup 2009). The build-up of iron deposits in the liver acts as a poison to the liver, and interferes with its function. Hepatoma is quite rare among GH sufferers, especially those diagnosed early, but occasionally can be found in those patients who present very late.

Joint disease

The cause of joint disease in the haemochromatosis patient is not well understood and as arthritis is common in the general population is can be difficult to ascertain whether the iron overload caused the joint problem or the patient would have developed it anyway. Sometimes the fact that the patient has joint disease can lead to a diagnosis of haemochromatosis. It is thought that iron deposition can cause progressive damage to the cells in the cartilage and joint lining (Justin *et al.* 2006; Warrell *et al.* 2005).

Types of arthritis include:

- *Rheumatoid arthritis*: a systemic illness affecting any joint in the body.
- *Osteoarthritis*: the most common type of joint disease, affecting the large weight-bearing joints, and is mainly local destruction caused by joint wear and tear.

- *Chrondrocalcinosis*: a build-up of calcium pyrophosphate crystals in the cartilage of a joint and accompanies osteoarthritis.
- *Osteonecrosis*: when joint tissue rapidly becomes necrosed causing much pain and deformity. The reason for this is not understood.
- *Osteoporosis*: means porous bones as bone density and mass is lost, making them especially vulnerable to fracture. This is very common in women and especially prevalent among haemochromatosis patients who are diagnosed in the later stages of the disease. However if a patient is susceptible to osteoporosis they seem to suffer even with moderate iron overload.

Endocrine system

The endocrine system consists of glands which secrete hormones directly into the circulatory blood system. When iron is deposited into these structures it interferes with their ability to secrete their speciality hormone, thus affecting various bodily functions (Warrell *et al*. 2005):

- *Pancreas*: iron deposits in the beta cells of the islets of Langerhans. These cells become damaged, resulting in lack of insulin production. This results in the patient developing diabetes mellitus. Diabetes can be diagnosed at a very early stage and independently of the haemochromatosis that may have caused it. Therefore it has been suggested that all newly diagnosed diabetics should be screened for GH. Treatment of diabetes is dependent on the severity of liver cirrhosis and the degree of iron accumulation.
- *Pituitary gland*: iron deposition leads to changes in cellular activity responsible for the gonads. The function of the ovaries and testes is impaired, which can lead to the loss of libido; men may become impotent and women may become amenorrhoeic. This is the result of a reduction of testosterone production in men and oestrogen production in women. Sexual dysfunction is the most common endocrine disorder for men with haemochromatosis and occurs in 10–40% of patients.
- *Thyroid gland*: haemochromatosis can affect the production of the hormone thyroxine. Treatment will be dependent on over (hyper) or under (hypo) production of the hormone. Males appear to be more susceptible than females.

Cardiovascular system

Cardiac problems usually occur when the iron levels have been grossly elevated over a prolonged period of time. Iron deposits in the cardiac muscle (myocardium), particularly in the inter-ventricular septal thickness, and problems include:

- Cardiomyopathy
- Cardiomegaly
- Cardiac arrythmias
- Ventricular dysfunction

Some improvement in cardiac function occurs as iron stores are depleted. Functionality is monitored by regular echocardiograms and electrocardiograms (ECGs).

Skin problems

Iron can deposit within the epidermis and around the sweat glands. This can cause pigmentation of the skin, giving the patient a bronzed and healthy looking appearance. However, as iron accumulates over time the colour becomes darker and heavy looking, before turning a slate grey colour. Old scars become highly pigmented and prominent, and the conjunctiva becomes stained. Additionally the facial, pubic and axillary hair becomes thin and there is often skin dryness associated with some itching, which varies in intensity from person to person. Patients can feel disfigured and may need psychological support. There is again some improvement as iron stores are depleted (Warrell *et al.* 2005).

Diagnostic testing

British Committee for Standards in Haematology guidance (2000) recommends that patients of European ancestry presenting with unexplained weakness or fatigue, abnormal liver function tests, arthralgia/arthritis, impotence, diabetes of late onset, cirrhosis, or bronze pigmentation should be investigated for haemochromatosis.

Blood tests

* Transferrin saturation
  Transferrin saturation (TS) is the ratio of two simple blood tests, which indicates iron accumulation. Serum iron is divided by total iron binding capacity (TIBC) to give the TS percentage. The test should be performed after an overnight fast. Normal average is 30% (slightly higher in men than women). Opinions differ on the levels of measure which determine the likelihood of GH, some mentioning over 40% saturation and others over 50–55% (BCSH 2000). However, the patient should be frequently monitored and a fasting TS should be performed.
* Serum ferritin
  This indicates the amount of iron stored in the body. Levels significantly over 300 µg/L (micrograms per litre) in men and 200 µg/L in women are further evidence of GH. It should be realised that in the early stages of iron accumulation, serum ferritin may be within the normal range. Raised TS with a normal serum ferritin level does not rule out a diagnosis of GH.
* Gene test
  A simple blood test for the HFE gene mutation is positive in over 90% of those affected. It will identify family members at risk.

Liver biopsy

A small sample of the liver is removed using a biopsy needle, which determines the degree of hepatic fibrosis and whether cirrhosis has developed. British Committee for Standards in Haematology guidelines (2000) recommend liver biopsy should be performed in any patient if:

* There is evidence of a raised transferrin saturation

- The serum ferritin reading is over 1000 µg/L
- There is evidence of abnormal liver function or damage, such as hepatomegaly

Because the risk of cirrhosis is low, no biopsy is necessary in patients where:

- There is a raised transferrin saturation
- But the serum ferritin reading is under 1000 µg/L
- No hepatomegaly present

If patients are diagnosed in the pre-cirrhotic, pre-diabetic stage and treated by venesection to remove the excess iron then life expectancy is normal (BCSH 2000). However, once cirrhosis and diabetes mellitus have developed, patients have a shortened life expectancy and, if cirrhosis is present, there is a very high risk of liver cancer developing even when iron depletion has been achieved. Therefore the necessity to make an early diagnosis cannot be emphasized enough.

Treatment for haemochromatosis

The mainstay of treatment for patients with haemochromatosis is therapeutic venesection. There are two phases to treatment, the reduction phase and the maintenance phase.

Therapeutic venesection is the act of removing blood from the circulatory system via a needle (venepuncture) as part of the treatment for certain blood disorders (Warrell *et al.* 2005) The volume obtained is approx 450–500 ml. By bleeding the patient, circulating iron is removed from the system, removing 225 mg of iron in the form of haemoglobin. Synthesis of new haemoglobin gradually depletes stored iron,, which is released into the circulation, thus reducing serum ferritin levels (BCSH 2000).

It is essential that regular monitoring of haemoglobin and ferritin is maintained, especially during the reduction phase. This is to prevent excessive anaemia, as the patient is initially bled once or twice a week, and to observe the rate of improvement in ferritin levels. It can take up to two years to achieve normal ferritin levels. The patient is then on maintenance phase with venesection performed 3–4 times per year to prevent recurrent ferritin build-up.

Figure 10.2 demonstrates how venesection, during the reduction phase, may affect iron levels during treatment. The serum ferritin decreases steadily, but the transferrin saturation levels remain high until iron deficiency occurs, then it falls sharply. This treatment is very straightforward. In most hospitals nurses or health care assistants who have attended the in-house IV study days and updates, and have completed the training and assessments for adult venepuncture may perform this procedure.

Commencing venesection as early as possible to prevent iron overload and the consequent damage to the liver is essential. Venesection therapy cannot reverse liver damage. It is necessary to monitor the liver by performing an annual liver ultrasound examination to exclude disease and ensure there is no iron build-up. Patients should be encouraged in moderate alcohol consumption as excessive drinking can make an already vulnerable liver very susceptible to disease. Monitoring should also include twice yearly liver function blood tests. Venesection may not restore normal organ

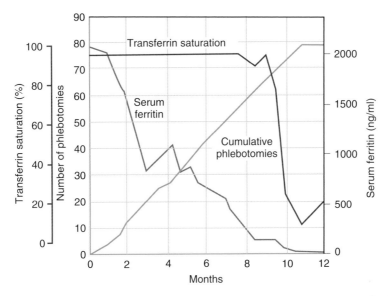

Figure 10.2 Effects of venesection. (with permission from the Haemochromatosis Society).

functions which have been compromised due to iron accumulation. If the patient has thyroid dysfunction, venesection rarely restores its functions, and once the patient has commenced on insulin therapy, the beta cells in the islets of Langerhans are irreversibly damaged.

Sexual dysfunction is a very common symptom of GH, which requires tactful, sensitive counselling. Venesection can sometimes restore the pituitary gland function if GH is diagnosed early. Hormonal intervention of testosterone for men and oestrogen for women is administered and Viagra can be useful to both sexes if there is loss of libido. Depending on the extent of iron accumulation in the myocardium, there may be some improvement, but patients may require cardiotrophic drugs. Skin pigmentation generally improves over time once venesection has commenced.

Venesection has limited positive impact on joint disease and patients may require non-steroidal anti-inflammatory drugs (NSAIDs) to ease their pain as well as psychological and practical help. This could include joining the Haemochromatosis Society and meeting with others who manage the same condition.

Blood donation for people with haemochromatosis

This is only available for those patients on maintenance therapy. The patient will have to meet all the criteria for being a blood donor (UKBTS 2005). This includes among other things:

- Not having had a previous transfusion (since 1980)
- Not on any heart or blood pressure medication
- Under 65 for a new donor

It would be helpful to encourage the hospital consultant, responsible for the ongoing care of the haemochromatosis patient, to liaise with the local NHS Blood and Tissues (NBSBT) consultant. This can be with a view to the patient becoming a donor once the patient is on maintenance and, provided of course, that they match all the blood donor criteria. It is the hospital's responsibility to monitor the patient. If the patient requires extra venesections over and above the number per annum NHSBT performs on routine donors (3–4 per year), then the hospital has to continue to provide a venesection service, as the NBS has no plans to run a therapeutic venesection service for patients with haemochromatosis at the present time.

Nursing care for venesection

Patient preparation

Patients, especially at disease management onset, are undoubtedly very anxious and in common with all treatment intervention will require support, explanation and careful monitoring. Although treatment is simple and straightforward in this condition, some patients find this impossible to believe. Patients who have been blood donors in the past are not as worried as they are confident with the procedure itself, but may well require reassurance in finding that treatment is so simple.

It is very helpful for patients requiring venesection to keep their extremities warm, especially in cold weather, so as to ensure good venous dilation which will assist in gaining painless venous access (Sado 2001). Therefore asking the patient to wear warm clothing and gloves in very cold weather is essential. Equally essential is ensuring the patient is well hydrated and should have eaten before the procedure as this will help with blood flow during the procedure and lessen the chances of them fainting. If dehydrated the patient may require fluid replacement during the procedure and assessment of the patient's needs must be carried out.

Equipment required

As with any procedure it is essential that all equipment is assembled before commencing (see Table 10.2 for a list of equipment considered necessary).

Venesection procedure

It may be useful to prepare a standard operating procedure (SOP) document or locally approved clinical guidelines to use as a basis for staff training and assessment. Additionally this will ensure all staff perform the procedure in the same manner and give the patient the same care and advice. The procedure can take anywhere between 5–30 minutes to perform, and is mainly dependent on achieving good venous access and patient bleeding time, which is variable (Warrell *et al.* 2005). Tables 10.3 and 10.4 give further information.

Table 10.2 Equipment required for venesection.

- Venesection bag with its attached needle and diversion pouches for blood sampling if required
- Additional cannulae and cannula dressing for fluid replacement if required
- Tourniquet for insertion of cannula for fluid replacement
- Giving set and prescribed fluid (usually 500 ml N/saline) if required and as prescribed on the patient drug chart
- Sphygmomanometer cuff
- Skin prep
- Tape
- Clamp and clamp squeezer for permanent line clamping
- Artery forceps for temporary line clamping
- Scissors
- Scales to measure volume of blood venesected
- Blood sampling bottles if required

Table 10.3 Guideline content.

An example of a local guideline could include:

Ensure the patient is either sitting in a reclining chair or lying on a bed.

Ensure limb which will have the procedure performed, is well supported.

Check the resting blood pressure and inform the appropriate health care practitioner if it is below 100/60 before proceeding as fluid replacement may be required.

If fluid replacement is a requirement then give 250–500 ml 0.9% sodium chloride as prescribed on the patient's drug chart, before the venesection commences, to ensure the patient is well hydrated.

If the patient needs cannulation to support fluid replacement then prepare and insert cannula.

Inflate the sphygmomanometer cuff to 60/80 mm/Hg. Select a good large vein in the antecubital fossa if possible and clean the skin.

Insert the needle, which is attached to the venesection bag. Blood will flow automatically when the needle is in the vein. The bag will fill by gravity.

Once the blood is flowing freely deflate the sphygmomanometer cuff to 40 mm/Hg and maintain this pressure until venesection is completed as this helps to maintain venous engorgement.

Sometimes obtaining venous access can be difficult. See Table 10.4 for tips to assist with venous access.

Secure the tubing firmly with tape so the weight of the bag will not dislodge the needle and make sure there is some slack in the tubing.

Use weighing scales to ascertain volume of blood removed (the scales must be regularly maintained by equipment department).

When venesection is completed, deflate cuff and apply forceps to the line to clamp off. Fold over the line and clamp off using the clamp and clamp squeezer.

Remove needle and dispose of in a sharps bin. Do not re-sheath needle.

Apply a sterile dressing and maintain pressure on the site for several minutes as this will help to prevent bruising.

If blood samples are required this can be obtained from the sampling diversion pouches.

Table 10.4 Tips to assist with obtaining venous access in 'difficult veins'.

If the veins are small and/or access is difficult inflate cuff to 80 mm/Hg.
Warm the patient's limb using a heat pad or water bath.
Stroke the vein to assist in dilation and ask the patient's permission to gently tap the vein.
Encourage the patient to shake their arm for 1–3 minutes, keeping the arm below the heart level.
Ask the patient to open and clench their fist gently.
Use a green or pink cannula for venous access if needle on venesection bag is too small.
Cut off the needle from the venesection bag and insert the tubing into the end of the cannula after venous access has been achieved.
Deflate cuff to 40 mm/Hg.

Aftercare

Aftercare is equally important for the patient and gives them confidence for future visits. Ensure all documentation and record keeping has been completed.

- Apply pressure to the dressing over the venepuncture site, for about five minutes. If there is a haematoma then apply a pressure dressing. Ensure bleeding has stopped before taping the dressing securely in place. Advise the patient they can remove the dressing the following day. Patients should not be discharged until the bleeding has stopped.
- Patients must be advised to seek urgent medical help if the bleeding recurs and does not stop after pressure has been applied for ten minutes. Patients should be advised to avoid carrying heavy objects with the affected arm for at least 24 hours. If the patient suffers with severe bruising, pain or numbness advise them to contact the hospital department where venesection has been performed.
- Ensure the patient is in a comfortable, reclining position, and does not feel faint. Offer the patient oral fluids. Allow the patient to rest for at least 10–20 minutes. Do not allow the patient to get up too quickly and if they feel faint ensure they rest for a further ten minutes with their feet raised. The patient should be encouraged to increase fluid intake over the next 24 hours to help replace lost volume.
- Advise the patient to avoid smoking or drinking alcohol for at least an hour after venesection.
- Return discarded unit for safe disposal in the rigid blood boxes supplied by the haematology department.
- Ensure the venesection record has been completed and any collected samples sent to the lab for processing.

Risks

The patient may experience dizziness and may faint during the procedure. It is the role of the practitioner to ensure the patient is well hydrated and has eaten before the procedure. As time goes on patients feel they can cope with the procedure but equally there may be some that find each experience of venepuncture and venesection worse. This patient will require increased support and understanding.

As with all invasive procedures there is small risk of infection, but this should be minimized by using aseptic techniques. There may be some mild bruising, which can be reduced by prolonging the time pressure is maintained after the needle has been removed. Soreness at the puncture site can be reduced by the use of EMLA cream applied to the site by the patient prior to attending for therapeutic venesection. This, however, can be a disadvantage as the site where the patient has applied the cream may not be the one that the operator would necessarily choose for access. It also has to be applied at least an hour before the venesection is performed to give adequate anaesthesia.

Screening and counselling

It is recommended that once a family member has been identified with the genetic mutation responsible for haemochromatosis, then all members of the family should be tested (BCSH 2000) including:

- Children over the age of 18
- Siblings

The screening test is a simple blood test which shows the patient's genetic risk and genetic status for the disease. With early diagnosis, effective and simple management, and monitoring of this disorder, patients live a normal lifespan.

Genetic testing can confirm a diagnosis of HFE-associated hereditary haemochromatosis (genetic iron overload) or it can show that the patient is at risk for developing it in the future, thereby giving the patient the opportunity to take preventive measures such as diet adjustment and blood donation (Adams *et al.* 1991; Adams & Barton 2010). Family support alongside genetic counselling is an important and often overlooked aspect of patient care. Genetic counselling is not primarily counselling in the psychological sense, but counsellors, or indeed the GP or nurse specialist in the context of GH, can provide information and support to families who may be at risk. Once a person within a family has been diagnosed with haemochromatosis, the GP or nurse specialist familiar with this disorder can support the rest of the family members who may be at risk, interpret information about the disorder, analyse inheritance patterns and review available testing options with the family.

It may be that the patient and their family will need more in-depth information and understanding than can be provided and then a medical referral to a genetic counsellor may be indicated. In the context of haemochromatosis common reasons for genetic counselling include wanting:

- To know the risks to themselves and their children
- In-depth specialist advice about the condition
- To know their risks and options

Training for practitioners and educational requirements

Each person wishing to undertake therapeutic venesection is responsible for ensuring their training requirements are met by the standards outlined in their local clinical guidelines for adult venepuncture before they can undertake the procedure of therapeutic venesection. Following on from therapeutic venesection training, the practitioner must undergo a period of supervised practice of the procedure, by a medical practitioner or trained nurse, who has performed this procedure and is able to train others.

Accountability

All practitioners should be aware of, and act within, their own scope of practice according to their professional governing bodies, relevant codes of conduct and within trust guidelines.

Conclusion

As described, GH is a complex hereditary condition which provided it is recognised and diagnosed early is easily treatable, with little or no side effects. Patients will have a normal healthy lifespan, but treatment is lifelong and ongoing, which can have an impact on the patient's mental well-being. Additionally it is important that, once diagnosed, the patient's family have access to genetic counselling and screening services.

References

Adams, P.C., Speechley, M. and Kertesz, A.E. (1991) Long-term survival analysis in hereditary hemochromatosis. *Gastroenterology*, 101, 368–372.

Adams, P.C. and Barton, J.C. (2010) How I treat hemochromatosis. *Blood*. 116 (3), 317–325.

British Committee for Standards in Haematology (BCSH) (2000) Genetic Haemochromatosis: Guidelines on diagnosis and therapy: http://www.bcshguidelines.com/pdf/chpt9B.pdf. Accessed February 2008.

Cancer Backup (2009) http://www.cancerbackup.org.uk/Cancertype/Liver/Primarylivercancer. Accessed March 2009.

Haemochromatosis Society (2008) http://www.haemochromatosis.org.uk/. Accessed February 2008.

Haemochromatosis Society (2009) Information for General Practitioners http://www. haemochromatosis.org.uk/. Accessed March 2009.

Justin, Q., Ly, M.D., Douglas, P., Beall, M.D., Jaspal, S. and Ahluwalia, B.S. (2006) Hemochromatosis Arthropathy. *Appl Radiol*, 35 (8). Posted online 19 September 2006. http://www.medscape.com/viewarticle/543512

Phatak, P., Bonkovsky, H. and Kowdley, K. (2008). Hereditary hemochromatosis: Time for targeted screening. *Annals of Internal Medicine*, 149 (4), 270–272.

Sado, D. (2001) Improving your blood taking skills. *Student BMJ*. 09:261–304 August ISSN 0966-6494.

Warrell, D.A., Cox, T.M., Firth, J.D. and Benz, E.J. (2005) *Oxford Textbook of Medicine*. Chapter 11 pages 91–101. Oxford University Press, Oxford.

United Kingdom Blood Transfusion Service (2005) *Guidelines for the Blood Transfusion Services in the United Kingdom*, 7th edition. Chapter 3 Care and selection of blood donors. http://www.transfusionguidelines.org.uk/index.aspx?Publication=WB&Section=5

Section 3

Myeloproliferative and lymphoproliferative disorders

Chapter 11

Polycythaemia: pathophysiology, care and management

Marvelle Brown

At the end of this chapter you will:
- Understand the pathophysiology of polycythaemia
- Be familiar with investigations to diagnose polycythaemia
- Know the therapeutic interventions and nursing care required for patients with polycythaemia

---

Introduction

Erythrocyte production is regulated under hormonal control, as discussed in Chapter 1 (Normal blood physiology), and the red cell count is controlled within very narrow margins. Therefore anything which affects the regulation and production of red blood cells will have an impact on this tightly controlled system. Polycythaemia (erythrocytosis) is a non-leukaemic myeloproliferative disorder and relates to excessive production of red blood cells. Depending on the cause, polycythaemia is classified as absolute or apparent polycythaemia and can occur in all ages, but it is predominately seen in adults.

Absolute polycythaemia

This is due to excessive production of erythrocytes and can be subgrouped as primary polycythaemia and secondary polycythaemia. The increase in erythrocyte production and haematocrit leads to a significant increase in blood volume, causing increased blood viscosity. The blood flow becomes sluggish, slow in flow and can block small capillary blood vessels (Pallister 2005). Primary polycythaemia can be inherited or acquired. Inherited primary polycythaemia is often known as primary familial and congenital polycythaemia (PFCP). This is an autosomal dominant inheritance that causes several mutations of the erythropoietin receptor (EPOR) gene, which leads to proliferation of erythrocyte production (Kralovics and Prchal 2001).

Haematology Nursing, First Edition. Marvelle Brown and Tracey J. Cutler.
© 2012 Blackwell Publishing Ltd. Published 2012 by Blackwell Publishing Ltd.

Acquired primary polycythaemia, often known as polycythaemia rubra vera (PRV) or polycythaemia vera (PV), is caused by a somatic mutation of a single stem cell, leading to an increase in erythrocyte production. The mutation prevents responses to normal hormonal controls leading to the proliferation of erythrocytes. This means the mutated stem cell no longer responds to hormonal controls and erythrocytes proliferate. In addition, a mutation of JAK2 is common in PV. It encodes for the enzyme tyrosine kinase, which increases erythrocyte precursor sensitivity to EPO, thereby also creating the environment for increasing erythrocyte production (Baxter *et al.* 2005). It is also common for an increase in granulocytes and platelets to occur with PV. Polycythaemia vera has a 10% risk of transforming to AML and a 30% risk of transforming to myelofibrosis (Hoffbrand and Moss 2011).

Secondary polycythaemia

This is generally related to external triggers which cause an increase in erythropoietin production. There are a number of factors which can cause secondary polycythaemia, which are outlined in Table 11.1.

Table 11.1   Factors related to secondary polycythaemia.

- Altitude – living in high altitude where atmospheric oxygen is low, the body compensates for this by increasing erythrocyte production.
- Hypoxia – congestive cardiac failure, chronic obstructive airways disease, emphysema, chronic sleep apnoea.
- Hormonal – the hormone testosterone enhances erythrocyte production.
- Tumours – renal and hepatic tumours which lead to an excess production of erythropoietin.
- Carbon monoxide exposure – haemoglobin has a great affinity for carbon monoxide. This will lead to a reduction in the haemoglobin ability to carry oxygen. As a consequence the resulting hypoxia leads to an increase in erythrocyte production. However, neither the haemoglobin level nor red cell count has actually been reduced. Therefore the increase in EPO activity to produce more red cells, leads to excess of erythrocytes. Any employment which exposes the individual to continued levels of carbon monoxide, such as garage car mechanics or tunnel workers, have a higher potential of developing PV.

Apparent polycythaemia

This is sometimes referred to by other terms such pseudo-polycythaemia, stress polycythaemia, relative polycythaemia, Gaisböck's syndrome. The cause relates to reduced plasma volume but there tends to be a normal red blood cell mass. It is primarily caused by factors such as dehydration stress, excessive smoking, excessive alcohol, hypertension, burns, diuretic therapy and cerebral ischemia attacks. It occurs more commonly in young and middle-aged men, particularly men who are obese and highly anxious.

Investigations and diagnosis

Diagnosis of polycythaemia is primarily based on haemoglobin and haematocrit levels, the presence or absence of JAK3 mutation, existence of splenomegaly and/or thrombosis. In men, if the haemoglobin is over 18.5 g/dL and the haematocrit is over 0.60 there is a suspicion of polycythaemia. In women, haemoglobin over 16.5 g/dL and a haematocrit of more than 0.52 would be suspicious of polycythaemia (WHO 2008).

In primary polycythaemia, 95% of patients have mutations of JAK 2. In PV, the neutrophils and thrombocyte counts tend to be increased, but not always in secondary polycythaemia (McMullin *et al.* 2005). In polycythaemia vera the bone marrow is hypercellular and the erythrocyte sedimentation rate (ESR) increased. In primary polycythaemia serum levels of EPO are low but if the polycythaemia is due to a secondary cause such as a renal tumour then serum levels will be increased (see Figure 11.1).

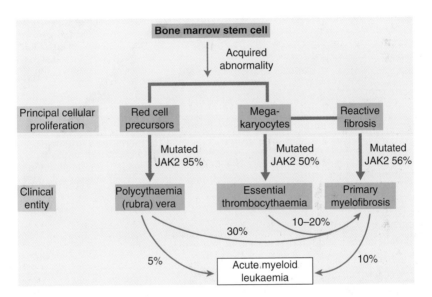

Figure 11.1 Relationship between the three myeloproliferative diseases (from Hoffbrand and Moss 2011). Reprinted with permission of John Wiley & Sons, Inc.

Signs and symptoms

Many patients can be asymptomatic, whereas other patients may have vague, non-specific symptoms (see Figure 11.2). Generally, patients may present with manifestations related to plasma viscosity and these include:

- Headaches
- Vertigo
- Blurred vision
- Hepatomegaly

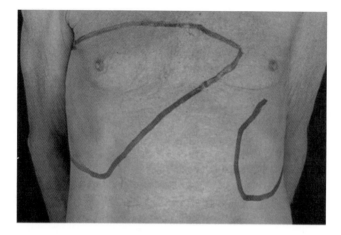

Figure 11.2   Splenomegaly (from Hoffbrand and Moss 2011) in a male with polycythaemia vera. Reprinted with permission of John Wiley & Sons, Inc.

- Splenomegaly
- Night sweats
- Hypertension
- Pruritus (especially following a hot bath); this is thought to be associated with the release of histamine and prostaglandins
- Gout (the excessive production of erythrocytes leads to increase in uric acid)
- Fatigue
- Weight loss
- Lack of concentration
- Ruddy complexion
- Peptic ulcer
- Erythromelalgia – sudden severe pain in hands and feet
- Haemorrhage – gastrointestinal, uterine and/or cerebral

Nursing care and management

Polycythaemia is incurable and treatment is aimed at reducing plasma volume, relieving symptoms and minimising risks of thrombosis and haemorrhage complications. Having an awareness of symptoms of PV, nurses should assess the patients for pain. Sensitively question the patient if they are experiencing headaches or joint pain. Timely administration of analgesia, if required, should be administered. If the patient is complaining of pain in the lower limbs, elevating the leg can help to relieve the pressure. Passive and active range of motion and ambulation are used to promote circulation and prevent thrombus formation. Application of a cold cloth or ice pack to the head can be soothing, or heat to joints can relieve discomfort. Assess if the patient is experiencing fatigue. Establish if the patient has difficulty with concentration. This should guide how much information the nurse should provide at any one time.

Venesection is the mainstay of treatment for PV. This is seen as the most effective and efficient way of reducing the haematocrit. The usual aim is to achieve a haematocrit level to 45% for men and 42% for women (McMullin *et al.* 2005). Commonly 250–500 ml of blood is removed. Nurses should be fully cognisant of procedures and practices with venepucturing and cannulation. See Chapter 10 for venesection procedure guidelines. Venesection is a rapid way of decreasing the blood volume and may be undertaken initially 2–3 days per week until normal haematocrit levels are achieved. Thereafter the maintenance management of planned venesection is undertaken. Care should be taken in monitoring the patient for iron deficiency anaemia, as this can be a consequence of venesection. Careful monitoring of intake and output during hydration therapy and phlebotomy to avoid over or under hydration should be undertaken.

Oral myelosuppressive drugs such as hydroxycarbamide (hydroxyurea) or busulfan can be prescribed if venesection is not reducing the haematocrit or if the patient has persistent splenomegaly. Prescribing chemotherapy drugs has some concerns of an increased risk of secondary AML and therefore is often delayed in use, particularly in young adults (Bjökholm *et al.* 2011). Low dose aspirin (75–81 mg) may be prescribed, which is aimed at reducing the risk of thrombotic tendencies to prevent strokes. The dose is considered low enough not to increase the risk of haemorrhage. Adjunctive therapy includes allopurinol to treat high levels of uric acid, antihistamines to reduce pruritus and antacids for gastric hyperacidity.

Phosphorus 32 (^{32}P) is a radioactive treatment that may be offered to older patients. Phosphorus 32 is used if venesection is not successful. It is highly effective and can keep a patient in remission for two years. However, the risk of it causing transformation to acute myeloid leukaemia does not make its use popular. Alpha interferon is another treatment option. It is administered as a subcutaneous injection, which is inconvenient, but more significantly the side effects of the drug can be unbearable for some patients. The side effects of alpha interferon are listed in Table 11.2.

Nurses have an important role in educating the patient about their illness, in particular stressing the chronic nature of the disease, the requirement for long-term venesection and being aware of the major complications if PV is not treated. Patients should be advised to drink plenty of fluids to reduce plasma viscosity. Unless prescribed, patients should be

Table 11.2   Side effects of alpha interferon.

Leukopenia
Thrombocytopenia
Erythrocytopenia
Fatigue
Petechia
Taste aberrations
Nausea
Flu-like symptoms
Diarrhoea
Loss of appetite
Pruritus
Hair thinning

discouraged from taking iron supplements as they will increase erythrocyte production. If the patient has splenomegaly, contact sport should be advised against to reduce the risk of damage or rupture. Treatment for secondary polycythaemia would depend on the cause. It may involve venesection, but not always.

Conclusion

The main concern regarding clinical complications which can cause morbidity and mortality is haemorrhage and thrombosis. The risk of haemorrhage is due to defective, dysfunctional platelets. Thrombosis is related to increased viscosity, vascular stasis and increase platelet count. Deep vein thrombosis, pulmonary embolism, cerebrovascular accidents and myocardial infarcts are major complications associated with PV.

Nurses should ensure patients are well informed about PV, be skilled in cannulation and continue to educate the patient in relation to any changes which may occur throughout the chronicity of the illness.

References

Baxter, E.J., Scott, M.A., Campbell, P.J. *et al.* (2005) Acquired mutation of the tryosine kinase JAK2 in human myeloprofilterative disorders. *Lancet*, 365 (9464), 1054–1061.

Bjökholm, M., Derolf, A.R., Hultcrantz, M. *et al.* (2011) Treatment-related risk factors for transformation to acute myeloid leukemia and myelodysplastic syndromes in myeloproliferative neoplasms. *Journal Clinical Oncology*, 34, 7542–7549.

Finazzi, G., Caruso, V., Marchioli, R. *et al.* (2005) Acute leukemia in polycythemia vera: an analysis of 1638 patients enrolled in a prospective observational study. *Blood*, 105 (7), 2664–2670.

Hoffbrand, A.V. and Moss, P.A.H. (2011) *Essential Haematology*, 6th edition. Wiley-Blackwell, Oxford.

Kralovics, R. and Prchal, J.T. (2001) Genetic heterogeneity of primary familial and congenital polycythemia. *American Journal of Hematology*, 68, 115–121.

McMullin, M.E., Bareford, D., Campbell, P. *et al.* (2005) General Haematology Task Force of the British Committee for Standards for Haematology Guidelines for the diagnosis, investigations and management of polycythaemia/erythrocytosis. *British Journal Haematology*, 130, 174–195.

Pallister C.J. (2005) *Haematology*, 2nd edition. Hodder Arnold, London.

World Health Organisation (2008) *WHO Classification of Tumours – Myeloproliferative Disorders.* WHO, Geneva.

Chapter 12

The myelodysplastic syndromes: pathophysiology, care and management

Jackie Green

After reading this chapter you will:

- Have an overview of the myelodysplastic syndromes (MDS)
- Be able to discuss the clinical progression of the disease and prognosis
- Be able to identify and discuss the nursing care issues and the supportive care required for this group of patients

---

Introduction

The myelodysplastic syndromes (MDS) are a group of haematological disorders characterised by disruption in the production of effective blood cells. Bone marrow, blood cell morphology and the number, structure and functional ability of all blood cells may be abnormal, resulting in anaemia, leucopenia and thrombocytopenia.

Myelodysplastic syndromes have the potential to transform into acute myeloid leukaemia (AML) although not all individuals diagnosed with MDS will develop AML. Myelodysplastic syndromes will transform in about 30% of patients, although the time interval from diagnosis to transformation varies tremendously (Gyger *et al.* 1988). However, MDS is frequently a chronic progressive disease, requiring a gradual increase in supportive care and treatment. This chapter examines MDS: the diseases, diagnosis, classification, treatment and specific nursing issues.

Myelodysplastic syndromes: the diseases

Myelodysplastic syndromes (MDS) are a group of disorders characterised by one or more peripheral blood cytopenias secondary to bone marrow dysfunction. Anaemia is common and usually dysplastic changes are present in more than one blood cell lineage. Bone marrow cellularity may be normal or become hypercellular. Both cell division and numbers of blast cells may be increased. Myelodysplastic syndrome is associated with

---

Haematology Nursing, First Edition. Marvelle Brown and Tracey J. Cutler.

impaired maturation of blood cells and increased apoptosis (programmed cell death). Blood cells may have functional deficits predisposing to infection or bleeding (Heaney and Golde 1999). Myelodysplastic syndromes may arise *de novo* and be considered an idiopathic disease, or secondarily after treatment with chemotherapy or radiation therapy for another disease. It is sometimes referred to as a 'pre-leukaemic' condition. However, not all patients progress to AML and many die from the effects of cytopenias or other co-morbid conditions common in an elderly population (Albitar *et al.* 2002; Greenburg *et al.* 2002). Accurate estimation of the incidence of MDS is difficult, because it may be asymptomatic and remain undetected for several years.

The causes of MDS remain unclear, although exposure to radiation, chemicals, cytotoxic drugs and benzene has been implicated (Heaney and Golde 1999). Myelodysplastic syndromes predominately affect the elderly (median age 70 years), although patients as young as two years have been reported (Tuncer *et al.* 1992). It has a non-age incidence of 3/100,000 rising to 20/100,000 in those over 70 years. Secondary MDS can arise as a result of chemotherapy/radiation for other malignancies. The incidence is not known but may represent as many as 10–15% of all cases of MDS diagnosed annually.

Clinical progression and prognosis of the disease is extremely variable. It may remain stable for many years or progress rapidly to AML. Secondary myelodysplasia usually has a poorer prognosis than *de novo* MDS (Cheson 1992). Survival and prognosis is directly related to the disease classification and prognostic indicators, including percentage of bone marrow blast cells, degree of peripheral blood cytopenias and cytogenetic abnormalities.

Diagnosis

Those affected by MDS frequently present with the features of bone marrow failure: symptoms of anaemia, repeated infections, bleeding and/or bruising. Approximately 10% of patients diagnosed with MDS present with splenomegaly (Mufti and Galton 1992).

The myelodysplastic syndromes are diagnosed primarily on the basis of characteristic full blood count assays, morphological abnormalities on the peripheral blood film, and characteristic bone marrow appearances. Although MDS may sometimes be diagnosed on the basis of a blood film alone, a bone marrow aspirate and trephine are needed to confidently diagnose and assess the severity of the disease (Bowen *et al.* 2003).

Diagnosis is easily made if morphological abnormalities are found in the three major blood cell lineages: erythroid (red cells), myeloid cells (granulocytes, including neutrophils) and megakaryocytes (platelets) (Oscier and Oscier 1997). However, morphological dysplasia is not necessarily indicative of MDS, as some similar morphological abnormalities to those found in early MDS may be seen in vitamin B_{12} deficiency, alcohol excess, after chemotherapy and HIV infection. Cytogenetic analysis is also recommended for all those who have bone marrow examination (Bowen *et al.* 2003).

Classification of myelodysplastic syndrome

Myelodysplastic syndrome has classically been subdivided into five categories according to the abnormalities found within the bone marrow. This classification is known as the French-American-British (FAB) system after the French, American and British haematologists who designed the system (Bennett *et al.* 1982) (Table 12.1). The FAB classification has been used as a prognostic indicator depending on the percentage of blast cells, ringed sideroblasts, monocytes and presence of Auer rods. Survival times and the prognosis of the disease vary significantly. However, the World Health Organisation (WHO) (Harris *et al.* 1999) has published a new classification system intended to supersede the FAB system (Table 12.2). In 2008 the World Health Organisation developed introduced another revised classification system, (Gupta, 2010).

Survival times and the prognosis of the disease vary significantly even among patients of the same subgroup (Mufti and Galton 1992). The above classification systems are used in conjunction with additional prognostic scoring systems such as the International Prognostic scoring system (IPSS) (Greenburg *et al.* 1997) (Table 12.3). The IPSS considers three parameters: bone marrow blast percentage, bone marrow cytogenetics and the number of blood lineages with cytopenia. The IPSS identifies four risk groups: low risk, intermediate 1, intermediate 2 and high risk. The higher the score the poorer the prognosis (Table 12.4). Other prognostic factors include age and gender, with males having slightly poorer survival than females (Greenburg *et al.* 1997; Verburgh *et al.* 2003).

Table 12.1   French American British (FAB) classification of MDS (Bennett *et al.* 1982).

FAB Type	Percentage of blasts	Percentage of blasts in peripheral blood
1. Refractory anaemia (RA)	<5	<1
2. RA with ringed sideroblasts (RARS)	<5 Ringed sideroblasts >15 of total erythrocytes	<1
3. RA with excess blasts (RAEB)	5–20	>5
4. RAEB in transformation (RAEB-t)	20–30 or presence of Auer rods	>5
5. Chronic myelomonocytic leukaemia	5–20 monocyte count >1.0 x 10^9/l	>5

Table 12.2   WHO histological classification of myelodysplastic syndromes (Harris *et al.* 1999).

Refractory anaemia (RA)
Refractory anaemia with ringed sideroblasts (RARS)
Refractory cytopenia with multilineage dysplasis (RCMD)
Refractory anaemia with excess blasts 1 (RAEB-1)
Refractory anaemia with excess blasts 2 (RAEB-2)
Myelodysplastic syndrome unclassified (MDS-U)
Myelodysplastic syndrome associated with isolated del(5q) chromosome abnormality

Table 12.3 International Prognostic Scoring System (IPSS) for MDS (Greenberg *et al.* 1997).

Prognostic variable	Survival and AML evolution score value				
	0	0.5	1.0	1.5	2.5
Bone marrow blasts%	<5	5–10	—	11–20	21–30
Karyotype	Good	Intermediate	Poor		
Cytopenias	0/1	2/3			

Scores for risk groups

Risk category	Combined score
Low	0
Intermediate 1 (Int-1)	0.5–1.0
Intermediate 2 (Int-2)	1.5–2.0
High	≥2.5

Karyotype: good = normal, -Y, del(5q), del(20q); Poor = complex (≥3 abnormalities) or chromosome 7 abnormalities
Intermediate = other abnormalities
Cytopenias: haemoglobin concentrate <10 g/dL, neutrophils <1.5 x 10^9/L and platelets <100 x 10^9/L

Table 12.4 Mean survival in relation to risk score (Greenberg *et al.* 1997).

Risk and score		Median survival (years)		
		Under 60	Over 60	Over 70
Low	0	11.8	4.8	3.9
Intermediate 1	0.5–1.0	5.2	2.7	2.4
Intermediate 2	1.2.0	1.8	1.1	1.2
High	>2.5	0.3	0.5	0.4

Although it is recommended that management of MDS should be based on the IPSS score (Bowen *et al.* 2003) it is important to remember that this system of scoring is only an indicator of prognosis. All patients with MDS have a reduced life expectancy, although patients react to their illness and treatment differently. An individual patient's prognosis will depend on their own specific circumstances and many patients live beyond their predicted survival time. The classification relates to adults as the disease follows a very different pattern in children.

Treatment and management of myelodysplastic syndromes

There is no consistently effective treatment that provides long-term improvements in hae-mopoiesis. Therefore, it is recommended that, where appropriate, management decisions are based on the patient's IPSS score and patient choice (Bowen *et al.* 2003; Cheson *et al.*

2000). Quality of life is important in decisions about treatment, and management decisions should be taken with the informed involvement of the patient. In order to facilitate patient involvement, the proposed management of MDS should be explained to the patient and supported with written information related to guidelines.

Supportive care

Supportive care remains the most important aspect of management for all patients with MDS. The aim is to reduce morbidity and mortality and provision of an acceptable quality of life (Bowen *et al.* 2003). Management of the various cytopenias is therefore essential.

Anaemia

At presentation, approximately two-thirds of patients will be anaemic and virtually all will experience anaemia at some point in their illness, due to ineffective erythropoiesis and other disease and treatment related influence, for example chemotherapy or haemorrhage (Casadevall *et al.* 2004). Anaemia may cause fatigue and breathlessness, affecting the individual's quality of life. Red cell transfusion is used to correct anaemia. It is not possible to identify a single optimal haemoglobin level, below which a red cell transfusion should be given, as it is dependent on the individual. However, in clinical practice transfusion is used if the individual is symptomatic. Guidelines also suggest haemoglobin is maintained >8 g/dL (Murphy *et al.* 2001). Disease progression may require an increasing number of red cell transfusions due to a chronic anaemia state. This may cause an increase in body iron stores and iron overload, as the body has no means of increasing iron excretion (Hughes *et al.* 2009). If iron stores become greatly increased, damage may occur to the heart, liver and endocrine organs. In order to monitor iron stores ferritin levels should be monitored and a target ferritin level of <1000 µg/L is recommended (Franchini and Gandini 2000).

To prevent iron overload it is recommended that once a patient has received 5 g iron (approximately 25 units of red cells) iron chelation should be considered for those patients who are likely to require long-term red cell transfusion (Bowen *et al.* 2003). However, iron chelation treatment in MDS is based on limited evidence. It is recommended that desferrioxamine (an iron-chelating compound) 20–40 mg/kg should be administered to patients who are likely to need long-term blood component transfusions. Desferrioxamine is usually administered subcutaneously over 8–12 hours, three times a week. Desferrioxamine (up to 2 g per unit of blood) can also be administered intravenously at the same time as the blood transfusion, provided it is not added to or given through the same line (British Medical Association 2004). Auditory and ophthalmic assessments are essential prior to commencing desferrioxamine because it is known to produce visual and hearing disturbances.

Erythropoietin (EPO) a colony stimulating factor (which promotes the growth and differentiation of blood cells may increase haemoglobin concentration and reduce the need for red cell transfusion in selected MDS patients, reducing the risk of iron overload (Table 12.5). Studies using EPO have been small, involving less than 120 patients and suggest that patients with refractory anaemia (RA) or RA with excess blasts

Table 12.5   Colony stimulating factors.

---

1. Granulocyte, macrophage colony-stimulating factor (GM-CSF) promotes growth and differentiation of granulocyte and macrophage progenitors.
2. Granuloycte colony-stimulating factors (G-CSF) stimulates neutrophil precursors to produce large amounts of circulating neutrophils.
3. Erythropoietin (EPO) promotes erythrocyte production.

(RAEB) are more likely to respond to EPO (Estey *et al.* 1997). It is recommended that patients with RA and RAEB who have minimal blood transfusion requirement (<2 units a month) and an EPO level <200 U/L should be considered for EPO (Hellstrom Lindberg *et al.* 1998).

A combination of G-CSF (granulocyte colony-stimulating factor) and EPO has been shown to have a synergistic effect and is recommended to improve anaemia for some individuals (Bowen *et al.* 2003). For patients with RARS, symptomatic anaemia, EPO serum levels <500 U/L and a transfusion requirement of less than two units of blood a month EPO + GCSF is recommended (Hellstrom Lindberg *et al.* 1998). However, not all patients with anaemia secondary to MDS respond to growth factors and clinical trials investigating their use continue. There is an assumption that improving anaemia will improve quality of life, although there is little data to support this. One randomised trial comparing EPO and GCSF with supportive care found that the combination was expensive and did not improve quality of life (Casadevall *et al.* 2004).

Thrombocytopenia

Spontaneous bleeding is a potentially serious complication of MDS and it is suggested that treatment is based on symptoms (Ancliff and Machin 1998). Patients may experience unexplained bruising, nose bleeds (epistaxis), a petechial rash or gum bleeding. Patients who experience spontaneous bleeding should be advised to seek medical and/or nursing advice and support immediately. Platelet transfusion may be required to both stop bleeding and reduce the risk of further bleeding.

Management of infection

White cell count and in particular the neutrophil count can be significantly lowered in MDS, increasing the risk of developing a life-threatening infection. The lower the neutrophil count the higher the risk of infection and the risk of infection rises as the neutrophil count falls. Immunosuppressed patients can become infected with pathogenic organisms and opportunistic organisms (Mimms 1993; Farshid *et al.* 2010).

The evidence base for symptomatic management of infection in MDS is limited. The use of prophylactic antibiotic therapy has not been proven and individuals with MDS may require hospital admission for intravenous antibiotic therapy. The use of colony stimulating factors (CSF) may be considered in the cases of severe neutropenia in order to maintain a neutrophil count $>1 \times 10^9/L$ (Negrin *et al.* 1996). Colony stimulating factors may improve the supportive therapy of patients with MDS by minimising the risk of infection, as fewer infections have been reported with their use (Ganser *et al.* 1989). Intermittent use of CSFs for patients with severe neutropenia and recurrent infections has been found to be beneficial (Ozer *et al.* 2000). However, prolonged use of CSFs is not recommended in MDS (Pagliuca *et al.* 2003). Long-term use may be considered for patients with recurring life-threatening infections.

Haemopoietic stem cell transplantation

A small percentage of patients with MDS may be eligible for haemopoietic stem cell transplantation (HSCT). It is suggested that allogeneic HSCT results in long-term survival in 30–55% of patients and has the best chance of cure (Anderson *et al.* 1996; Deeg *et al.* 2000).

Eligibility for HSCT is dependent on several factors:

- Stage and duration of the disease
- The individual's general health (including previous medical history, lung, renal and cardiac status) and physical ability to tolerate treatment
- Availability of a histocompatible sibling or unrelated donor
- Psychological state
- Age

Good risk factors for transplant for the individual with MDS are considered to be <10% blasts and good cytogenetics (Anderson *et al.* 1993; Sutton *et al.* 1996). An example of good cytogenetics is chromosomal abnormalities 5q, where there is a deletion of the long arm of chromosome 5q. This is associated with macrocytic anaemia in elderly women and has a low risk of transformation to AML, whereas loss of short arm p chromosome 17 is found in advanced disease and associated with drug resistance and short-term survival.

It is also suggested that autologous HSCT may prolong survival (De Witte *et al.* 1997). Factors associated with improved outcome are shorter disease duration, age, primary MDS with <10 blasts in the bone marrow (Deeg *et al.* 2000). The type of HSCT is usually determined by the likely survival outcome, donor availability and well-being of the individual.

Intensive chemotherapy

Individuals with MDS over 65 and those under 65 who are not eligible for HSCT should be considered for intensive chemotherapy (Bowen *et al.* 2003). Prospective studies have compared supportive therapy versus intensive chemotherapy (Hellstrom Lindberg *et al.* 1992; Miller *et al.* 1992). Such studies suggest that of all high-risk MDS patients (IPSS>2), those with RAEB in transformation and lacking independent adverse risk factors may respond to intensive chemotherapy. Independent adverse risk factors can be considered as karyotype, age, performance status and duration of disease (Estey *et al.* 1997). There does not appear to be any superior chemotherapy combination. However, a combination such as that used in AML treatment is commonly used. Estey *et al.* (2001)

suggests that regimens containing cytosine arabinoside, idarubicin, with or without fludarabine are likely to produce the best outcome at present. If MDS transforms to AML the treatment is that of AML, usually high intensity combination chemotherapy with or without HSCT. This is dependent on the individual's views, beliefs, and physical and mental well-being (Estey *et al.* 1997).

Specific nursing issues

The nursing care of an individual with MDS requires specific skills in order to maximise their quality of life whilst living with the disease. As MDS may significantly reduce life expectancy great emphasis is placed on quality of life. Good symptom management is therefore imperative to achieve and improve outcomes for patients. It is essential that nurses caring for these patients understand the disease process, treatment options and side effects. Psychological and social factors and education are also important nursing considerations due to the unpredictability of the disease process and reduced life expectancy. Nurses need to provide the individual and their families with specific information and education related to bone marrow depression and living with MDS.

Specific education and information needs

Nurses should observe for signs of anaemia, such as fatigue, shortness of breath, pallor and reduction in activity due to excessive tiredness. Expert nursing care can help the individual prioritise activities in order to ensure that they have sufficient energy for the activities that are most valuable to them. For individuals who require blood transfusion it is essential that the British Committee for Standards in Haematology (BCSH) guidelines (Treleaven *et al.* 2010) and local hospital policy are followed to ensure the transfusion is administered safely. Individuals require information and understanding of the need for transfusion as well as the associated risks. It is recommended that written information is given to support verbal information and consent is obtained (Department of Health 2001). It is also important for patients to be aware of how they can help themselves to cope with anaemia. Information and education about appropriate diet, fluid intake and managing their breathlessness and lethargy should be provided.

Nurses must also be aware of signs and symptoms of thrombocytopenia. Bleeding can be a frightening experience. Patients and their families require explicit information about what to do if bleeding occurs. Emergency contact numbers of the ward or the day care unit are generally very helpful and provide reassurance. Verbal and written information outlining what to do during office hours and out of hours is important. Education is extremely important and individuals should be made aware of risk factors associated with bleeding and bruising. Advice should be given about activities that increase the risk of bleeding and bruising such as contact sports, climbing at high altitudes, flying in aeroplanes, avoiding cuts and scratches whilst gardening. It is acknowledged that not all those with MDS will participate in such activities, and advice should be adapted to the individual's needs. If any surgical intervention or dental work is required, the haematology team caring for the individual should be notified prior to such an event so that the risks of bleeding can be reduced and clotting factors and platelet levels are maintained at a safe volume.

The individual with MDS requires education to understand the infection risks associated with the disease. Being able to identify early signs of infection is significant and can help reduce the risk of severe infection. Infection may have a significant impact on an individual's lifestyle, such as hospital admissions due to septic episodes, the need to avoid crowded places, antibiotic therapy and potentially time off work due to infection. Individuals therefore require support from both the haematology team and in the social setting from employers, family and any social organisations they may attend.

Nurses have an important role in educating individuals about what to do in the event of an infection and measures to minimise the risk of an infective process. Patients should be informed both verbally and in written format of the actions they should take, if they become unwell, have hot and cold episodes, shivers or a high temperature (>38°C). Information should include who to contact and what to do. The need to act promptly and not ignore these signs should be emphasised.

Psychological impact

A diagnosis of MDS potentially has a great psychological impact on individuals. The unpredictability of the disease, frequent hospital attendance and potentially frequent hospital admissions can have an enormous impact on an individual's life and psychological needs should be considered at all times. Some individuals and their carers will require professional counselling to help them live with the disease. Others may benefit from the support and understanding provided by the multidisciplinary team. Nurses can help considerably by ensuring that treatments and hospital appointments, as far as possible, are made flexible in order to minimise the disruption to the individual's lifestyle and particularly the working environment. It is possible that the individual may require medical information to be given to employers in order to assist them in retaining employment. Other individuals may wish to give up work and may need some assistance with financial support.

The psychological impact of living with this group of diseases should not be underestimated. In order to identify what living with MDS means to the patient the nurse requires excellent communication skills and the ability to listen. It is important that nurses recognise the need to refer appropriately to other colleagues. Seeking advice from multidisciplinary team members and recognising when referral to a counsellor is appropriate is an essential aspect of care.

Social implications

The diseases also have significant social implications and nurses must be aware of these. Although nurses may not be the most appropriate person to deal with some of the issues, such as completing forms for financial support or advising on writing a will; they are in an ideal position to act as a coordinator and refer the individual to appropriate personnel.

Conclusion

Myelodysplastic syndrome varies in its manifestations, disease classification, treatment options and life expectancy. It is essential that individuals with MDS are fully informed about their disease. Nurses have a very specialist role in supporting individuals with MDS to live their lives to the full within the constraints placed upon them by the disease. Clearly there are differing treatment options available, ranging from supportive therapy to intensive chemotherapy and stem cell transplantation. Nursing care aims to meet individual needs at all stages in the disease pathway. This demands experienced/expert nurses with the skills and knowledge to meet these needs.

References

Albitar, M., Manshouri, T., Shen, Y. *et al.* (2002) Myelodysplastic syndrome is not merely 'preleukaemia'. *Blood*, 100 (3), 791–798.

Ancliff, P. and Machin, S. (1998) Trigger factors for the prophylactic platelet transfusion. *Blood Reviews*, 12, 234–238.

Anderson, J.E., Appelbaum, F.R., Fischer, L.D. *et al.* (1993) Allogeneic bone marrow transplantation for 93 patients with myelodysplastic syndrome. *Blood*, 82, 677–681.

Anderson, J.E., Appelbaum, F.R., Schoch, G. *et al.* (1996) Allogeneic bone marrow transplantation for refractory anaemia: a comparison of two preparative regimes and analysis of prognostic factors. *Blood*, 87, 51–58.

Bennett, J.M., Catousky, D., Daniel, M.T. *et al.* (1982) Proposals for the classification of the myelodysplastic syndromes. *British Journal of Haematology*, 51 (2), 189–199.

Bowen, D., Culligan, D., Jowitt, S. and the UK MDS Guidelines Group (2003) Guidelines for the diagnosis and therapy of adult myelodysplastic syndrome. *British Journal of Haematology*, 120, 187–200.

British Committee for Standards in Haematology (1999) Guidelines for the administration of blood and blood components in the management of transfused patients. *Transfusion Medicine*, 9, 227–238.

British Medical Association (2004) *British National Formulary 48*. British Medical Association, London.

Casadevall, N., Durieux, P., Dubois, S. *et al.* (2004) Health, economic and quality of life effects of erythropoietin and granulocyte colony-stimulating factor for the treatment of myelodysplastic syndromes: a randomised controlled trial. *Blood*, 104 (2), 321–327.

Cheson, B.D. (1992) Chemotherapy and bone marrow transplantation for myelodysplastic syndromes. *Seminars in Oncology*, 19 (1), 85–94.

Cheson, B.D., Bennett, J.M., Kantarjian, H. *et al.* (2000) Report of an international working group to standardise criteria for myelodysplastic syndromes. *Blood*, 96, 3671–3674.

Deeg, H., Shulman, H.M., Anderson, J.E. *et al.* (2000) Allogeneic and syngeneic marrow transplantation for myelodysplastic syndromes in patients 55–66 years of age. *Blood*, 95 (10), 1188–1194.

Department of Health (2001) Good practice in consent: achieving the NHS plan commitment to patient centred consent practice. *Health Service Circular (HSC) 2001/023*. DoH, London.

De Witte, T., Van Biezen, A., Hermans, J. *et al.* (1997) Autologous bone marrow transplantation for patients with myelodysplastic syndromes (MDS) or acute myeloid leukaemia following MDS.

Chronic or Acute Leukaemia Working Parties of the European Group for Blood and Marrow Transplantation. *Blood*, 90 (10), 3853–3857.

Estey, E., Thall, P. and Beran, M. (1997) Effect of diagnosis: refractory anaemia with excess blasts, refractory anaemia with excess blasts in transformation or AML on outcome of AML type chemotherapy. *Blood*, 90 (8), 2969–2977.

Estey, E., Thall, P.F., Cortes, J.E. *et al.* (2001) Comparison of idaurubicin + ara-C-, fludarabine + ara-C and topotocan + ara-C based regimes in treatment of newly diagnosed acute myeloid leukaemia, refractory anaemia with excess blasts in transformation, or refractory anaemia with excess blasts. *Blood*, 98, 3575–3583.

Franchini, M. and Gandini, G. (2000) Safety and efficacy of subcutaneous bolous injection of desferoxamine in adult patients with iron overload. *Blood*, 95, 2776–2779.

Farshid, D., Conley, A.P., Strom, S.S., Stevenson, W., Cortes, J.E., Borthakur, G., Faderl, S., O'Brien, S., Pierce, S., Kantarjian, H., Garcia-Manero G. (2010) Cause of death in patients with lower-risk myelodysplastic syndrome. *Cancer*, Vol 116, 9; 2174–2179.

Ganser, A., Volkers, B., Greher, J. *et al.* (1989) Recombinant human granulocyte macrophage colony stimulating factor in patients with myelodysplastic syndromes – a phase I/II trial. *Blood*, 73, 31–37.

Greenberg, P., Cox, C., Le Beau, M. *et al.* (1997) International scoring system for evaluating prognosis in myelodysplastic syndromes. *Blood*, 89 (6), 2079–2088.

Greenberg, PL, Young, N.S. and Gattermann, N. (2002) Myelodysplastic syndromes. *Hematology*, 1, 136–161.

Gyger, M., Infante-Rivard, C. and D'Angelo, G. (1988) Prognostic value or clonal chromosomal abnormalities in patients with myelodysplastic syndromes. *American Journal of Haematology*, 28 (1), 13–20.

Gupta, G., Singh, R., Kotasthane, D.S. & Kotasthane, V.D. (2010) Myelodysplastic syndromes/neoplasms: recent classification system based on World Health Organisation Classification of Tumors – International Agency for Research on Cancer for Hematopoietic and Lymphoid Tissues. *Journal of Blood Medicine*: 1. 171–182.

Harris, N.L., Jaffe, E.S., Diebold, J. *et al.* (1999) World Health Organisation classification of neoplastic diseases of the haematopoietic and lymphoid tissue: report of the Clinical Advisory Committee meeting (1997) Airline House, Virginia. *Journal of Clinical Oncology*, 17, 3835–3849.

Heaney, M.L. and Golde, D.W. (1999) Medical progress: myelodysplasia. *New England Journal of Medicine*, 340 (21), 1649–1660.

Hellstrom Lindberg, E., Robert, K.H., Gahrton, G. *et al.* (1992) A predictive model for clinical response to low dose ara-C: a study of 102 patients with myelodysplastic syndromes or acute leukaemia. *British Journal of Haematology of Haematology*, 81, 503–511.

Hellstrom Lindberg, E., Ahlgren, T., Beguin, T. *et al.* (1998) Treatment of anaemia in myelodysplastic syndromes with granulocyte stimulating factor plus erythropoietin: results from a randomised phase II study and long-term follow-up of 71 patients. *Blood*, 92, 68–75.

Hughes-Jones, N.C., Wickramasinghe, S.N., Hatton, C.S.R. (2009) *Lecture notes on haematology*, 8th ed. Wiley-Blackwell, Oxford.

Miller, K.B., Head, D.R., Cassileth, P.A. *et al.* (1993) The evaluation of low-dose cytarabine in treatment of myelodysplastic syndromes: a phase-III international group study. *Annals of Hematology*, 65, 162–168.

Mimms, C., Playfair, J., Roitt, I., Wakelin, D. and Williams, R. (1993) *Medical Microbiology*. Mosby, St Louis.

Mufti, G. and Galton, D. (1992) *The Myelodysplastic Syndromes*. Churchill Livingstone, Edinburgh.

Murphy, M.F., Wallington, T.B., Kelsey, P. *et al.* (2001) British Committee for Standards in Haematology, Blood Transfusion Task Force. Guidelines for clinical use of red cell transfusions. *British Journal of Haematology*, 113 (1), 24–31.

Negrin, R., Haeuber, D.H., Nagler, A. *et al.* (1989) Treatment of myelodysplastic syndromes with recombinant human granulocyte colony-stimulating factor: a phase I–II trial. *Annals of International Medicine*, 110, 976–984.

Negrin, R., Stein, R. and Doherty, K. (1996) Maintenance treatment of the anaemia of myelodysplastic syndromes with recombinant human granulocyte colony stimulatory factor and *in vitro* surgery, *Blood*, 87 (10), 4076–4081.

Oscier, C. and Oscier, D. (1997) ABC of haematology, the myelodysplastic syndromes. *British Journal of Medicine*, 314, 883–886.

Ozer, H., Armitage, J.O., Bennett, C.L. *et al.* (2000) 2000 update of recommendations for the use of hematopoietic colony stimulating factors: evidence-based, clinical practice guidelines. American Society of Clinical Oncology Growth Factors Expert Panel. *Journal of Clinical Oncology*, 18, 3558–3585.

Pagliuca, A., Carrington, P.A., Pettingell, R. *et al.* (2003) Guidelines on the use of colony-stimulating factors in haematological malignancies. *British Journal of Haematology*, 123, 22–33.

Sutton, L., Chastang, C. and Ribaud, P. (1996) Factors influencing outcomes in *de novo* MDS treated by allogenic BMT. *Blood*, 88, 358–365.

Treleaven, J., Gennery, A., Marsh, J., Norfolk, D., Page, L., Parker, A., Saran, F., Thurston, J. and Webb, D. (2010) Guidelines on the use of irradiated blood components prepared by the British Committee for Standards in Haematology bloodtransfusion task force. *British Journal of Haematology*, 152, 35–51.

Tricot, G. and Laver, R. (1987) Management of the myelodysplastic syndrome. *Seminars in Oncology*, 14 (4), 444–453.

Tuncer, M., Pagliuca, A. and Hicsonmez, G. (1992) Primary myelodysplastic syndrome in children: the clinical experience in 33 cases. *British Journal of Haematology*, 82 (2), 347–353.

Verburgh, E., Achten, R., Maes, B. *et al.* (2003) Additional prognostic value of bone marrow histology in patients with sub-classified according to the international prognostic scoring system for myelodysplastci syndromes. *Journal of Clinical Oncology*, 21 (2), 273–282.

Chapter 13

Acute leukaemia: pathophysiology, care and management

Jackie Green

After reading this chapter you will:

- Have an overview of the acute leukaemias
- Be able to identify the current classification systems
- Be able to consider the nursing care issues and the need for inter-professional working

---

Introduction

Acute leukaemias are a subclassification of leukaemia. They are subdivided into acute myeloid leukaemia (AML) and acute lymphoblastic leukaemia (ALL). Acute leukaemia is defined by the presence of greater than 20% blasts in the bone marrow at clinical presentation (Jaffe *et al.* 2001). This chapter will look at AML and ALL, its classification, aetiology and the nursing intervention in caring for patients with acute leukaemia.

Acute myeloid leukaemia

Acute myeloid leukaemia occurs due to a proliferation of immature myeloid progenitor cells. There is a presence of 30% myeloid blast cells in the bone marrow (Jaffe *et al.* 2001). It is a disease where the normal controls for cell division and maturation or cell death (apoptosis) is lost. Leukaemia is described as a neoplastic proliferation of cells following haematopoietic origin, which following mutation arises in a single haematopoietic cell. These abnormal cells cause symptoms due to bone marrow failure and infiltration of organs. Increased cell proliferation has metabolic consequences and infiltrating cells also disturb tissue function. Anaemia, neutropenia and thrombocytopenia are important consequences of the bone marrow failure, which may lead to infection, haemorrhage and organ damage.

Classification

Classification of AML is based on morphological and immunological markers. The French American British (FAB) classification is commonly used (see Table 13.1).

Haematology Nursing, First Edition. Marvelle Brown and Tracey J. Cutler.
© 2012 Blackwell Publishing Ltd. Published 2012 by Blackwell Publishing Ltd.

Table 13.1   FAB classification for acute myeloid leukaemia.

M0	Undifferentiated
M1	Without maturation
M2	With granulocytic maturation
M3	Acute promyelocytic
M4	Granulocytic and monocytic maturation
M5	(M5a) monoblastic (M5b) monocytic
M6	Erythroleukaemia
M7	Megakaryoblastic

The FAB classification was originally based on morphological appearance. In 1993 the FAB classification for AML was revised to include the identification of surface markers and cytogenetics, which provide important and prognostic information (Jaffe *et al.* 2001). The World Health Organisation (2008) adopted the Revised European American Lymphoma (REAL) classification system, which acknowledges the importance of cytogenetic changes within cells, this classification is currently being integrated into diagnostic and prognostic classification (Atkinson and Richardson 2006).

Epidemiology and aetiology

Acute myeloid leukaemia is the common form of leukaemia in adults and forms only a minor fraction in children (10–15%). It represents 30% of cancer incidence internationally. However, published incidence indicates AML varies widely. It is not age, gender or ethnicity specific, although the AML incident data for England and Wales indicates that the incidence increases with age (Quinn 2001).

The cause of AML is largely unknown. However, common factors that have been considered are radiation, familial, viruses, genetics, chemicals and drugs. It appears to arise *de novo* and secondarily. It may develop from myelodysplasia and other haematological disease, or develop due to previous treatment with cytotoxic chemotherapy for other diseases. *De novo* and secondary AML are associated with distinct genetic markers and have differing prognosis. Prognosis can be defined as dependent on cell markers and cytogenetics, and also response to initial treatment. All have an influence on prognosis (see Table 13.2).

Diagnostic investigations

Peripheral blood film

- White cell count may be low or high.
- Platelet count may be low.
- Reduced red cell production may be evident.
- Clotting may be abnormal (especially in APML).
- Peripheral blasts may be seen.

Table 13.2   Prognostic indicators in acute myeloid leukaemia.

	Favourable	Unfavourable
Cytogenetics	t(15;17) t(8;21) inv (16)	Deletions of chromosome 5 or 7 Flt – 3 mutation 11q 23 t(6;9) abn (3q) Complex rearrangements
Bone marrow response to remission induction	<5% blasts after first course	>20% blasts after first course
Age	<60 years	>60 years

Bone marrow biopsy (aspirate and trephine)

- This facilitates the ability to subclassify the AML.
- Cytogentics, immunological markers and cytochemistry are required to clearly identify the sub-classification.

Acute myeloid leukaemia subtypes are different genetic diseases, but grouping AML together is accepted as treatment and prognosis is similar, with the exception of acute promyelocytic leukaemia (APML).

Clinical features

Presenting symptoms are variable. Usually individuals present with a short history, frequently days or weeks, with varying symptoms. These symptoms commonly include bone marrow failure. Patients often have had repeated infections, such as urinary tract infection and oral infection. Patients frequently complain of feeling tired, with reduced exercise tolerance, bleeding or bruising and occasionally weight loss. It is also important to recognise that patients may present with no symptoms and the disease is picked up through a routine blood test, which may be done as part of occupational health clearance or a well-person health check.

Treatment

Specific therapy for AML is the use of intensive chemotherapy. This is usually a combination of cytotoxic chemotherapy. The commonly used drugs include: cytosine arabinoside, daunorubicin, idarubicin, etoposide and mitoxantrone. It is usually given over 5–10 days per course and often the patient requires four courses (two inductions and two consolidations). Table 13.3 shows a common example of AML treatment. The chemotherapeutic strategy is to achieve complete remission (CR) by eradicating the blast cells from the bone marrow, allowing healthy cells to regenerate. A complete remission is defined as less than 5% blasts (Lowenberg 1999). The current MRC trials are AML 15 and AML 16 for the over 60-year-old patients; AML 17 has now opened for AML patients from 18 to 60 years old.

Table 13.3 Example of intensive cytotoxic chemotherapy treatment plan for acute myeloid leukaemia.

Course 1 DA 3 + 10

(ARA-C and daunorubicin)

↓

Less than 20% blasts following course 1

Course 2 DA 3 + 8

↓

Complete remission

(<5% blasts in bone marrow)

Course 3 MACE

(amsacrine, cytarabine, etoposide)

↓

Course 4 MIDAC

(mitoxantrone, idarubicin, cytarabine)

↓

Course 5 BMT if eligible

Acute promyelocytic leukaemia (AML M3) variant is associated with t(15:17) transformation. It often presents with disseminated intravascular coagulation (DIC). This is potentially an emergency situation. Patients with this condition may have excessive bleeding. This is caused by the clotting factors being used up from the micro-thrombin in the capillaries and arterioles so there are none remaining in the circulating blood. Essentially the patient is bleeding and clotting simultaneously. It is imperative that the clotting abnormality is corrected. Fresh frozen plasma, platelets and cryoprecipitate is given. The FBC and clotting screen should be monitored at least twice a day and the appropriate clotting products are used. All-trans retinoic acid (ATRA) is given to mature the blast cells and is given in conjunction with cytotoxic chemotherapy.

Haemopoietic stem cell transplantation

Autologous haemopoietic stem cell transplants (HSCT) may reduce the rate of relapse but its role continues to cause debate. There are two schools of thought; some would say that autologous HSCT adds value following consolidation in sustaining CR and others believe that autologous HSCT should be reserved for good risk cases until relapse. Allogeneic HSCT (HLA matched sibling donor) or matched unrelated donor HSCT is used for patients who are clinically and age suitable. The usual agreed age limit is 60, but this is a matter to be considered on an individual basis at the multidisciplinary team meeting. The aim of the allogeneic HSCT is curative intent.

There are studies considering suitable treatment regimes for those over 60. Historically AML therapy for the elderly has demonstrated poor outcomes, because of primary disease resistance, multiple pathology and poor tolerability of intensive treatment protocols.

Clinical trials have considered therapeutic treatment options for over 60s (Melchert 2006). The official outcomes of these AML trials have yet to be published.

Acute lymphoblastic leukaemia

This is a malignant blood disorder caused by the proliferation of lymphoblasts. It is the most common malignancy in childhood, accounting for an estimated 25% of childhood malignancies (Cancer Research UK 2003). Highest incidence age is 3–7 and the incident reduces significantly after the age of 10. There is a secondary rise after the age of 40 (Howard and Hamilton 2002).

Classification

The French American British (FAB) classification is based morphology or immunological phenotype. The FAB classification subdivides ALL into 3 L1, L2 and L3 (see Table 13.4). However, the WHO classification in 2008, outlined two major classifications types: precursor B lymphoblastic leukaemia and precursor T lymphoblastic leukaemia.

Clinical features

Patients with ALL present with variable features depending on the degree of bone marrow failure and other organs affected by the disease. It is not uncommon at presentation that the patient diagnosed with ALL has an accumulation of malignant lymphoblasts in the bone marrow. As a result, like AML, the patients may present with bone infection, anaemia and bleeding. Acute lymphoblastic leukaemia patients frequently complain of joint pain at presentation. This is largely due to the proliferation of blast cells. Other presenting

Table 13.4 ALL classification.

L1	Blasts cells small, uniform high nuclear to cytoplasmic ratio
L2	Blasts cells larger, heterogeneous, lower nuclear cytoplasmic ratio
L3	Vaculolated blasts, basophilic, cytoplasma, usually B cell-ALL

ALL prognostic indicator		
	Good	**Poor**
WBC	Low	High >50 x 109/l
Sex	Girls	Boys
Immunophenotype	c-ALL(CD10+)	B-ALL
Age	Child	Adult or infant <2
Cytogenetics	Normal or hyperdiploidy, >50	Ph +, 11q23
Time to clear blasts from blood	<week	>week
Time to remission	<4 weeks	>4 weeks
CNS disease at presentation	Absent	Present
Minimal residual disease	– at 1–3 months	Still + at 3–6 months

symptoms are abdominal distension, with hepatosplenomegaly and lymphadenopathy (Lieser and Goldstone 1997).

Diagnostic investigations

Acute lymphoblastic leukaemia is diagnosed based on clinical features and blood tests. It is expected that the WBC will be raised, but only 20% of patients have an excess of WBC >50 × 10⁹/L (Howard and Hamilton 2002). The diagnosis is confirmed by a bone marrow biopsy. Cytogenetics and cell markers are helpful prognostic indicators (Reilly 1996). An example is patients who are said to be Philadelphia positive (Ph +ive); this cytogenetic translocation of chromosome 9 and 22 indicates a poorer prognosis.

Treatment

Treatment is similar to that in AML, a combination intensive cytotoxic chemotherapy with or without bone marrow transplant. Combinations of drugs are variable according to protocol. Most combinations will include a steroid, vinca-alkaloid, asparaginase and cytarabine (Bratt-Wyton 2000). High-risk patients will usually receive intrathecal chemotherapy prophylaxis.

Haemopoietic stem cell transplants should be considered for all patients with ALL once remission is achieved. The HSCT of choice would be allogeneic: cells donated form a sibling, with an expected 40% long-term survival (Duncombe 1997). The evidence for improved survival outcomes using autologous HSCT (cells from the patient) is not clear (NICE 2003). Autologous HSCT may be used to allow administration of high doses of cytotoxic chemotherapy (Howard and Hamilton 2002).

Nursing intervention and care of patients with acute leukaemia

The nursing intervention required is predominately focused on chemotherapy administration and its side effects, quality of life issues and symptom management of the disease.

Nursing care of the side effects of chemotherapy

Intensive chemotherapy regimes required to treat acute leukaemia have specific side effects requiring specialised nursing care.

Myelosuppression

It is often considered that the myelosuppression of the bone marrow is the most life-threatening toxicity (Spence and Johnson 2001).

Anaemia and thrombocytopenia

Patients may require blood product support following treatment for acute leukaemia. British Committee for Standards in Haematology guidelines (BSCH 2010) for the administration of blood products should form the template for local transfusion policy. Individuals require information and understanding of the need for transfusion as well as the associated risks. It is recommended that written information is given to support verbal information and consent is obtained (Department of Health 2001). Red blood cells (RBC) and platelets should be ordered, prescribed and administered in line with local policy.

Nurses should observe for signs of anaemia, such as fatigue, shortness of breath, pallor and reduction in activity due to excessive tiredness. Any evidence, and/or a drop in haemoglobin levels should prompt consideration of a red blood cell transfusion. The rationale for use of blood products should be clearly identified and documented. Blood product transfusions are not without their risk (Department of Health 2002).

Nurses must also be aware of signs and symptoms of thrombocytopenia. Spontaneous bleeding is a risk for patients with acute leukaemia (Ancliff and Machin 1998). Bleeding gums, epistaxis, unexplained bruising and a petechial rash are often signs that a patient's platelet count is low. Bleeding can be a frightening experience. Patients and their families require explicit information about what to do if bleeding occurs. It is considered that risk of symptoms related to thrombocytopenia occurs when a patient is febrile. Local policy should be followed as to when to administer a platelet transfusion (BSCH 2003).

Infection risk

Infection risk is a major and potential life-threatening issue for patients with leukaemia (Glauser and Clalandra 2000). This is because they are immunocompromised. Successful and effective management of infection is related to early detection and treatment. Nurses have a key role to play in the identifying infection early. This requires careful assessment of patients. Listen to how they feel; consider whether they are less alert and cheerful, than when you last spoke with them. What are their vital signs; have they altered from previous recordings? Consider potential infection risks, for example intravenous access devices, wound sites, buccal cavity, any loose or offensive bowel action and any burning sensation when passing urine.

If the nursing assessment highlights any potential cause for concern, infection should be suspected and a total infection screen should be undertaken. This should include an MSU, stool specimen, swab from wound sites and intravenous access devices, and blood cultures. Routine full blood count, chemistry, including a C-reactive protein (CRP) may be useful. Antibiotic therapy should be considered and commenced before identifying the source. The source of infection in this patient group is rarely identified (Auner *et al.* 2002). For those patients who are neutropenic, local neutropenic policy should be followed. Working closely with the microbiology team is important to ensure prompt and appropriate treatment. Monitoring this vulnerable patient group closely is essential. Nursing care needs to include strict fluid balance and regular vital signs monitoring, in order to reduce the risk of other organ damage.

Alopecia

Loss of hair can be traumatic for patients, but for this group of patients it is inevitable, due to the combination chemotherapy (Dougherty and Bailey 2001). Nursing staff caring for this group of patients need to prepare them for hair loss. Identifying access to wigs is important and will vary depending on local arrangements.

Fertility

The treatment for acute leukaemia can impact on the individual's fertility. It is essential that as part of the consent to treatment fertility issues are discussed. It is important that patients are given the appropriate support with fertility issues and access to a fertility specialist should be considered (Dannie 2000). Intensive chemotherapy treatment frequently leaves patients infertile. Consideration to sperm banking and ova collection should be given, although it is acknowledged that often the patient's condition does not allow time to arrange sperm banking or ova collection. Ova collection is strictly regulated and not all females may be eligible. The key point is that when patients diagnosed with acute leukaemia are about to embark on intensive cytotoxic chemotherapy, fertility issues must be discussed.

Intravenous access devices

Without exception all patients with leukaemia will require intravenous venous access at some stage. A central venous access device (CVAD) is commonly used, in order to administer the drug therapy and blood products. The care and management of any venous access device should be in accordance with local policy. It should also be considered and the patient assessed for the most appropriate device. The device should be removed immediately it is no longer required, in order to reduce infection risk.

Nausea and vomiting

A side effect of chemotherapy is potential nausea and vomiting. It should not be underestimated that this can cause a debilitating effect. It can lead to low mood or depression, poor nutritional status, non-compliance to treatment and consequently a poorer quality of life (Martin *et al.* 2003). Nursing management of nausea and vomiting is key to minimising the effect it has on the patient. Consideration should be given to administration of an appropriate antiemetic for the administered chemotherapy regime (Roila 1996). With a more moderately emetic regime, such as that used for the treatment of acute leukaemia, a potent antiemetic cover may be required (Doherty 1999), such as a 5HT3 antagonist . Nursing care should also consider non-pharmacological intervention for patients, such as relaxation techniques, discussion about diet and fluid intake.

Symptom management and palliative care

For poor risk patients, patients who have not responded to initial induction therapy or choose not to have intensive cytotoxic chemotherapy, symptom management and palliative care is the option of choice (Booth and Bruera 2003). The concentration of such intervention is not in achieving a remission or a cure for the acute leukaemia, but managing the symptoms of the disease. The reader is guided to chapter 21 which discusses palliative care in haematology.

Bone marrow failure is a significant symptom of acute leukaemia. It may cause lethargy and reduced mobility due a low haemoglobin and lack of oxygenation to the tissue can cause further tissue damage. Low platelets may cause excessive bleeding or bruising. In the short term blood product support may help reduce these symptoms. However, unless you treat the underlying cause of the bone marrow failure at some point blood product support may not be effective or appropriate. Consideration to stopping blood product support must be given. This is often a difficult decision for the patient, family and the clinicians. The important point is that the topic is discussed and plans for care and support put in place when blood product support is no longer effective. It is a significant discussion and one that should take place in an appropriate setting and using breaking bad news communication principles.

Risk of reoccurring infection due to low white cell count and neutropenia requires careful management. Infective episodes in the patient with leukaemia can be life threatening and impact on quality of life. Antibiotic therapy may be appropriate for this group of patients. Consideration should be given when considering admitting patients to hospital for intravenous antibiotics versus the amount of time the person may have at home. We need to consider what the patient wants and what we are trying to achieve. The use of growth factors may be considered to minimise the risk of infection. The use of granulocyte colony stimulating factor (G-CSF) remains a topic of debate. It is considered by some that the use of G-SCF may stimulate further production of the abnormal myeloid cell. There are clinical trials that have looked at the use of G-SCF in preventing infection (AML 15, AML 16). In the case of patients who are not receiving intensive treatment it is usually a decision made with the clinician in charge of the patient's care, the patient and family. Infection screening should be undertaken if suspected in order to identify the potential cause and appropriate antibiotic sensitivity.

Managing a high white cell count

Patients may present with a high white cell count (WCC), usually over 100×10^9/L. This will need intervention to reduce the WCC before commencing intensive chemotherapy. This can be achieved usually in one of two ways: (1) Use of hydroxycarbamide (2) Leucopheresis (this means using a cell separator machine). The machine separates the blood into components and the white blood cells are removed via venous access; the remainder is returned to the patient via another venous access device. The significant point with a high WCC that nurses need to be aware of is that increased WCC means that the circulating blood is very thick and viscous, leading to leucostasis (blockage). This can cause a stroke, renal or lung problems. In order to help reduce the thickness of the blood the patient needs to be well hydrated. An accurate fluid balance chart must be maintained and the patient requires at least 2–3 litres of fluid every 24 hours. This can be a combination of oral and intravenous. It is also important that blood product prescriptions are queried with the prescriber as these blood products can increase the viscosity of the circulating blood and should be avoided until the WCC has been successfully reduced.

Specific nursing intervention

Nursing plays a significant role in the treatment, care and management of patients diagnosed with acute leukaemia. A diagnosis of leukaemia may be perceived by many as a 'death sentence', it certainly leaves newly diagnosed patients and their family considering their mortality. Nurses may be best placed to help patients explore how they feel and to create opportunities for patients and their family to ask questions. Nurses should consider appropriate referral to an accredited counsellor. Patients who are kept informed of diagnostic tests, interventions required and have the opportunity to express feelings and ask questions may adjust to the diagnosis and are better placed to make informed choices. Nurses are in a good position to facilitate this.

Nursing intervention requires support, care and management of the side effects of cytotoxic chemotherapy: bone marrow failure as previously discussed, nausea, vomiting, mucositis, hair loss, biochemical imbalance, and skin and taste changes, which may lead to poor nutritional intake.

Intensive cytotoxic chemotherapy for patients diagnosed with acute leukaemia requires long stays in hospital, usually 4–5 weeks at a time. The impact of this for the patient can be immense. It may lead to loss of role identity, for example a mother diagnosed with acute leukaemia who usually walks her children to school and helps them with their homework may be unable to do this due to her hospital admission. Nursing staff are in an ideal position to encourage the patient to discuss role changes and the impact this may have. It is possible that through discussion solutions may be identified, for example getting the children to bring in their homework for their mother to look at and help with, as appropriate.

Due to the fact that the patient requires a prolonged length of hospital stay the nurses caring for this cohort of patients are in a privileged position, and should be able to build up a good relationship. This relationship should allow the opportunity for frank and open discussions. As part of the nursing role a supportive strategy should be agreed and should include: fluid intake (at least two litres daily), observing for bruising and bleeding, monitoring for signs of infection, and consideration to appropriate dietary intake should be given, as well as considering quality of life issues.

Patients may be eligible for entry into a clinical trial looking at the treatment for acute leukaemia. Clinical trials are a significant part of health care development and nurses acting as the patient's advocate at the multidisciplinary team meetings play a pivotal role in identifying patients who are eligible to be considered for entry into a clinical trial. Nurses have a key role in allowing patients to participate in treatment decisions. This means that the nurse has a role to ensure that information, both verbal and written, is offered to the patients about their illness and treatment. It should be remembered that 'too little' information or information being given 'at the wrong time' are frequent complaints highlighted by patients.

The clinical nurse specialist is usually considered the patient's key worker, a point of contact and an advocate. It is important that patients and relatives are given contact details, both during working hours and outside working hours in case they have any concerns. There needs to be clear instructions and guidance as to what to do in an emergency. The multidisciplinary team are instrumental in considering the patient's treatment plan. The nurse is a core member of the multidisciplinary team in considering the patients physical, psychological and spiritual care.

Conclusion

Acute leukaemia is a potentially life-threatening diagnosis. It is a disease that is not age specific. Treatment intent is to achieve complete remission and a potential cure. Expert care and knowledge is required to care for this group of patients. The nursing role in the care and management of the patient is pivotal to achieving this. Expert nursing care is required to manage the side effects of intensive cytotoxic chemotherapy, help identify the patient's psychological and social needs, and create opportunities for patients to discuss fears and concerns. This is an important aspect of nursing care. Acute leukaemia is treatable and the prognosis of acute leukaemia has been improving steadily over the years. Clinical trials play an important role in achieving this. Treatment for those diagnosed over 60 years of age has improved and clinical trials have begun to address the difficult questions of treatment choice.

References

Ancliff, P. and Machin, S. (1998) Trigger factors for the prophylactic platelet transfusion. *Blood Reviews*, 12, 234–238.

Atkinson, J. and Richardson, C. (2006) The leukaemias. In: *Nursing in Haematological Oncology* (ed. M. Grundy). Chapter 4, pp. 61–83. Baillière Tindall, Edinburgh.

Auner, H., Sil, H., Mulabecirovic, A. *et al.* (2002) Infectious complications after autologous hematopeitic stem cell transplantation: comparison of patients with acute myeloid leukaemia, malignant lymphoma and multiple myeloma. *Annals of Haematology*, 81 (7), 374–377.

Booth, S. and Bruera, E. (2003) *Palliative Care Consultations in Haemato-oncology*. Oxford University Press, Oxford.

Bratt-Wyton, R. (2000) The leukaemias. In: *Nursing in Haematological Oncology* (ed. M. Grundy). pp. 44–59. Baillière Tindall, Edinburgh.

British Committee for Standards in Haematology (1999) Guidelines for the administration of blood components and the management of transfused patients. *Transfusion Medicine*, 227–238.

British Committee for Standards in Haematology (2003) Guidelines for platelet transfusion. *British Journal of Haematology*, 122, 10–23.

Cancer Research UK (2003) *Cancer Stats – Leukaemia – UK*. CRUK, London.

Dannie, E. (2000) Fertility issues. In: *Nursing in Haematological Oncology* (ed. M. Grundy). pp. 236–249. Baillière Tindall, Edinburgh.

Department of Health (2001) Good practice in consent implantation guideline: consent to examination or treatment. *Health Service Circular* 2001/023. DoH, London.

Department of Health (2002) Better blood transfusion – appropriate use of blood. *Health Service Circular* 2002/009 (England). DoH, London.

Doherty, K. (1999) Closing the gap in prophylatic antiemetic therapy: patient factors in calculating the emetogentic potential of chemotherapy. *Clinical Journal of Oncology Nursing*, 3 (3), 113–119.

Dougherty, L. and Bailey, C. (2001) Chemotherpay. In: *Cancer Nursing: Care in Context* (eds J. Corner and C. Bailey). pp. 179–221. Blackwell Publishing Ltd, Oxford.

Duncombe, A. (1997) ABC of clinical haematology bone marrow and stem cell transplantation. *British Medical Journal*, 126, 1179–1191.

Field, D., Douglous, C., Jagger, C. *et al.* (1995) Terminal Illness: views of patients and their lay carers. *Palliative Medicine*, 9, 45–54.

Glauser, M. and Clalandra, T. (2000) Infections in patients with haematologic malignancies. In: *Management of Infections in Immunocompromised Patients* (eds M. Glauser and P. Pizzo). pp. 141–188. WB Saunders, London.

Howard, M. and Hamilton, P. (2002) *Haematology: an Illustrated Colour Text*, 2nd edition. Churchill Livingstone, Edinburgh.

Jaffe, E., Harris, N., Stein, H. *et al.* (2001) *Pathology and Genetics of Tumours of Haempoetic and Lymphoid Tissues*. IARC Press, Lyon.

Lieser, R. and Goldstone, A. (1997) ABC clinical haematology: acute leukaemias. *British Medical Journal*, 314, 1103–1113.

Lowenberg, B., Downing, J. and Burnett, A. (1999) Acute myeloid leukaemia. *New England Journal of Medicine*, 341, 1051–1062.

Martin, C., Rubenstein, E., Elting, L. *et al.* (2003) Measuring chemotherapy induced nausea and emesis. *Cancer*, 98, 645–655.

Melchert, M. (2006) Managing acute myeloid leukaemia in the elderly. *Oncology*, 20 (13).

National Institute of Clinical Excellence (2003) *Improving Outcomes Guidance in Haematological Cancers: the Manual*. NICE, London.

Quinn, M., Babb, P., Brock, A. *et al.* (2001) *Cancer Trends in England and Wales 1950–1999*, Vol. SMPS no. 66. TSO, London.

Reilly, J. (1996) The role of cytology, cytochemistry, immunophenotyping and cytogenetic analysis in the diagnosis of haematological neoplasms, *Clinical Lab Haem*, 108, 19–30.

Roila, F., Tomato, M., Ballatori, E. *et al.* (1996) Comparative studies of various antiemetic regimes. *Supportive Care in Cancer*, 4, 270–280.

Spence, R. and Johnson, P. (2001) *Oncology*. Oxford University Press, Oxford.

World Health Organisation (2008) *Pathology and Genetics. Tumors of Haematopoietic and Lymphoid Tissue*. 4th edition. WHO, Geneva.

Chapter 14

Chronic leukaemia: pathophysiology, care and management

Samantha Toland

After reading this chapter you will be able to:

- Describe the presenting features of both chronic myeloid leukaemia and chronic lymphocytic leukaemia
- Understand the diagnostic techniques used in identifying chronic leukaemias
- Identify the current treatment options available for patients with chronic leukaemias

---

Chronic myeloid leukaemia

Chronic myeloid leukaemia (CML) is a clonal malignant myeloproliferative disorder, originating from an abnormal pluripotent stem cell. The progeny of this abnormal stem cell proliferate over months or years, so that by the time leukaemia is diagnosed, the bone marrow is filled with numerous abnormal cells and peripheral blood contains large numbers of leucocytes (Goldman 2007). Chronic myeloid leukaemia has three clinical phases – a relatively benign 'chronic phase', followed by the more advanced, ominous 'accelerated phase' and finally an almost invariably fatal acute leukaemic phase termed 'blast crisis' (Howard and Hamilton 2008). The disease accounts for around 15% of leukaemias and may occur at any age. Annual incidence is around 1 per 100,000 with presentation most common in the fifth and sixth decades of life (Atkinson and Richardson 2006). Diagnosis is increasingly made in asymptomatic patients having routine blood tests (Howard and Hamilton 2008).

Diagnosis

The major diagnostic tool is a full blood count and peripheral blood film, which will point to the diagnosis of CML; bone marrow is also examined as confirmation (Atkinson and Richardson 2006). Blood film shows greatly increased numbers of leucocytes, with many immature forms. Marrow examination shows increased cellularity and distribution of immature leucocytes resembling that seen in the blood film (Goldman 2007). Chronic myeloid leukaemia is characterised by the presence of a Philadelphia (Ph)

Haematology Nursing, First Edition. Marvelle Brown and Tracey J. Cutler.
© 2012 Blackwell Publishing Ltd. Published 2012 by Blackwell Publishing Ltd.

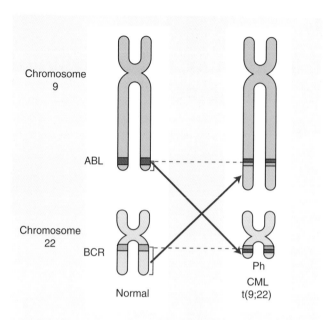

Figure 14.1 Philadelphia chromosome (from Hoffbrand *et al.* 2006). Reprinted with permission of John Wiley & Sons, Inc.

chromosome – the t(9:22) (q34:q11) chromosomal translocation. This translocation results in part of the proto-oncogene c-ABL moving to the BCR gene on chromosome 22, and part of chromosome 22 moving to chromosome 9. The abnormal chromosome 22 is the Philadelphia chromosome. The resulting chimeric BCR-ABL gene codes for a fusion protein that has excessive tyrosine kinase activity (Hoffbrand *et al.* 2006) (see Figure 14.1). Over 95% of classical CML cases are Ph positive.

Presentation

Patients usually present in the chronic phase, when they will display typical symptoms of anaemia, anorexia, weight loss and splenomegaly. Occasionally patients present with gout or hyperviscosity associated with high serum uric acid and a high white cell count (Howard and Hamilton 2008). Often the disease is detected as a result of routine blood tests performed for unrelated reasons – up to 50% of patients are completely asymptomatic at time of diagnosis. Rarer features include non-specific fever, lymphadenopathy, visual disturbances due to leucostasis, retinal haemorrhages, splenic pain, gout and occasionally priapism (Goldman 2007).

Treatment

Hydroxyurea can be used to rapidly reduce a high white cell count in chronic phase CML. It is useful as a short-term measure for newly diagnosed patients or an interim measure for patients resistant to imatinib, while other more definitive treatments are being considered (Goldman 2007). Tyrosine kinase inhibitors (TKIs) such as imatinib, are specific inhibitors of the BCR-ABL fusion protein, and block tyrosine kinase activity. Imatinib is the first-line drug in the management of chronic phase disease and is able to produce a complete haematological response in virtually all previously untreated patients (Hoffbrand *et al.* 2006). Of patients who respond, 70–80% will achieve complete cytogenetic remission (Goldman 2007). At a continuous oral dose of 400 mg daily, very high rates of haematological, cytogenetic and molecular responses can be obtained with limited toxicity. These impressive response rates are accompanied by high levels of short-term, progression-free survival, particularly for patients with the greatest reduction in BCR-ABL transcripts. Longer term results are uncertain as patients may develop resistance to imatinib but may still respond to other tyrosine kinase inhibitors (Howard and Hamilton 2008).

There are various possibilities for managing patients who become resistant to imatinib and whose disease is still in chronic phase. Allogeneic HSCT is a possibility if the patient is relatively young and has an HLA-identical sibling or well-matched unrelated donor. A reasonable option for patients without any matched donor would be to switch to a second generation TKI, namely dasatinib, or nilotinib (Goldman 2007).

Haemopoietic stem cell transplant

Allogeneic haemopoietic stem cell transplant (HSCT) is at present the only proven curative treatment for CML. Patients have survived for over ten years after HSCT, with no detectable BCR-ABL transcripts in blood or bone marrow. Five-year, leukaemia-free survival after HLA identical sibling HSCT is around 60%. Use of low intensity conditioning prior to allogeneic HSCT allows the procedure in older patients. In younger patients, use of HLA-matched unrelated donor is possible, but results are poorer than for sibling donor HSCT. Autologous HSCT can induce Philadelphia negative haematopoiesis, but therapeutic value is unproven (Howard and Hamilton 2008).

Advanced phase disease

Acute transformation (20% or more blasts in the marrow) may occur rapidly over days or weeks. More commonly, there is an accelerated phase with anaemia, thrombocytopenia and an increase in basophils, eosinophils or blast cells in the blood and marrow which can last for several months and is less easy to control. In most cases, transformation is to AML or mixed types – in one-fifth of cases transformation is lymphoblastic and patients may be treated in a similar way to acute lymphoblastic leukaemia (Hoffbrand *et al.* 2006). Imatinib may derive short-term benefit for patients in accelerated phase, which can re-establish chronic phase disease and even Ph negative haemopoeisis in some cases (Goldman 2007). Imatinib is also valuable in blastic transformation, but resistance usually occurs within a few weeks (Hoffbrand *et al.* 2006). However, imatinib has no role in the management of patients who received this for prior chronic disease (Goldman 2007). Blast crises can be treated with combination chemotherapy regimens used in acute leukaemia. Haemopoietic stem cell transplant is usually offered to younger patients with an HLA-matched donor, but results are less good than in chronic phase (Hoffbrand *et al.* 2006).

Chronic lymphocytic leukaemia

Chronic lymphocytic leukaemia (CLL) is characterised by clonal proliferation of mature lymphocytes (Howard and Hamilton 2008). There is considerable overlap with the lymphomas (Hoffbrand *et al.* 2006). It is the most common form of leukaemia in the Western world and mostly affects the elderly – almost all patients are over 50 years of age at the time of diagnosis with a peak incidence at between 60 and 80 years. There is a seven-fold increase in the risk of CLL in close relatives of patients (Hoffbrand *et al.* 2006). Overall, incidence is about 3/100000 per year and it makes up 40% of all leukaemia patients over 65 years of age (Leukaemia Research 2007). There is great variation in presentation – many patients survive long periods of time with minimal symptoms, whilst others have rapid demise with marrow failure, bulky lymphadenopathy and hepatosplenomegaly. The majority of patients are fortunately the former and diagnosis is increasingly being made by chance on routine blood counts (Howard and Hamilton 2008).

Diagnosis

Diagnosis is often made during routine blood count and is suggested by a raised lymphocyte count (Elphee 2008). Symmetrical enlargement of cervical, axillary or inguinal lymph nodes is a frequent clinical sign and tonsillar enlargement may be a feature (Hoffbrand *et al.* 2006). Chronic lymphocytic leukaemia is diagnosed by elevated lymphocyte count (from 5–500 x 10^9/L) and by flow cytometry, which will identify surface antigens, indicating that it is a monoclonal population. Bone marrow aspirate shows an increase in the number of small lymphocytes, and trephine biopsy is used to identify lymphocyte infiltration (Howard and Hamilton 2008). Blood film will show 70–99% of white blood cells to be small lymphocytes, and smudge or smear cells are also present (see Figure 14.2). Immunophenotyping shows these lymphocytes to be B-cells, surface CD19+, weakly expressing surface immunoglobulin (IgM or IgD) (Hoffbrand *et al.* 2006).

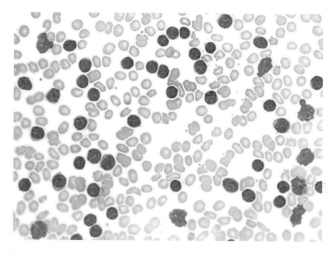

Figure 14.2   Smudge cell for CLL (from Hoffbrand *et al.* 2006). Reprinted with permission of John Wiley & Sons, Inc.

Presentation

As previously mentioned, diagnosis is often made through routine blood tests and therefore patients are asymptomatic at this time. Other classic signs include enlarged lymph nodes, hepatomegaly, splenomegaly, anaemia and thrombocytopenia (Hoffbrand *et al.* 2006). Around 15% of patients will present with 'B' symptoms, including weight loss, night sweats, fatigue and fever (Elphee 2008). Immunosuppression can be a significant problem, with bacterial infections predominating early in the disease, and viral/fungal infections such as herpes zoster appearing in advanced disease (Hoffbrand *et al.* 2006).

Staging

There are two staging systems for CLL, the Rai and the Binet systems (see Tables 14.1 and 14.2). These are useful in helping to make decisions as to instituting treatment, and for assessing prognosis (Elphee 2008).

Table 14.1   Rai classification.

Stage	
0	Absolute lymphocytosis >15 x 10^9/L
I	As stage 0 + enlarged lymph nodes (adenopathy)
II	As stage 0 + enlarged liver and/or spleen ± adenopathy
III	As stage 0 + anaemia (Hb<10 g/dL) ± adenopathy ± organomegaly
IV	As stage 0 + thrombocytopenia (platelets <100 x 10^9/l) ± adenopathy ± organomegaly

Table 14.2   Binet classification.

Stage (% affected)	Organ enlargement	Haemoglobin (g/dL)	Platelets (x 10^9/L)
A (50–60%)	0, 1 or 2 areas		
B (30%)	3, 4 or 5 areas	≥10	≥100
C (<20%)	Not considered	<10	and/or<100

Treatment

Treatment for CLL is generally aimed at slowing disease progression and managing symptoms, rather than a cure (Elphee 2008). Patients who are well, with stable disease, may be watched without treatment – chemotherapy given too early can actually shorten rather than prolong life expectancy. Treatment is generally given for troublesome organomegaly, haemolytic episodes and bone marrow suppression (Hoffbrand *et al.* 2006).

Chemotherapy

Purine antagonists such as fludarabine have been suggested to be more effective than the more traditionally used alkylating agents such as chlorambucil. However, a Cochrane review by Steurer *et al.* (2009) found that fludarabine results in higher response rates, but there was inconclusive evidence as to whether this improves overall survival. Fludarabine is now frequently used in combination with cyclophosphamide (Elphee 2008). More recently, the National Institute for Clinical Excellence (NICE) (2009) have released guidance relating to the use of rituximab in combination with fludarabine and cyclophosphamide, recommending this combination for first-line treatment of CLL in patients for whom fludarabine and cyclophosphamide treatment is appropriate (NICE 2009). Bendamustine is another alkylating agent which is recommended as an option for first-line treatment of CLL in patients for whom fludarabine combination chemotherapy is not appropriate (NICE 2011). Alemtuzumab (Campath, Mabcampath) is an anti-CD52 monoclonal antibody which targets a surface protein on CLL B-cells as well as normal T and B-cells (Wierda *et al.* 2005). It may be used early on in treatment but also has a valuable role in resistant and relapsed disease. However, it is highly immunosuppressive, so antiviral and antibacterial prophylaxis is advisable (Hoffbrand *et al.* 2006). Studies evaluating the effectiveness of alemtuzumab alone or in combination with chemotherapy are currently under way (Elter *et al.* 2009).

Allogeneic HSCT can offer a possible cure or prolonged disease free survival. However, it comes with considerable mortality risk and is not appropriate for all patients. Patients under 65 who have not had success with conventional treatment and otherwise have a poor prognosis may be the best candidates for this procedure (Elphee 2008).

Course of disease

Many patients in Binet stage A or Rai stage 0 or I may never need therapy. For those who do need treatment, a typical pattern is of a disease that is responsive to several courses of chemotherapy before gradual onset of extensive marrow infiltration, bulky lymphadenopathy and recurrent infection. The disease may transform into a localised high grade lymphoma or the disease may become more refractory to treatment over time (Hoffbrand *et al.* 2006).

The nursing care for patients with chronic leukaemia share similarities outlined in chapters 13, 18 and 20, depending on treatment interventions.

Conclusion

Chronic leukaemias predominately occur in adults and for a significant number of patients diagnosis is incidental.

Is important that nurses have a sound understanding of treatment interventions to best advise and support the patient. Concerns regarding the unpredictable nature of the disease becoming aggressive can be very stressful and therefore providing opportunities for patients to discuss the anxieties and if necessary to make appropriates referral is essential.

References

Atkinson, J. and Richardson, C. (2006) Acute leukaemias. In: *Nursing in Haematological Oncology* (ed. M. Grundy). Baillière Tindall, Edinburgh.

Elphee, E.E. (2008) Caring for patients with chronic lymphocytic leukemia. *Clinical Journal of Oncology Nursing*, 12 (3).

Elter. T., Weingar, T.O., Bauer, K. *et al.* (2009) *Alemtuzumab for Chronic Lymphocytic Leukaemia (Protocol) Cochrane review*. Wiley, London.

Goldman, J.M. (2007) Chronic myeloid leukaemia. In: *ABC of Clinical Haematology* (ed. D. Provan). Blackwell, Oxford.

Hoffbrand, A.V., Moss, P.A.H. and Pettit, J.E. (2006) *Essential Haematology*, 5th edition. Blackwell Publishing Ltd, Oxford.

Howard, M.R. and Hamilton, P.J. (2008) *Haematology: an Illustrated Colour Text*, 3rd edition. Churchill Livingstone Elsevier, London.

Leukaemia Research (2007) *Chronic Lymphocytic Leukaemia (CLL)*. Leukaemia Research, London.

National Institute for Health and Clinical Excellence (NICE) (2009) *Rituximab for the First-line Treatment of Chronic Lymphocytic Leukaemia*. National Institute for Health and Clinical Excellence, London.

National Institute for Health and Clinical Excellence (NICE) (2011) *Bendamustine for the First-line Treatment of Chronic Lymphocytic Leukaemia*. National Institute for Health and Clinical Excellence, London.

Steurer, M., Paul, G., Richards, S., Schwarzer, G., Bohlius, J. and Greil, R. (2006) *Purine Antagonists for Chronic Lymphocytic Leukaemia (Review) Cochrane Review*. Wiley, London.

Wierda, W., O'Brien, S., Wen, S. *et al.* (2005) Chemoimmunotherapy with fludarabine, cyclophosphamide and rituximab for relapsed and refractory chronic lymphocytic leukaemia. *Journal of clinical Oncology*, 20, 23 (18), 4070–4078.

Chapter 15

Multiple myeloma: pathophysiology, care and management

Marvelle Brown

At the end of reading this chapter you should:

- Have an understanding of which marrow cell causes MM
- Be able to describe the pathology of MM
- Have an awareness of the treatment options
- Be familiar with nursing care for the patient with MM

Introduction

Multiple myeloma (MM), also known as myelomatosis or Kahler's disease (named after the Austrian physician who first described MM (Raab *et al.* 2009)), accounts for 1% of all cancers and is the second commonest haemato-oncological disease in the United Kingdom (Devenney and Erickson 2004). It is an incurable disease and nurses need to be very aware of the emotional challenges patients and their family face. This chapter will discuss the pathology of MM, the role cytokines play in its development, the staging systems used to determine severity and guide treatment options, and explore key nursing skills and management interventions.

Pathology of multiple myeloma

B-cells begin their development and subsequent maturity in the bone marrow. As described in Chapter 1, B-cells go through several stages of differentiation, eventually maturing into plasma cells. Plasma cells are the functional mature cell of B-cell differentiation and secrete immunoglobulins (antibodies), which provide humoral immunity. Immunoglobulins are classified into five categories, outlined in Table 15.1. Immunoglobulins have a 'Y' monomer structure, composed of light chains, which form the upper part of the immunoglobulin, and heavy chains, which form the lower half. It is the heavy chain which determines the classification of the immunoglobulin. The light chain structure of the immunoglobulin is

---

Haematology Nursing, First Edition. Marvelle Brown and Tracey J. Cutler.

Table 15.1   Classification of immunoglobulins.

IgA – alpha
IgD – delta
IgE – Epsilon
IgG – gamma
IgM – mu

Table 15.2   Conditions producing M-proteins (adapted from King 2006; Hoffbrand and Moss 2011).

Monoclonal gammopathy of undetermined origin (MGUS)
Solitary plasmacytoma
Non-Hodgkins lymphoma
Chronic lymphocytic leukaemia
Waldenström's macroglobulinaemia
Heavy chain disease
Gaucher's disease
Plasma cell leukaemia
Non-secretary myeloma
Smouldering (asymptomatic) myeloma
Primary amyloidosis
Osteosclerotic myeloma (POEMS syndrome)

either kappa or Lambda. The gene for kappa is found on chromosome 2, the Lambda gene is found on chromosome 22 and chromosome 14 carries the gene for the heavy chain (Ross *et al*. 2005; Shaughnessy Jr and Stewart 2004).

See Chapter 1 'Normal blood physiology and Chapter 2 'Immunology', for more details of B-cell and antibody development and functions.

Multiple myeloma is a malignancy of plasma cells, leading to the proliferation of mono-clonal immunoglobulin's (M-protein), which are non-functioning cells. The abundance of immunoglobulins are known as paraproteins and they have the same structure as their normal counterpart and therefore produce an M-band on protein electrophoresis. Malignant plasma cells can also produce incomplete antibodies which are light chains known as Bence-Jones proteins (BJPs) (Hughes-Jones *et al*. 2009).

There are a number of illnesses which can produce M-band proteins which are investi-gated to enable confirmation or exclusion of a MM diagnosis. These are outlined in Table 15.2.

Monoclonal gammopathy of underdetermined significance (MGUS) is a benign condi-tion, but can be a potentially prolonged prophase to MM, and evidence suggests that almost all patients with MM previously had MGUS (Bladé *et al*. 2009; Rajkumar 2005).

Our increased knowledge of the microenvironment or the 'niche', of the bone marrow, enables a greater understanding of how myeloma cells are able to thrive in the bone mar-row, causing bone destruction, pain, compromisation of the immune system and leading to haematopoietic dysfunction. Podar *et al*. (2009, p. 61) describe niches as: 'the physical entities composed of stromal cells which maintain haematopoietic cells, quiescence,

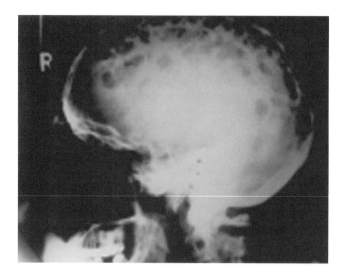

Figure 15.1 Radiograph of the skull of a patient with multiple myeloma showing multiple discrete osteolytic lesions with no sclerosis at the margin (from Hughes-Jones *et al.* 2009). Reprinted with permission of John Wiley & Sons, Inc.

maintenance, expansion and survival as well as enable their migration'. These activities are tightly controlled by mechanisms involved in cell-to-cell interactions, which control cellular, extracellular and fluid compartment activities, supported by a complex circulatory system. How MM causes significant disturbances in the microenvironment of the bone marrow, leading to major problems will be discussed, but first it is worth noting the normal mechanisms involved in bone remodelling to form the basis for understanding what happens the skeleton system in MM.

The normal process of bone remodelling involves a balance between osteoclast and osteoblast activities. When the bone is 'tired' or fatigued, it attracts osteoclasts, which remove the fatigued bone by resorption, creating a cavity. Osteoblasts are attracted to the cavity, filling it with a matrix framework, eventually forming new bone. This is referred to as bone remodelling. This process is essential in maintaining the mechanical integrity of the skeleton and helps with calcium homeostasis. In MM there is an imbalance between osteoclasts and osteoblasts in which osteoclasts resorption is occurring faster than osteoblasts can carry out bone formation and hence results in weakening the bone by causing osteolytic lesions. A significant cause of this disturbance is due to interactions and altered behaviours of a number of cytokines (Klein *et al.* 2007).

The increased osteoclast activity is caused by osteoclast activating factors, (OAFs) such as interleukin-1 (IL-1) and tumor necrosis factor (TNF). Osteoclast activating factors stimulate the BM to produce another growth factor RANKL (receptor activator for nuclear factor K B ligand), also known as TNF-related activation-induced cytokine (TRANCE), TRANCE (RANKL) (Klein *et al.* 2011). This encourages the development of osteoclasts, leading to an increase in their activity, enabling increased destruction of the bone. As a result of the increased osteoclast activity and a reduction in osteoblasts to repair the bone, osteolytic lesions occur, leading to the release of calcium, causing hypercalcaemia (see Figure 15.1). Other cytokines including, insulin-like growth factor (IGF-1), vascular endothelial growth factor (VEGF), tumour growth factor –β (TGF-β) and stromal derived growth factor -1α (SDG-1α), are also involved in the progression of the disease (Podar *et al*. 2009).

In addition to cytokine interactions, myeloma cells have an adhesive molecular structure on their surfaces which allows them to bind onto VCAM-1 (vascular cell adhesion molecule -1), found on stromal cells which are on the structural cells of the BM (Podar *et al*. 2009). Increased production of interleukin 6 (IL-6) by the stromal cells plays a key role in MM. Interleukin 6 stimulates myeloma growth and prevents apoptosis. It is unclear whether IL-6 is a paracrine growth factor (produced by the tumour environment of the BM) or an autocrine growth factor (produced by the myeloma cells) (Dankbar *et al*. 2000).

The interactions of cytokines and the binding ability of the myeloma cells disturbs the BM microenvironment in MM leading to:

- Increased tumour growth and expansion
- Inhibition of apoptosis (natural cell death)
- Promotion of angiogenesis (development of new blood vessels) and promotion of bone resorption (Cao *et al*. 2010)

Ultimately, the impact of MM is impaired haemopoiesis, inadequate immunity and renal dysfunction.

Epidemiology, aetiology, genetics and incidence

There are approximately 4000 new cases per year in the UK (Cancer Research UK 2007). It primarily occurs from the fifth decade; however, MM has been diagnosed in younger adults. The incidence of MM will potentially increase due to an aging population and earlier recognition and diagnosis. The incidence of MM is higher in black men and there appears to be no explanation for this difference in incidence between black men and other ethnic communities (Alexander *et al*. 2007).

The aetiology is unknown but there has been some suggested associations with occupational exposure to certain chemicals such as benzene and pesticides; dieldrin, chlorothalonil, dichlorodiphenyltrichloroethane (DDT), but nothing has been proven conclusively (Landgren *et al*. 2009). In addition, it has been suggested there is a possible link with a dysfunctional immune system and the lack of effective surveillance to detect and destroy malignant cells (Morgan *et al*. 2002). Many patients with MM have chromosomal and genetic abnormalities. Deletion of chromosome 13, translocations of chromosome 14, t(4;14), t(14;16) have been found to carry a poor prognosis and mutation of the RAS oncogene increases IL-6 activity (Hideshima *et al*. 2007; IMWG 2009).

Signs and symptoms

The signs and symptoms of multiple myeloma are shown in Table 15.3.

Table 15.3   Signs and symptoms of multiple myeloma.

Bone marrow failure	Anaemia is usually normocytic or macrocytic. Mucosal haemorrhage may occur due to antibody interference and platelet dysfunction.
Skeletal damage	Bone destruction, particularly lumbar spine, is a common site for skeletal damage and pain. The osteolytic lesions causes weakness and potential for pathological compression fractures of the vertebra can cause spinal cord damage.
Renal dysfunction	Hypercalcaemia, amyloid deposits in the glomeruli and light chain can lead to renal dysfunction. Chronic renal failure can result from protein deposits (BJPs) damaging distal renal tubules leading to tubular atrophy and interstitial fibrosis known as the myeloma kidney. Dehydration and hyperuricaemia can be a precipitate of acute renal failure.
Infections	Respiratory infections are common in MM. This is due to lack of normal antibodies which increase the risk of infections from bacterial organisms such as *Streptococcus pneumoniae*, *Staphylococcus aureus* and *Haemophilus influenzae*. *Escherichia coli (E. coli)* is a common cause of pyelonephritis.
Hypercalcaemia	Leads to vomiting, anorexia, lethargy stupor and coma. Patients may present with polyuria and polydipsia.
Hyperviscosity syndrome	Increased viscosity due to the paraproteins, Ig A the main cause of plasma hyperviscosity, which is characterised by neurological disturbances (dizziness, somnolence, headaches, coma), cardiac failure and haemorrhagic manifestations.
Amyloidosis	Peripheral neuropathy, macroglossia, cardiomegaly, diarrhoea and carpal tunnel syndrome.
Neurological disturbances	Mental confusion, weakness or numbness of the legs and arms.

Investigations

Skeletal X-ray, CAT (computer assisted tomography) and MRI (magnetic resonance imaging) can be undertaken. Bone marrow aspiration may show an increase in plasma cells, which may be pleomorphic (various shaped cells). The increase in antibodies leads to a raised erythrocyte sedimentation rate (ESR) (Hoffbrand and Moss 2011). Haematological investigations would demonstrate impaired haemopoiesis, reduced haemoglobin concentration and plasma cell count of > 20%. Erythrocytes tend to be rouleaux in shape. Rouleaux is the stacking up of red blood cells, caused by extra or abnormal proteins in the blood that decrease the normal distance red cells maintain between each other (Greer *et al.* 2009). Protein electrophoresis will determine abnormal M-proteins in serum. The most common paraprotein is IgG, with 50% of patients presenting with this, followed by approximately 25% of patients with IgA paraproteins. Paraproteins of IgD and IgE are rare. IgM paraprotein is more commonly associated with Waldenström's macroglobulinemia.

Urinalysis is undertaken to identify Bence-Jones proteins. Renal function tests to determine any renal damage forms part of the investigation process. Blood urea above 14 mmol/L and serum creatinine above 20% would be suspicious of renal damage. The β_2-microglobulin (β_2M) levels measure proteins, which are shed by B-cells and correlates with a myeloma cell mass and is a useful aid in prognosis (Bataille *et al.* 1992). A β_2-microglobulin (β_2M) level of below 4 mg/L offers a good prognosis (Hoffbrand and Moss 2011). In some patients, serum calcium levels may also be raised (>9–10.5 mg/dL).

Diagnosis

Following investigations, diagnosis is based on the following findings:

1   Skeletal survey demonstrating osteolytic lesions; fractures are a common presentation
2   Bone marrow – plasma cells above 4–30%, containing myeloma cells; immunological tests, which confirmed M-proteins
3   M-proteins found in serum and urine or both
4   BJPs found in urine

Staging of multiple myeloma

Once a diagnosis confirms MM, staging of the disease is undertaken, using either Durie-Salmon staging (DSS) (Durie and Salmon 1975) or the more recently developed, International Staging System (ISS) (Greipp *et al.* 2005). Neither method has proven superior over the other and both use different prognostic parameters and are therefore commonly used in combination. The DSS predicts tumour mass and survival based on the levels of immunoglobin proteins, haemoglobin, calcium concentrations, level of anaemia, platelet count and number of bone lesions (see Table 15.4). The ISS, on the other hand, is based on levels of serum β_2 microglobulin and albumin proteins (Grieep *et al.* 2005) (see Table 15.5).

Table 15.4   Durie-Salmon staging (DSS) system.

Stage 1 all below	Stage 2	Stage 3 one or more below
Hb >10 g/dL normal calcium Skeletal survey: normal or single plasmacytoma or osteoporosis Serum paraprotein level <5 g/dL if IgG, <3 g/dL if IgA Urinary light chain excretion <4 g/24 h	Fulfilling the criteria of neither I nor III	Hb <8.5 g/dL high calcium >12 mg/dL Skeletal survey: three or more lytic bone lesions Serum paraprotein >7 g/dL if IgG, >5 g/dL if IgA Urinary light chain excretion >12 g/24 h

Table 15.5   International Staging System (adapted from Griepp *et al.* 2005).

Stage I: β_2-microglobulin (β_2M) <3.5 mg/L, albumin ≥3.5 g/dL Stage II: β_2M <3.5 and albumin <3.5; or β_2M ≥3.5 and <5.5 Stage III: β_2M ≥5.5

Plasma cell labeling index (PCLI) is also used as a useful additional prognostic indicator. This indicates the percentage of plasma cells that are actively dividing and therefore provides evidence of the level of plasma proliferation (Steensma *et al.* 2001).

In addition, stages I, II and III of the Durie-Salmon staging system can be divided into A or B depending on serum creatinine:

- A: serum creatinine <2 mg/dL (<177 umol/L)
- B: serum creatinine >2 mg/dL (>177 umol/L)

Treatment and nursing care in multiple myeloma

Although myeloma remains incurable, increased understanding of the disease has made it highly treatable. Enhancing the patient's quality of life for as long as possible, is the hallmark of treatment and nursing care. Primarily the aim of treatment is to:

- Extend the plateau phase of the disease
- Reduce the disease bulk
- Reduce M-protein levels
- Increase haemoglobin level
- Relieve the anaemia
- Provide effective management of pain and other symptoms associated with both the disease and treatment.
- Improve and maintain good quality of life

Treatment

A greater understanding of the behaviour of myeloma cells and the role cytokines play in the disease, has been aided by the use of novel and immunomodulatory therapies. The type of treatment offered will be determined by the results of the staging process. The treatment options are outlined in Table 15.6, and Figure15.2 outlines the algorithm of the treatment options.

If the patient is asymptomatic, no treatment is usually administered as this could lead to increased resistance to chemotherapy, particularly resistance to alkylating agents. The patient is regularly monitored to ascertain when treatment may be required. For patients over 65 years, non-intensive therapy using chemotherapy options such as, melphalan or cyclophosphamide with or without prednisolone, or melphalan, prednisolone and thalidomide (MPT), may be used. In younger patients a more intensive therapy approach is undertaken, with options including combination chemotherapy such as

Table 15.6 Treatment options.

Chemotherapy	**1** Melphalan +/- prednisolone (MP) **2** Vincristine, adriamycin dexamethasone (VAD) **3** Adriamycin, BCNU, cyclophosphamide, melphalan (ABCM) **4** Vincristine, adriamycin, methylprednisolone (VAMP) **5** Cyclophosphamide+VAMP **6** Idarubicin+dexamethasone (Z-Dex)
Radiotherapy	Useful in localised sites reducing pain, prevention of pathological fractures, paraspinal masses
Surgery	Decompression laminectomy Pinning of potential fractures
Bisphosphonates	Strengthens bones, reduces pain, prevents further destruction. Common drugs are: • Clodronate • Pamidronate • Zoledronic acid It is suggested that bisphosphonates inhibit the activity of osteoclast through: • Inhibiting production of cytokines • Inhibiting the development of osteoclast cells • Inhibiting attachment of osteoclasts to bone surfaces
Immunomodulatory therapies	Thalidomide – used in newly diagnosed and relapsed patients Thalidomide analogues – lenalidomide is used in patients who have relapsed; normally used in combination with dexamethasone
Proteasome inhibitors	Bortezomib (Velcade) – used in patients who have relapsed or where treatment has not brought about remission
Autologous haemopoietic stem cell transplantation	Not curative, helps in prolonging life
Allogenic haemopoietic stem cell transplant	Potentially curative, rarely undertaken, may be offered to patients <45 years, high mortality

Adapted from (Hoffbrand and Moss 2011; Rajkumar and Kyle 2005).

vincristine, adriamycin dexamethasone (VAD). Thalidomide or its analogue such as lenalidomide combined with cyclophosphamide or dexamethasone, or both is also seen as an alternative treatment (Kumar 2010).

Following first-line therapy, haemopoietic stem cells may be harvested and high dose melphalan followed by autologous haemopoietic stem cell transplant might be considered. Autologous haemopoietic stem cell transplant is not curative, but aimed at prolonging life. Allogeneic haemopoietic stem cell transplant may be offered to patients under 45 years and offers the possibility of a cure but this is not commonly undertaken as mortality is very high. Myeloma cells are particularly radiosensitive and radiotherapy can therefore be effective for managing bone pain and reducing tumour mass. Spinal cord compression, vertebral collapse or paravertebral mass may necessitate decompression laminectomy. Pinning and plating as surgical procedures may be undertaken for pathological factures.

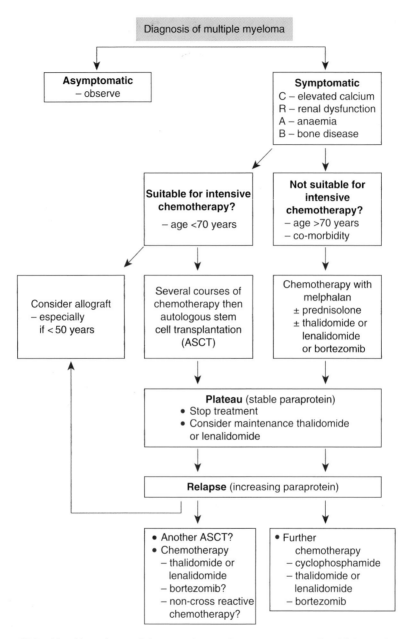

Figure 15.2   Algorithm of potential approaches to the management of multiple myeloma (from Hoffbrand and Moss 2011). Reprinted with permission of John Wiley & Sons, Inc.

Immunomodulatory drugs

These are a group of drugs which work by either modifying or regulating the functioning of the immune system. They have various actions which are thought to include:

- Disrupting angiogenesis (blood vessel growth)
- Inhibiting growth factors involved in angiogenesis (vascular endothelial growth factor (VEGF) and basic fibroblast growth factor (bFGF))
- Directly causing myeloma cell death (apoptosis)
- Affecting the binding of myeloma cells to stromal cells
- Interfering with cytokine production of IL-6
- Stimulating immunity (T and NK cells) (Moehler and Goldschmidt 2011)

Proteasome inhibitors

Proteasome inhibitors such as bortezomib (Velcade) are responsible for helping to regulate cell growth, and myeloma cells are particularly dependent on proteasomes to grow. Selected proteasome inhibitors can induce myeloma cell death and bortezomib has been found to cause myeloma cell death. Bortezomib acts on the bone marrow microenvironment and inhibits NFkB (a messenger protein essential for cell growth, adhesion molecules for MM cells). Dexamethasone is thought to have a synergistic effect on bortezomib, enhancing its effectiveness (Krauze and Roodman 2010).

Thalidomide

The role of thalidomide is unknown but it is thought to have an anti-angiogeneic effect (Kumar *et al.* 2004). Thalidomide has a number of side effects, which include constipation, somnolence, venous thromboembolism (VTE) and neuropathy. A serious side effect of thalidomide is phocomelia (birth abnormality in which a portion of the forearm, arm, leg or thigh is absent, and parts of the limb) (Rogerson 1962). It is essential that contraceptive advice is given to patients on thalidomide. Men should be advised to wear condoms even if they have had a vasectomy. It is considered good practice to advise the patient to commence contraception at least four weeks before treatment and to continue with contraceptive use four weeks after completion of the thalidomide treatment. To increase safety precautions the patient has to sign a consent form and be part of a risk management programme.

Maintenance therapy

This is a difficult area for clinicians to decide on (see Table 15.7). Traditionally, alpha interferon has been used but evidence suggests that although there are some clinical benefits, the side effects make it a difficult drug to tolerate and outweigh any benefits. Currently it has been suggested that thalidomide alone or in combination with corticosteroids has more positive benefits (Ashraf 2008). An optimum dose of thalidomide needs to be determined and can vary from 50–600 mg.

Treatment of relapse or patients who are refractory to treatment is very difficult. Treatment will depend on the timing of the relapse, the clinical state of the relapse and the nature of the previous chemotherapy treatment. Further chemotherapy is usually the main option, or the possibility of autologous haemopoietic stem cell transplant. Thalidomide with or without chemotherapy and steroids may also be considered.

Table 15.7   Poor prognostic features.

Low haemoglobin concentration
Hypercalcaemia
Advanced lytic bone disease
High M protein production rates
Renal dysfunction
High plasma cell proliferation
High C-reactive proteins
Low serum albumin concentration
High β_{-2} microglobukin >6 mg/ml

Adapted from Hughes-Jones *et al*. (2009).

Nursing care

Multiple myeloma is significantly associated with pain and it is essential that pain assessment and effective pain management is an important cornerstone of nursing care. The need for emotional and psychological support is essential. The realisation that the disease is incurable inevitability results in patients having to come to terms with their mortality. The fear of debilitation, pain, the difficulty with mobility the impact of being unable to carry out daily activities, can have a devastating effect, both mentally and emotionally, on the patient. Education is the key in helping the patient and their family to cope with the challenges of MM. Providing patients with accurate information in a user-friendly way in a sensitive manner, in a variety of formats, can empower patients to make decisions for themselves. Helping patients to establish realistic goals for themselves, helps to give the patient a sense of control.

Ongoing assessment to identify the changes occurring at different stages of the disease is necessary. Gaining an understanding of how MM is impacting of daily life is essential to know what interventions are required. Close monitoring for earlier signs of relapse, managing the symptoms of the disease and liaising with members of the multidisciplinary team are important management activities for nurses. The nurse is pivotal to coordinating the services required by the patient. Kelly and Dowling's (2011) study of patients' experiences of living with multiple myeloma eloquently demonstrates the need for nurses to take the time to actively listen to patients to gain an understanding of the impact of the disease on patients' lives in order to identify the needs of the patient and the appropriate interventions required. Palliative specialist services should be part of early care interventions to assist with symptom management, particularly with pain, mobility and emesis management.

Effective use of pain assessment tools such as visual, numerical or facial analogue tools, brief pain inventory tools, should form a routine part of nursing assessment in MM. It is important to ascertain the impact pain may be having on daily activities such as dressing, washing, eating, mobility, exercise, sleep, mood, relationships and work. Opiates are commonly used alongside adjuvants such as amitriptyline, carbamazepine or gabapentin, which can help with neuropathic pain. Non-steroidal anti-inflammatory drugs (NSAIDS) may be used with caution, because of the risk of renal effects and gastric irritation. Some patients may find alternative therapies such as relaxation, aromatherapy and hypnotherapy helpful in controlling or relieving their pain.

Equally important is renal function monitoring. Accurate recording of fluids and urine output is critical in establishing early signs of renal failure. Encouraging fluids helps to reduce dehydration, plasma viscosity and renal impairment. Patients should be encouraged to drink at least 2–3 litres daily. If the patient is having difficulty with oral fluids, intravenous fluids should be commenced. Assessing for the signs of increased hypercalcaemia is important as this could be an indication of increasing progression of the disease, as well as causing renal dysfunction. Signs and symptoms of hypercalcaemia include polydipsia and polyuria, constipation, loss of appetite, nausea and vomiting, increased bone pain and neurological signs such as depression and mental confusion (Mehta and Singhal 2003).

Assessing for neurological problems such as numbness, tingling, back or neck pain, pain in the arms and legs (peripheral neuropathy), loss of bowel and bladder control, are common effects of spinal cord compression (SCC). Spinal cord compression warrants rapid intervention and must be treated as a neurological emergency to minimise long-term complications or mortality (Dougherty and Lister 2004). The National Institute for Clinical Excellence (NICE) (2008) document, *Metastatic Spinal Cord Compression: Diagnosis and Management of Patients at Risk of or with Metastatic Spinal Cord Compression*, provides detailed aspects of the nursing care for SCC. Monitor the patient for symptoms such as epistasis, blurred vision, bruising or numbness, and tingling of arms and legs, as these may be significant symptoms of hyperviscosity syndrome. Plasma exchange through apheresis may be required to manage hyperviscosity syndrome in severe cases.

Infections are common and frequent and can be a cause of mortality. It is crucial that vital signs are monitored every four hours, including observations for signs of sepsis. Patients should be educated about the importance of early reporting of any signs of infection to instigate prompt antimicrobial management. This is of particular importance if the patient has been prescribed corticosteroids as they can mask infections.

Fatigue can play a crucial role in compromising daily activities (Murphy and Murphy 2004). Having a balance of rest and activity is essential. It can be helpful for patients to keep a diary of activities to ascertain any patterns that appear to lead to fatigue which can then be addressed. Advise patients to plan ahead with activities to ensure they give themselves a balance between rest and activity. Fatigue can also have an effect on concentration, therefore assessing how much information to give at any one time to ensure the patient is able to absorb it is also important. Anaemia can compound the fatigue and be exacerbated by increasing renal failure. If prolonged, the patient maybe commenced on erythropoietin and in severe anaemia blood transfusion maybe necessary. Encouraging a balanced diet may help to increase energy levels, which is important in enhancing the patient's quality of life. Nurses should also be aware that culturally it is quite common for black patients to use herbs for medicinal purposes. It is therefore important that nurses advise patients against taking herbal remedies unless advised by the specialist nurse or consultant as herbal therapy could act adversely with the chemotherapy regimen.

Prevention and management of constipation must form part of nursing care practice (King 2006). Constipation can become a problem due to side effects of treatment such as thalidomide, dehydration, reduced mobility and hypercalcaemia. The gut also has morphine receptor sites and if the patient is receiving opiates for pain, this can affect peristalsis activity leading to constipation. Patients requiring opiate analgesia or those receiving thalidomide should be have stool softeners or laxatives to help with bowel movement. Nurses need to establish the patient's usual bowel habits to have a benchmark from which to assess the patient and encourage the patient to report any changes in bowel habits and function.

Mobility is an important part of patient care. Keeping active can help to strengthen bones, so patients should be advised by the specialist nurse or consultant regarding the type of activity which is safe to do and to help with any pain which is restricting movement. Walking and swimming can be beneficial and improve muscle tone. Pathological fractures can occur spontaneously and therefore advising the patient not to have sudden jolting movements to minimise fractures is essential. Patients should be advised that myeloma can cause shortening of the spine, which leads to height reduction and as a consequence length of clothes will need to be altered.

Patients should be advised not to have immunisations with live vaccines while they are undergoing treatment. This is because the vaccine will trigger B-cells to produce antibodies against the vaccine; as a consequence this could lead to proliferation on myeloma cells. Live vaccines are not advisable for six months after treatment, if the level of neutrophils is low. Advice from specialist nurses or the consultant regarding safety of different types of vaccines should be sought.

Sexuality and intimacy are aspects of patients' quality of life that should not be forgotten (Brown 2010). The older age of the patient should not lead to an assumption that these issues are not important aspects of someone's life. Good interpersonal skills are required and taking the time to listen to the patient, providing opportunities for the patient to ask questions in a safe, relaxing environment is important. Using questions such as: 'Has the treatment affected the way you feel as a husband, wife, partner?' can be a non-threatening approach to identifying with the patient if there are sexuality concerns.

Conclusion

Myeloma is an incurable disease, but in recent years there has been increased interest in the disease, with new and novel therapies being developed. This means that nurses need to keep abreast of developments to help support patients and gain an understanding of what may be specific side effects of treatment to know how best to manage the patient. Nurses should advise patients of support groups such as Myeloma UK to help patients gain further information as well as support from other patients. Pain is a significant feature of MM and it is fundamental that effective, expert pain management is provided. A multidisciplinary team approach to management is essential, as is having accurate up-to-date information to support and care for the patient.

References

Alexander, D.D., Mink, P.J., Adami, H.O. *et al.* (2007) Multiple myeloma: a review of the epidemiologic literature. *Int. J Cancer*, 120 (Suppl 12), 40–61.

Ashraf, B. (2008) Thalidomide in patients with relapsed myeloma. In: *Contemporary Hematology – Myeloma Therapy – Pursuing the Plasma Cell* (ed. S. Lonial). Humana Press, Atlanta.

Bataille, R., Boccadoro, M., Klein, B., Durie, B. and Pileri, A. (1992) C-reactive protein and beta-2 microglobulin produce a simple and powerful myeloma staging system. *Blood*, 80 (3), 733–737.

Bladé, J., Rosiñol, L. and Ciberia, M.T. (2009) Are all myelomas preceded by MGUS? *Blood*, 113 (22), 5370.

British Committee for Standards in Haematology in conjunction with the UK Myeloma Forum (UKMF) (2010) *Guidelines on the Diagnosis and Management of Multiple Myeloma*. BCSH, London.

Brown, M. (2010) Nursing care of patients undergoing allogeneic stem cell transplantation. *Nursing Standard*, 25 (11), 47–56.

Cancer Research UK. Myeloma Statistics (2007) http://info.cancerresearchuk/cancerstats/type/multiplemyeloma. Accessed 20 March 2011.

Cao, Y., Luetkens, T., Kobold, S. *et al.* (2010) The cytokine/chemokine pattern in the bone marrow environment of multiple myeloma patients. *Exp Hematology*, 38 (10), 860–867.

Chng, W.J. (2010) Genetic abnormalities in multiple myeloma. In: *Multiple Myeloma* (ed. S. Kumar*)*. Demos Medical Publishing, New York.

Dankbar, B., Padró, T., Leo, R. *et al.* (2000) Vascular endothelial growth factor and interleukin-6 in paracrine tumor-stromal cell interactions in multiple myeloma. *Blood*, 15, 95 (8), 2630–2636.

Devenney, B.W. and Erickson, C. (2004) Multiple myeloma, an overview. *Clinical Journal of Oncology Nursing*, 8 (4), 401–405.

Dougherty, L. and Lister, S. (2008) *The Royal Marsden Hospital Manual of Clinical Nursing Procedures*, 7th edition. Wiley-Blackwell, Oxford.

Durie, B.G. and Salmon, S.E. (1975) A clinical staging system for multiple myeloma. Correlation of measured myeloma cell mass with presenting clinical features, response to treatment, and survival. *Cancer*, 36 (3), 842–854.

Goldman, L., Ausiello, D., Kyle, R.A. and Rajkumar, S.V. (2004) Plasma cell disorders. In: *Cecil Textbook of Medicine*, 22nd edition (eds L. Goldman and D. Ausiello D). pp. 1184–1195. Saunders, Philadelphia.

Görgün, G., Calabrese, E., Soydan, E. *et al.* (2010) Immunomodulatory effects of lenalidomide and pomalidomide on interaction of tumor and bone marrow accessory cells in multiple myeloma. *Blood*, 116 (17), 3227–3237.

Greer, J.P., Foerster, J., Rodgers, G.M., Paraskevas, F., Arber, D.S. and Mears Jr, R.T. (2009) *Winrrobe's Clinical Hematology*. Vol.1. Lippincott, Williams and Wilkins, Philadephlia.

Griepp, P.R., San Miguel, J., Durie, B.G. *et al.* (2005). International staging system for multiple myeloma . *Journal Clinical Oncology*, 23, 3412–3420.

Hideshmia, T., Miisiades, C., Tonon, G., Richardson, P.G. and Anderson, K.C. (2007) Understanding multiple myeloma pathogenesis in the bone marrow to identify new therapeutic targets. *Nature Reviews Cancer*, 7, 585–598.

Hoffbrand, A.V. and Moss, P.A.H. (2011) *Essential Haematology*, 6th edition. Wiley-Blackwell, Oxford.

Hughes-Jones, N.C., Wickramasinghe, S.N. and Hatton, C.S.R. (2009) *Lecture Notes in Haematology*, 8th edition. Wiley-Blackwell, Oxford.

International Myeloma Working Group (2009) Molecular classification of multiple myeloma: spotlight review. *Leukemia*, 23, 2210–2221.

Joy Ho, P. (2002) Chromosomal and genetic abnormalities in myeloma. Clin Lab Haematol, 24 (5), 259–269.

Kelly, M. and Dowling, M. (2011) Patients' lived experience of multiple myeloma. *Nursing Standard*, 25 (28), 38–44.

King, T. (2006) Myeloma. In: *Nursing in Haematological Oncology*, 2nd edition (ed. M. Grundy). Chapter 5. pp. 86–107. Elsevier, Oxford.

Klein, B., Seckinger, A., Moehler, T. and Hose, D. (2011) molecular pathogenesis of multiple myeloma: chromosomal aberrations, changes in gene expression, cytokine networks, and the bone marrow microenvironment. Multiple myeloma. *Recent Results in Cancer Research*, 183 (part 2), 39–86.

Kline, M., Donovan, K., Wellik, L. *et al.* (2007) Cytokine and chemokine profiles in multiple myeloma; significance of stromal interaction and correlation of IL-8 production with disease progression. *Leukaemia Research Journal*, 31 (5), 591–598.

Krauze, M.T. and Roodman, G.D. (2010) Bortezomib and osteoclasts and osteoblasts In: *Bortezomib in the Treatment of Multiple Myeloma* (eds I. Ghobrial, P.G. Richardson and K.C. Anderson). pp. 43–52. Springer, Berlin.

Kumar, S., Witzig, T.E., Dispenzieri, A. *et al.* (2004) Effect of thalidomide therapy on bone marrow angiogenesis in multiple myeloma. *Leukemia*, 18, 624–627.

Kumar, S. (2010) Lenalidomide for initial therapy of newly diagnosed multiple myeloma. In: *Contemporary Hematology – Multiple Therapy* (ed. S. Lonial). pp. 279–288. Humana Press, Atlanta.

Landgren, O., Kyle, R.A., Hoppin, J.A. *et al.* (2009) Pesticide exposure and risk of monoclonal gammopathy of undetermined significance in the Agricultural Health Study. *Blood*, 113 (6), 6386–6391.

Mehta, J. and Singhal, S. (2003) Hyperviscosity syndrome in plasma cell dyscrasias. *Semin Thromb Hemost*, Oct, 29 (5), 467–471.

Moehler, T. and Goldschmidt, H. (2011) Therapy of relapsed and refractory multiple myeloma. In: *Multiple Myeloma* (eds T. Moehler and H. Goldschmidt). Chapter 11, pp. 239–260. Springer, Berlin.

Morgan, G.J., Davies, F.E. and Linet, M. (2002) Myeloma aetiology and epidemiology. *Biomed Pharmacother*, 56, 223–234.

Murphy, L. and Murphy, F. (2004) The role of fatigue in multiple myeloma. *Cancer Nursing Practice*, 3 (9), 29–33.

National Institute for Clinical Excellence (2008) *Metastatic Spinal Cord Compression: Diagnosis and Management of Patients at Risk of or with Metastatic Spinal Cord Compression. Full Guideline*. National Collaborating Centre for Cancer, Cardiff.

Podar, K., Chauhan, D. and Anderson, K.C. (2009) Bone marrow microenviroment and the identification of new targets for myeloma therapy. *Leukaemia*, 23, 10–24.

Raab, M.S., Podar, K., Breitkreutz, I., Richardson, P.G. and Anderson, K.C. (2009) Multiple myeloma. *Lancet*, 374 (9686), 324–339.

Rajkumar , S.V. (2005) MGUS and smoldering multiple myeloma: update on pathogenesis, natural history, and management. *Hematology*, 2005 (1), 340–345.

Rajkumar, S.V. and Kyle, R.A. (2005) Multiple myeloma: diagnosis and treatment. *Mayo Clinic Proceedings*, 80, 1371–1382.

Rogerson, G. (1962) Thalidomide and congental abnormalities. *Lancet*, (1), 691.

Ross, F.M., Ibrahim, A.H., Villain-Holmes, A. *et al.* (2005) Age has a profound effect on the incidence and significance of chromosome abnormalities in myeloma. *Leukemia*, 19, 1634–1642.

Shaughnessy Jr, J.D. and Stewart, A.K. (2004) Gene expression profiling and multiple myeloma. In: *Myeloma; Biology and Management*, 3rd edition (ed. J.S. Malpas). Chapter 6, pp. 83–96. Elsevier Health Sciences, Philadelphia.

Steensma, D.P., Gertz, M.A., Greipp, P.R. *et al.* (2001) A high bone marrow plasma cell labeling index in stable plateau-phase multiple myeloma is a marker for early disease progression and death. Brief report. *Blood* (15 April), 97 (8), 2522–2523.

Chapter 16

Lymphoma: pathophysiology, care and management

Tracey Cutler

> *Within this chapter the aetiology, epidemiology and pathogenesis of lymphoma will be explored and current classification and staging tools will be identified which will identify the differences between the subtypes of lymphoma. Nursing management will be discussed towards the end of the chapter.*
>
> *By the end of reading this chapter, you will:*
>
> - Have an overview of the types of lymphoma
> - Be familiar with standard diagnostic investigations
> - Be aware of the classification, staging and prognostic tools
> - Have an insight into the treatment options available

The term 'lymphoma' identifies a variety of disorders affecting the lymphatic tissue; unlike other haematological diseases these disorders are diagnosed and managed in a variety of in-patient and outpatient settings. This diversity presents a challenge to the multiprofessional team and it is therefore important that the identification of the specific subtype is undertaken which will aid correct classification, staging and prognosis.

Role of the lymphocyte

As identified in Chapter 2 (Immunology) the lymphatic tissues and cells (lymphocytes) play an important role in immune response to invading antigens. If these tissues or cells become damaged in any way their function will be affected. This includes damage to cellular function caused by malignant proliferation of lymphocytes in the case of lymphoma.

Lymphomas are classically divided into two subtypes, Hodgkin's lymphoma (HL) or non-Hodgkin's lymphoma (NHL), based on the histological presence or absence of the Reed-Sternberg (RS) cell in Hodgkin's lymphoma (Hoffbrand *et al.* 2001). Clinical symptoms at time of presentation are usually lymphadenopathy related and will be

Haematology Nursing, First Edition. Marvelle Brown and Tracey J. Cutler.
© 2012 Blackwell Publishing Ltd. Published 2012 by Blackwell Publishing Ltd.

dependent on which cell (T or B-lymphocyte) is involved, and usually relate to a protracted journey where the patient has presented progressive symptoms to their GP.

Diagnostic investigations

The gold standard diagnostic investigation is by excision biopsy, removing the affected node. It may be necessary to perform multiple site biopsies. Cytogenetics and immunophenotyping will identify cell type and any diagnostic markers. Physical examination includes palpation of lymph nodes and clinical examination for splenomegaly and hepatomegaly.

Laboratory tests include full blood count with differential, erythrocyte sedimentation rate (ESR) renal and liver function, serum alkaline phosphatase and lactate dehydrogenase (LDH). If abnormalities are noted in liver function a biopsy may be necessary; alkaline phosphatase can indicate bone involvement and may indicate the need for X-rays and bone scans. Viral screening may also be requested depending on the suspected diagnosis.

Imaging

Chest X-ray, computed tomography (CT) scans of neck, chest, abdomen and pelvis are now gold standard and an ultrasound of testes if involvement is found on clinical examination. If the patient is presenting with any numbness in limbs then a spinal magnetic resonance imaging (MRI) scan may be required. Bone marrow aspirate and trephine is required in patients presenting with stage IIB or higher and a cerebral spinal fluid (CSF) sample may be requested in patients suspected of having CSF involvement.

Revised European American Lymphoma Classification adopted by the World Health Organisation

The WHO classification of tumours of haematopoietic and lymphoid tissues originated from the lymphoma classification project which commenced in 1997. This project produced the Revised European American Lymphoma Classification (REAL), which is widely accepted as the preferred classification tool (Hoffbrand *et al.* 2006) and has now been adopted by the WHO (see Table 16.1).

Clinical staging

Stage is ascertained after clinical examination and results from laboratory and imaging tests have been considered. The recommended staging scheme is Ann Arbor (see Figure 16.1). Stage I is node involvement in one region of lymph nodes or extranodal area. Stage II is disease involving two or more lymph node areas on the same side of the diaphragm. Stage III is lymph node disease above and below the diaphragm, possibly in several sites. Stage IV is disease outside the lymph node areas, including disease in the bone marrow, liver and other extranodal sites. A or B after the stage number indicates absence (A) or presence (B) of one or more of the symptoms: unexplained fever above 38°C, drenching night sweats or loss of more than 10% of the body weight within six months. Localised extranodal extension from a mass of nodes is indicated by E (Griffin *et al.* 2003; Hoffbrand *et al.* 2001).

Table 16.1   The WHO classification of lymphomas (from Hoffbrand *et al.* 2005).

Mature B-cell neoplasms
Chronic lymphocytic leukaernia/small lymphocytic lymphoma
B-cell prolymphocytic leukaemia
Splenic B-cell marginal zone lymphoma
Hairy cell leukaemia
Splenic lymphoma/leukaemia unclassifiable
Splenic diffuse red pulp small B-cell lymphoma
Hairy cell leukaemia variant
Lymphoplasmacytic lymphoma/ Waldenström macroglobulinaemia
Heavy chain diseases
Plasma cell myelorna
Solitary plasmacytoma of bone
Extraosseous plasmacytoma
Extranodal marginal zone lymphoma of mucosa-associated lymphoid tissue (MALT lymphoma)
Nodal marginal zone lymphoma
Paediatric nodal marginal zone lymphoma
Follicular lymphoma
Paediatric follicular lymphoma
Primary cutaneous follide centre lymphoma
Mantle cell lymhoma
Dissuse large B-cell lymphoma (DLBCL), not otherwise specified
T-cell/histiocyte-rich large B-cell lymphoma
Primary DLBCL of the CNS
Primary cutaneous DLBCL, leg type
EBV-positive DLBCL of the elderly
DLBCL associated with chronic inflammation
Lymphomatoid granulomatosis
Primary mediastinal (thymic) large B-cell lymphoma
Intravascular large B-cell lymphoma
ALK-positive large B-cell lymphoma
Plasmablastic lymphoma
Large B-cell lymphomas arising in HHV8-associated multicentric Castleman disease
Primary effusion lymphoma
Burkitt lymphoma
B-cell lymphoma, unclassifiable, with features intermediate between DLBCL and Burkitt lymphoma

B-cell lymphoma, unclassifiable, with features intermediate between DLBCL and classical Hodgkin lymphoma
Mature T-cell and NK-cell neoplasms
T-cell prolymphocytic leukaemia
T-cell large granular lymphocytic leukaernia
Chronic lymphoproliferative disorder of NK cells
Aggressive NK-cell leukaemia
Systemic EBV-positive T-cell lymphoproliferative disease of childhood
Hydroa vacciniforme-like lymphoma
Adult T-cell leukaernia/lymphoma
Extranodal NK/T-cell lymphoma, nasal type
Enteropathy-asociated T-cell lymphoma
Hepatosplenic T-cell lymphoma
Subcutaneous panniculitis-like T-cell lymphoma
Mycosis fungoides
Sézary syndrome
Primary cutaneous CD30-positive T-cell lymphoproliferative disorders
Lymphomatoid papulosis
Primary cutaneous anaplastic large-cell lymphoma
Primary cutaneous $\gamma\delta$ T-cell lymphoma
Primary cutaneous CD8-positive aggressive epidermotropic cytotoxic T-cell lymphoma
Primary cutaneous CD4-positive small/ medium T-cell lymphoma
Peripheral T-cell lymphoma, unspecified
Angioimmunoblastic T-cell lymphoma
Anaplastic large-cell lymphoma, ALK positive
Anaplastic large-cell lymphoma, ALK negative
Hodgkin lymphoma
Nodular lymphocyte predominant Hodgkin lymphoma
Classical Hodgkin lymphoma
Nodular sclerosis classical Hodgkin lymphoma
Lymphocyte-rich classical Hodgkin lymphoma
Mixed cellularity classical Hodgkin lymphoma
Lymphocyte-depleted classical Hodgkin lymphoma

Source: Swerdlow *et al.* (2008) with permission.

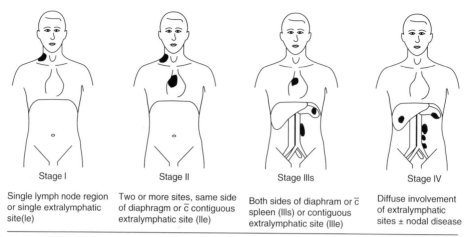

Stage I	Stage II	Stage IIIs	Stage IV
Single lymph node region or single extralymphatic site(Ie)	Two or more sites, same side of diaphragm or c̄ contiguous extralymphatic site (IIe)	Both sides of diaphram or c̄ spleen (IIIs) or contiguous extralymphatic site (IIIe)	Diffuse involvement of extralymphatic sites ± nodal disease

Stage subdivision: A-asymptomatic B-unexplained weight loss> 10% in 6m and/or fever and/or night sweats
Extralymphatic = tissue other than lymph nodes, thymus, spleen, waldeyer's ring, appendix & peyer's patches

Figure 16.1 Staging of lymphoma using the Ann Arbor staging tool (from Hoffbrand *et al.* 2001). Reprinted with permission of John Wiley & Sons, Inc.

International prognostic index (IPI)

The IPI is a tool used to identify adverse prognostic indicators (See Table 16.2).The IPI identifies adverse indicators if patients are of an older age group, have advanced Ann Arbor stage, higher than normal LDH, a poor performance status and more than two extranodal sites (Hughes-Jones *et al.* 2004).

Table 16.2 International Prognostic Index (from Mehta and Hoffbrand 2009).

	Adverse prognosis
Age	≥60 yr
Ann Arbor stage	III or IV
Serum LDH	Above normal
Number of extranodal sites	≥2
Performance status	ECOG2 or equivalent

Hodgkin's lymphoma

This was first described by Thomas Hodgkin in 1832. Hodgkin's lymphoma (HL) is a malignant condition which infiltrates the lymph nodes; these large binucleated cells are called Reed-Sternberg (RS) cells. The presence of these cells leads to the diagnosis of HL (see Figure 16.2).

RS cell

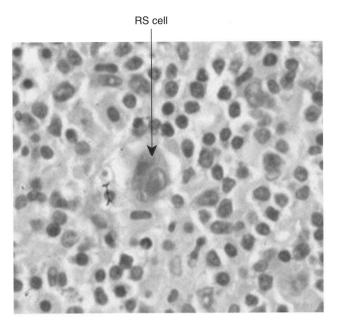

Figure 16.2 Histopathological sample demonstrating a Reed-Sternberg cell (from Bower and Waxman 2006). Reprinted with permission of John Wiley & Sons, Inc.

Incidence

The latest statistics available from Cancer Research UK (2010) are that 1673 people in the UK were diagnosed with HL in 2007 and of these 302 died in 2008.

There are 3.2 per 100,000 males diagnosed yearly and 2.3 per 100,000 females, giving a nearly 2:1 male predominance. The incidence is classed as age specific, with a peak of diagnoses in the thirties and a second in old age.

Aetiology

The causes of HL are as yet unknown, but current thought is that there may be links to familial factors, environmental factors, viruses and smoking (Yahalom and Straus 2009).

Familial factors

Provan *et al.* (2004) and Yahalom and Straus (2009) identify that there is a 99 times higher risk of identical twins developing HL and that siblings of diagnosed young adults have a seven times higher risk factor.

Environmental factors

Higher socioeconomic status, only children and social isolation are also noted as risk factors, indicating that a decrease in contact with common infectious diseases at a young age prevents activation of the immune system.

Viruses

The Epstein Barr virus (EBV) has been identified as a risk factor in individuals with a history of infectious mononucleosis (26–50% of cases positive for EBV) (Provan *et al.* 2004).

Smoking

Yahalom and Straus (2009) state that the incidence is increased two-fold in smokers.

Pathophysiology

Diagnosis is by biopsy of the affected lymph nodes and the identification of the RS cell. The RS cell is considered the malignant (tumour) cell and may only be present in less than 1% of the specimen; the majority of the other cells will be reactive inflammatory cells (Hoffbrand *et al.* 2001). The RS cell is large, with a binucleated structure, the cells express antigens such as CD25 or CD30 leading to the opinion that HL is a lymphoid malignancy and that the cells of origin are B-lymphocytes (Behringer *et al.* 2005).

Presentation

Patients present with lymphadenopathy which is above the diaphragm in more than 80% of patients (Yahalom and Strauss 2009). The nodes are painless and feel rubbery on palpation (Provan *et al.* 2004). The mode of progression is contiguous node chains. See Table 16.3 Presenting symptoms, and Figure 16.2 for sites of nodal involvement at presentation.

Table 16.3   Presenting symptoms (adapted from Provan *et al.* 2004 and Yahalom and Straus 2009).

Presenting symptom	
Peripheral lymphadenopathy – cervical, supraclavicular, axillary	Common
Anterior mediastinum, with or without superior vena cava obstruction	Common
Splenic involvement	30%
Lymphadenopathy below diaphragm	Less than 10–20%
Hepatomegaly	5%
Pleural effusions	20%
Systemic symptoms (B symptoms) fever, drenching night sweats, weight loss, itching	30%
Extranodal involvement (E) lungs, liver, bone and bone marrow	1–4%

Histological subtypes of Hodgkin's lymphoma

The WHO identifies five categories, which each have a different incidence and prognosis (see Table 16.4). Between 80% and 90% of cases are diagnosed as either nodular sclerosis or mixed cellularity (Tobias and Hochhauser 2010). Nodular sclerosis is seen

Table 16.4   WHO classification of HL (adapted from Hoffbrand *et al.* 2001 and Yahalom and Straus 2010).

Classification	Histological examination
Nodular/lymphocyte predominant	Unique form accounting for a very small percentage of cases. RS cells are absent, abnormal polymorphic B cells.
Classical Hodgkin's lymphoma Nodular sclerosis	Collagen bands extend from the node capsule; lacunar cells (RS cell variant) are present. Infiltrate may be lymphocyte predominant, mixed cellularity or lymphocyte depleted.
Mixed cellularity	Numerous RS cells.
Lymphocyte depleted	Either diffuse fibrosis or reticular with many RS cells.
Lymphocyte rich	Small lymphocytes with very few RS cells.

predominantly in young adults, whilst the other types are bimodal, with a second peak in old age and lymphocyte predominant has the most favourable prognosis (Hoffbrand *et al.* 2001).

Treatment of Hodgkin's lymphoma

Hodgkin's lymphoma is a treatable malignancy which is highly sensitive to chemotherapy and radiotherapy. The stage at diagnosis is the deciding factor which influences treatment choices. Patients with early stage disease I and II have three treatment options, radiation therapy, chemotherapy or combination therapy (including both chemotherapy and radiation). Although patients with non-bulky stage IA, IB or IIA can be treated with radiation alone this in no longer the treatment of choice due to the long-term side effects and carcinogenic risk associated with radiotherapy (Peranski 2007; Yahalom and Straus 2010). However, this treatment can be utilised for patients who are unable to receive chemotherapy because of co-morbidities. Chemotherapy regimens for HL have developed and are now tailored to stage of disease, age and performance status. There are a number of protocols utilised (see Table 16.5).

In the past MOPP was the treatment of choice but now only tends to be used in older patients with poor lung and cardiac function. The current gold standard therapy is ABVD; this is due to the reduced risk of secondary malignancy and a lower rate of infertility.

A regimen called BEACOPP has been trialled and although more toxic than ABVD results show it to be beneficial in younger patients or those with advanced disease.

Patients diagnosed with stage III, IV, B symptoms or bulky disease are classed as having advanced disease and ABVD is the treatment of choice, followed by involved field radiotherapy (mantle radiation or inverted Y).The overall five-year survival is 73%.

Patients who relapse post-standard therapy will be offered haemopoietic stem cell transplant (see Chapter 20). There are a number of trials investigating the use of monoclonal antibodies which target the CD30 antigen.

Table 16.5 Chemotherapy regimens for HL (adapted from Peranski 2007).

Regimen	Drugs included
MOPP	Mechlorethamine (Mustargen) Vincristine (Oncovin) Procarbazine Prednisolone
ABVD	Doxorubicin (Adriamycin) Bleomycin Vinblastine Dacarbazine
Ch1VPP	Chlorambucil Vinblastine Procarbazine Prednisolone
PABLOE	Prednisolone Doxorubicin (Adriamycin) Bleomycin Vincristine (Oncovin) Etoposide (VP16)
CHOPE	Cyclophosphamide Doxorubicin (Hydroxi-doxorubicin) Vincristine Prednisolone Etoposide
BEACOPP	Bleomycin Etoposide Doxorubicin (Adriamycin) Cyclophosphamide Vincristine Procarbazine Prednisolone
Stanford V	Mechlorethamine (Mustargen) Doxorubicin Vinblastine Vincristine Bleomycin Etoposide Prednisolone

Side effects

Side effects to chemotherapy are discussed in Chapter 19. However, mantle radiotherapy can cause a dry mouth, taste changes, pharyngitis, nausea, dry cough, dermatitis and fatigue. Inverted Y radiotherapy causes loss of appetite, nausea and diarrhoea (Yahalom and Straus 2010). The complications of treatment for HL are: a risk of pulmonary fibrosis due to the bleomycin; cardiac dysfunction due to anthracyclin chemotherapy and mantle radiotherapy; hyperthyroidism if the radiation involves the neck; infertility and early menopause; and the risk of secondary malignancy.

The most common secondary malignancy is acute myeloid leukaemia, followed by lung cancer, thyroid cancer, non-Hodgkin lymphoma and breast cancer (this occurs in 20–50% 15 years post-treatment and is more common if mantle radiation is given to females under the age of 30) (Peranski 2007).

Non-Hodgkin's lymphoma

Non-Hodgkin's lymphoma (NHL) refers to a wide range of T-cell and B-cell lymphoproliferative disorders. These disorders do not present with the RS cell and are therefore named NHL.

Incidence

The latest statistics available from Cancer Research UK (2010) are that 10,917 people in the UK were diagnosed with NHL in 2007. There are 19.7 per 100,000 males diagnosed and 16.2 per 100,000 females. It is more common in adults than children, but there is a steady increase with age; the average age at diagnosis is 45–50 years.

Aetiology

Risk factors

The aetiology of NHL is unknown but there are a variety of risk factors associated with immunodeficiency. The normal regulation of over proliferation is altered by the disorder or treatment. This will reduce the immune response and lead to large numbers of proliferating cells. Acquired and congenital immunodeficiencies are known to increase the risk factors. Those acquired would be after immunosuppression therapy, such as chemotherapy, radiation and transplantation (organ or haemopoietic stem cell), also acquired immunodeficiency syndrome (AIDS). Congenital immunodeficiency disorders also increase the risk, for example ataxia-telengiectasia and Wiscott-Aldrich syndrome. Autoimmune disorders such as Sjögren's syndrome, rheumatoid arthritis and inflammatory bowel disease also increase the risk (Peranski 2007).

Chromosomal translocations and molecular rearrangements

The chromosomal abnormality most often seen in NHL is t(14;18) (q32;q21); this translocation is reported by Evens *et al.* (2011) to be found in 85% of diagnosed follicular lymphoma and 25–30% of higher grade NHLs (2011). The mutation t(11;14) is associated with mantle cell lymphoma (Hoffbrand *et al.* 2001) and t(3;16) is seen in diffuse large B-cell lymphoma (Evens *et al.* 2009). In Burkitt's lymphoma 75% present with t(8;14) a translocation of c-myc gene; this causes proliferation and absence of regulated cell death (apoptosis). The other 25% are either t(2;8) or t(8;22) (Hughes-Jones *et al.* 2004).

Environmental factors

There are known environmental factors which increase the risk in certain professions: farmers due to the use of pesticides, wood and forestry workers due to wood treatments

Table 16.6   Infectious agents and types of lymphoma.

Infectious agent	Type of lymphoma
Epstein-Barr virus (EBV)	Burkitt's lymphoma, Hodgkin's lymphoma
Human T-cell leukaemia virus type 1 (HTLV-1)	Adult T-cell lymphoma and leukaemia
Helicobacter pylori	Gastric mucosa-associated lymphoid tissue (MALT) lymphoma
Hepatitis C virus	B-cell lymphoma especially marginal zone
Kaposi's sarcoma associated virus (KSHV)	Body cavity based lymphomas in patients with HIV and Castleman's disease
Human herpes virus-8 (HHV-8)	
Lyme disease (*Borrelia burgdorferi*)	Cutaneous B-cell lymphoma

Adapted from Evens *et al.* (2011) and Peranski (2007).

and mechanics, petrol refinery workers and those working with rubber, plastics and solvents, due to chemicals such as benzene (Evens *et al.* 2011; Peranski 2007).

Viruses and infections

Due to the stimulation of the immune response, infections with certain bacteria and viruses can increase the risk (see Table 16.6).

Pathophysiology

As stated earlier, NHL covers the range of lymphomas which are not Hodgkin's lymphoma. Therefore the diagnosis will depend on immunophenotype, morphologic features, genetic features and clinical features. These results will indicate if the cell of origin is a proliferation of T-lymphocytes or B-lymphocytes. Diagnosis is by biopsy of the affected lymph nodes; cytogenetic analysis will determine any chromosomal abnormalities and a bone marrow aspirate and trephine will identify progression to the bone marrow. Serum LDH is a useful marker and is used as a prognostic indicator alongside subtype of disease and age (Hoffbrand *et al.* 2006).

Presentation

Although the disease is thought to arise from one lymph node region it is reported that patients (approximately 90%) present with stage III or IV with generalised lymphadenopathy and widely disseminated disease, including in some cases bone marrow involvement (Peranski 2007; Watson *et al.* 2006). Presenting symptoms will vary, depending on the diagnosis (see Table 16.7).

Histological subtypes of non-Hodgkin's lymphoma

The WHO has identified the subtypes of NHL which each have a different incidence and prognosis (see Table 16.8). Non-Hodgkin's lymphoma is further subdivided into low grade, intermediate and high grade. Low grade NHL subtypes account for 20–40% of NHL and affect patients over 50 years old (Peranski 2007). The disease tends to be

Table 16.7   Non-Hodgkin's lymphoma presenting symptoms (adapted from Watson *et al.* 2006 and Evens *et al.* 2011).

Presenting symptom	
Peripheral lymphadenopathy – cervical, supraclavicular, axillary	May come and go in low grade disease
Anterior mediastinal mass, with or without superior vena cava obstruction	Lymphoblastic
Splenic involvement	40% in low grade
Lymphadenopathy below diaphragm	Burkitt's lymphoma
Systemic symptoms (B symptoms) fever, drenching night sweats, weight loss, itching	More common in disseminated disease (30–40%)
Extranodal involvement (E) bone marrow, gastrointestinal, skin, thyroid, CNS	>30% in high grade

Table 16.8   The WHO classification of NHL (from Hoffbrand *et al.* 2006).

Precursor B-cell neoplasm B-lymphoblastic leukaemia/lymphoma (precursor B-cell ALL, B-ALL/LBL)	*Precursor T-cell neoplasms* T-cell lymphoblastic lymphoma/leukaemia (T-ALL/LBL)
Mature B-cell neoplasms B-cell chronic lymphocytic leukaemia/small lymphocytic lymphoma B-cell prolymphocytic leukaemia Lymphoplasmacytic lymphoma Splenic marginal zone B-cell lymphoma (±villous lymphocytes) Hairy cell leukaemia Plasma cell myeloma/plasmacytoma	*Mature T-cell and NK cell neoplasms* T-cell prolymphocytic leukaemia T-cell granular lymphocytic leukaemia Aggressive NK-cell leukaemia Adult T-cell lymphoma/leukaemia (HTLV-1+)
Extranodal marginal zone B-cell lymphoma of MALT type	Extranodal NK/T-cell lymphoma, nasal type Enteropathy-type T-cell lymphoma Mycosis fungoides/Sézary syndrome Anaplastic large cell lymphoma, primary cutaneous type
Mantle cell lymphoma Follicular lymphoma Nodal marginal zone B-cell lymphoma Diffuse large B-cell lymphoma Burkitt's lymphoma/Burkitt's cell leukaemia Primary effusion lymphoma Mediastinal large B-cell lymphoma	Peripheral T-cell lymphoma, unspecified Angioimmunoblastic T-cell lymphoma Anaplastic large cell lymphoma, primary systemic type

ALL, acute lymphoblastic leukaemia; HTLV, human T-cell leukaemia/lymphoma virus; LBL, lymphoblastic lymphoma; MALT, mucosa-associated lymphoid tissue; NK, natural killer.

indolent but disseminated in nature, often going into remission spontaneously; treatment is often conservative with oral chemotherapy and/or radiotherapy. These types of NHL will transform at some stage to a high grade lymphoma and at this stage will require more aggressive treatment (Griffin *et al.* 2003). Intermediate and high grade NHL will require urgent treatment with chemotherapy and/or radiotherapy and may go on to need haemopoietic stem cell transplant (see Table 16.9 for the types of NHL).

Table 16.9 Types of non-Hodgkin's lymphoma.

Type	Grade	Markers	Presentation	Age
B-cell lymphomas				
Follicular lymphoma	Low but stage III–IV at diagnosis	t(14;18) translocation CD20+	Benign/indolent course with painless lymphadenopathy	Middle to older age group
Lymphocytic lymphoma	Low		Slow progressive disease (thought to be tissue phase of CLL)	Older age group
Lymphoplasmacytoid lymphoma – Waldenström's macroglobulinaemia		CD19, CD20, CD22 and CD79a	Anaemia and hyperviscosity syndrome	Older age group
Mantle cell lymphoma	Low	CD19+, CD5+, CD22+ but CD23- T(11;14) (q13;q23)	Lymphadenopathy with bone marrow infiltration common	Middle to older age
Marginal zone lymphoma – Mucosa-associated lymphoid tissue (MALT)		CD20+, CD79a+, CD5-, CD10-and CD23- t(11;18) (q21;q21)	Resulting from pre-existing inflammatory or autoimmune disorder	
Burkitt's lymphoma	High	c-myc translocation t(8;14)	Massive lymphadenopathy of jaw or abdomen	Children and young adults
Diffuse large B-cell lymphoma	High	CD10 and CD20+ in most cases	Rapid progressive lymphadenopathy	Middle age
Lymphoblastic lymphoma	High		Merge with acute lymphoblastic leukaemia	Children and young adults
T-cell lymphomas				
Peripheral T-cell lymphoma	High	CD4+	Lymphadenopathy, hepatosplenamegaly, skin rash	Middle to older age
Mycosis fungoides	Low	CD3+, CD4+, CD45RO+ and CD8-	Cutaneous with severe pruritus and psoriasis type lesions	
Sézary syndrome	Low	CD4+	Dermatitis, generalised lymphadenopathy	
Adult T-cell leukaemia/ lymphoma	High	HTLV-1	Lymphadenopathy, hepatosplenamegaly. Cutaneous infiltration	
Anaplastic large cell lymphoma	High	CD30+ t(2;5)	B symptoms and extranodal involvement	Children

Adapted from Hoffbrand *et al.* (2001) and Evens *et al.* (2011).

Table 16.10 Treatment regimens.

Type	First-line treatment	Second-line to treat relapse
Follicular lymphoma	• Watchful waiting • Radiotherapy (localised) • Chlorambucil • COP – cyclophosphamide, vincristine, prednisolone • Rituximab	• CHOP – cyclophosphamide, doxorubicin, vincristine prednisolone • Fludarabine • Fludarabine, cyclophosphamide/mitozantrone and dexamethasone (FMD) • Haemopoietic stem cell transplant
MALT	• Antibiotic to treat *Helicobacter pylori*	• Chemotherapy if non-responsive to antibiotics
Burkitt's lymphoma	• Hyper CVAD • CODOX-M/IVAC – cyclophosphamide, vincristine, doxorubicin, methotrexate/Ifosphamide, etoposide, Ara C	
Diffuse large B-cell lymphoma	• R-CHOP – rituximab, cyclophosphamide, doxorubicin, vincristine prednisolone • Haemopoietic stem cell transplant	• ESHAP – etoposide, methylprednisolone, cytarabine, cisplatin • DHAP – cisplatin, cytarabine, dexamethasone • Fludarabine
Waldenström's	• Chlorambucil • Fludarabine • Plasma exchange to reduce hyperviscosity	

Adapted from Hoffbrand *et al.* (2006), Evens *et al.* (2011).

Treatment of non-Hodgkin's lymphoma

The choice of treatment regimen will be decided after diagnosis. Consideration of prognostic indicators and physical fitness of the patient should also be considered.

Treatment for low grade lymphoma

The low grade lymphomas are classed as incurable. This is due to the slow nature of their progression and the spontaneous remissions which can occur. The indolent nature of this type of lymphoma means that many of the chemotherapy regimes will be ineffective until the time the disease transforms into a more aggressive phase. However, there are a range of strategies utilised depending on the patient's symptoms. As the majority of patients diagnosed have advanced stage disease (stage III–IV) the current treatment is either 'watchful waiting' or chemotherapy, and in patients who are symptomatic haemopoietic stem cell transplantation is considered. High grade lymphoma is classed as a curable disease and for this reason the treatment strategies are more aggressive. Due to the diversity of NHL there are a range of treatments available; please see Table 16.10 for some examples of treatment regimens.

Side effects

Side effects to chemotherapy, monoclonal antibodies and HSCT are discussed in Chapter 19 and 20. It is important to consider that each patient will undergo individualised treatment based on their diagnosis, prognosis and prognostic indicators. Therefore their side effects will differ. Any malignancy affecting the lymphocytes will also have an impact on the patient's ability to fight infection. For this reason some patients may require ongoing monitoring to ensure that their immune system is recovering post-treatment.

Conclusion

This chapter has provided an overview of Hodgkin's and non-Hodgkin's lymphoma.

It is evident in the chapter how diverse lymphoma is and that the mainstay of treating this disease is early diagnosis and specific classification of subtype. Nurses need to be aware of this diversity in order to understand why there are so many treatment regimens and how important it is to administer the protocol best suited to the diagnosis.

References

Behringer, K., Diehl, V. and Engert, A. (2005) Hodgkin lymphoma. In: *Textbook of Malignant Hematology*, 2nd edition (eds L. Degos, D.C. Linch and B. Lowenberg). Taylor and Francis, London.

Bower, B. and Waxman, J. (2006) Hodgkin's disease. In: *Lecture Notes: Oncology* (eds B. Bower B. and J. Waxman). Chapter 35, pp. 170–173. Wiley-Blackwell, Oxford.

Cancer Research UK (2010) Incidence of Hodgkin's lymphoma. http://info.cancerresearchuk.org/cancerstats/types/hodgkinslymphoma/index.htm. Accessed 21 June 2010.

Evens, A.M., Winter, J.N., Gordon, L.I., Chiu, B.C.H., Tsang, R. and Rosen, S.T. (2009a) Non-Hodgkin lymphoma. In: *Cancer Management: A Multidisciplinary Approach. Medical, Surgical and Radiation Oncology*, 12th edition (eds R. Pazdur, L.D. Wagman, K.A. Camphausen and W.J. Hoskins). Chapter 27. CMP Healthcare Media, New York.

Evens, A.M., Winter, J.N., Gordon, L.I., Chiu, B.C.H., Tsang, R. and Rosen, S.T. (2009b) Non-Hodgkin lymphoma. In: *Cancer Management: A Multidisciplinary Approach. Medical, Surgical and Radiation Oncology*, 13th edition (eds R. Pazdur, L.D. Wagman, K.A. Camphausen and W.J. Hoskins). CMP Healthcare Media, New York.

Griffin, J., Arif, S. and Mufti, A. (2003) White blood cells. In: *Immunology and Haematology*, 2nd edition (eds G. Kitchen and J. Griffin). Chapter 5, pp. 99–113. Mosby, London.

Hoffbrand, A.V., Pettit J.E. and Moss, P.A.H. (2001) *Essential Haematology*, 4th edition. Blackwell Science, Oxford.

Hoffbrand, A.V., Catovski, D. and Tuddenham, E.G.D. (2005) *Post Graduate Haematology*, 5th edition. Blackwell Publishing Ltd, Oxford.

Hoffbrand, A.V., Moss, P.A.H. and Pettit, J.E. (2006) *Essential Haematology*, 5th edition. Blackwell Science, Oxford.

Hughes-Jones, N.C., Wickramasinghe, S.N. and Hatton, C. (2004) Lymphomas: general principles. In: *Lecture Notes Haematology*, 7th edition. (eds N.C. Hughes S.N. Wickramasinghe and C. Hatton). Chapter 8, pp. 105–118. Blackwell Publishing, Oxford.

Isaacson, P.G. (2005) The classification of lymphomas. In: *Post Graduate Haematology*, 5th edition (eds A.V. Hoffbrand, D. Catovski, E.G.D. Tuddenham). Chapter 43. Blackwell Science, Oxford.

Mehta, A.B. and Hoffbrand A.V. (2009) Lymphoma III non-Hodgkin's lymphoma: clinical and laboratory features of commoner subtypes. In: *Haematology at a Glance*, 3rd edition (eds A.B. Mehta and A.V. Hoffbrand). Chapter 33, pp. 72–73. Blackwell Science, Oxford.

Peranski, K. (2007) Malignant lymphoma. In: *Oncology Nursing*, 5th edition (eds M.E. Langhorne, J.S. Fulton and S.E. Otto). Chapter 15, page 275–289. Mosby, London.

Provan, D., Singer, C.R.J., Baglin, T. and Lilleyman, J. (2004) *Oxford Handbook of Clinical Haematology*, 2nd edition. Oxford University Press, Oxford.

Tobias, J. and Hochhauser, D. (2010) Hodgkin's lymphoma. In: *Cancer and its Management*, 6th edition (eds J. Tobias and D. Hochhauser). Chapter 25, pp. 455–472. Wiley-Blackwell, Oxford.

Watson, M., Barrett A., Spence R.A.J. and Twelves, C. (2006) Patients with common haematological malignancies. In: *Oncology*, 2nd edition (M. Watson, A. Barrett, R.A.J. Spence and C. Twelves). Chapter 15, pp.134–150. Oxford University Press, Oxford.

Yahalom, J. and Straus, D. (2009) Hodgkin lymphoma. In: *Cancer Management: A Multidisciplinary Approach. Medical, Surgical and Radiation Oncology*, 12th edition (eds R. Pazdur, L.D. Wagman, K.A. Camphausen and W.J. Hoskins). Chapter 26. CMP Healthcare Media, New York.

Section 4

Nursing care interventions

Chapter 17

Blood transfusion

Jan Green

By the end of this chapter readers should have a working knowledge of:

- The levels of risk for receiving a blood transfusion
- The different blood groups, including the clinically significant Rh D system
- Blood components and products
- The difference between blood components and blood products
- The different blood components and their indications for use
- The different blood products and their indications for use
- Special requirements; what they are and their indications for use
- Nursing care of the patient undergoing blood transfusion therapy
- Traceability requirements
- Complications of blood transfusion
- Governance, regulation and legislation

Introduction

In the United Kingdom blood is considered to be a scarce resource and thus health care professionals should give due care and consideration to the appropriateness of transfusion in the first instance. The number of donors has been steadily reducing over recent years, with 1.9 million active donors in 2000 and 1.377 million active by late 2007. This equates to 27.5% reduction in the donor base (NHSBT data). However, it is possible that at some point in the future if no further work is done in reducing demand and increasing donor numbers then blood may become even scarcer. Following a concerted effort led by the National Blood Transfusion Committee (NBTC) and its counterparts across the United Kingdom with their associated Regional Blood Transfusion Committees (RTC), the UK Better Blood Transfusion Teams have worked with health care professionals to bring about a reduction of over 15% in the number of red cells transfused to UK patients over the same period of time.

Blood transfusion, as with all procedures and therapies, carries risks for patients. The biggest risk from receiving a blood transfusion is being given the wrong blood

---

Haematology Nursing, First Edition. Marvelle Brown and Tracey J. Cutler.
© 2012 Blackwell Publishing Ltd. Published 2012 by Blackwell Publishing Ltd.

(NHSBT 2007). The UK haemovigilance system, Serious Hazards of Transfusion (SHOT) (2008) and the National Comparative Audit of bedside transfusion practice (Parris and Grant-Casey 2007) show that patients are more at risk from misidentification and poor monitoring rather than the blood itself. Although there is much public concern about contracting an infection from a blood transfusion, compared to other everyday risks the likelihood is very low (see Box 17.1).

Box 17.1 Levels of risk in blood transfusion

The risk of transfusion transmitted infection due to:

Hepatitis B	1 in 500,000
Hepatitis C	1 in 30 million
HIV	1 in 5 million
HTLV	1 in 5 million
vCJD	probably very low with a single transfusion but the risk of any infection will increase with additional blood transfusions.

National Health Service Blood and Transplant (NHSBT) and National Blood Service (NBS) (2007).

Each health care professional plays a role in minimising the risks associated with transfusion. The knowledge required to do this includes an understanding of the ABO and D blood grouping systems and how components of blood should be stored, handled, checked and administered. Health care professionals must also be aware of possible adverse events during or after transfusion, how to monitor patients to detect these events and how to investigate and treat adverse events should they occur, including haemovigilance reporting. Indeed, all staff involved at any stage of the transfusion process must be aware of their local hospital policies and procedures and be trained and assessed as competent in their role (BCSH 1998, NPSA 2006).

Remember that a blood transfusion is a transplant of living cells from a donor to a recipient and as such must be treated with due regard and appropriate diligence.

Blood groups

Blood groups are genetically determined and there are many blood group systems characterised by the presence (or sometimes absence) of a particular structure on the surface of a red blood cell. These are known as antigens. The most important blood grouping, for the purposes of transfusion, is the ABO blood group system. There are four main types of red blood cells (RBC): RBC of group A carry the A antigen, group B, the B antigen, group AB both A and B antigens and group O neither antigen (McClelland 2007). From early childhood, all individuals produce antibodies against the A or B antigens that are not represented on their own RBC (Hearnshaw 2007). These antibodies do not affect the persons own RBC but attack and rapidly destroy RBC containing the relevant antigen. So anti-A attacks RBC of blood from groups A or AB, anti-B attacks RBC of groups B or AB.

Table 17.1 Antigens and antibodies.

Patient blood group	Patients plasma	Compatible red cells
A	Anti-B	A, O
B	Anti-A	B, O
AB	None	A, B, AB or O
O	Anti-A and anti-B	O

Red blood cells for transfusion must be selected to be ABO compatible with the recipient. If incompatible RBC are transfused into a patient, they are immediately attacked and destroyed by the antibodies in the patient's plasma, resulting in intravascular haemolysis, a catastrophic condition which causes the recipient to collapse, developing acute renal failure and disseminated intravascular coagulation (DIC) (McClelland 2007). This reaction can be fatal. The transfusion of even a few millilitres of ABO incompatible blood can cause serious problems and a reaction will occur within a few minutes. Table 17.1 shows the antigens and antibodies in the different blood groups and their compatibility and incompatibility with other groups.

There are many other antigens on red cells. Transfusion can cause antibodies (alloantibodies) to develop in a recipient if the donor cells have an antigen that the recipient does not possess. Antibodies to red cells are usually detected in patients who have been given a blood transfusion in the past, or women who have been pregnant and some of the baby's blood has crossed into the mother's circulation.

The blood group system that can result in the development of potentially harmful RBC antibodies is the Rh system and within this system the D antigen is very important. Approximately 85% of the population is Rh D positive (previously known as rhesus positive) and 15% lack the D antigen. These Rh D negative (previously known as rhesus negative) individuals will form the antibody anti-D if they are exposed to the D antigen. This does not cause an immediate problem but if they are transfused with Rh D positive blood again, a delayed haemolytic transfusion reaction occurs. Transfused red cells are destroyed, causing jaundice and a fall in haemoglobin level. This transfusion reaction does not cause the same acute illness as ABO incompatibility, but should be avoided, particularly in women of childbearing age.

Thus, before blood transfusion it is essential take a blood sample from the recipient for a blood group (ABO and Rh D group) and antibody screen to detect potentially harmful alloantibodies. Suitable RBC can then be selected by the transfusion laboratory and cross-matched against the patient's plasma so that compatible RBC can be issued for transfusion (McClelland 2007).

For the nurse or other clinical staff member administering a transfusion it is important that the blood group on the blood pack matches the patient's blood group. If there is any discrepancy the blood should not be transfused until the laboratory has been contacted and confirmed that the unit may or may not be transfused. For further information and to learn more go to www.learnbloodtransfusion.org.uk

Blood components and products

A blood donor usually donates a unit of whole blood which is then processed by the National Blood Service to produce different blood components. These blood components are red blood cells, platelets and plasma (OPSI 2005). All blood components collected by the UK Blood Services have had the white cells removed prior to issuing. Universal leucodepletion across the UK Blood Services was fully implemented 1999, as a precautionary measure to minimise the risk of variant Creutzfeldt-Jakob disease (vCJD). No further filtration of blood components at the bedside is required.

By contrast, blood products are any therapeutic product derived from plasma (OPSI 2005). These include human albumin solution, the various clotting factor concentrates to treat inherited bleeding disorders (for example haemophilia), anti-D to prevent haemolytic disease of the foetus and newborn and other therapeutic immunoglobulins (Massey *et al.* 2008). For a full detailed list of all blood components supplied by the National Blood Service go to http://hospital.blood.co.uk/products/blood_components/

Red cells

Red blood cells are biconcave, disc-shaped cells without a nucleus (see Figure 17.1). Red cells contain haemoglobin (Hb) which carries oxygen to the tissues. Transfusion of RBC to an anaemic, or bleeding patient will improve the oxygen carrying capacity of blood by raising the haemoglobin concentration. Patients with acute or chronic anaemia develop a number of symptoms related to lack of oxygen, or organ ischaemia when the Hb drops below a critical level (see Table 17.2).

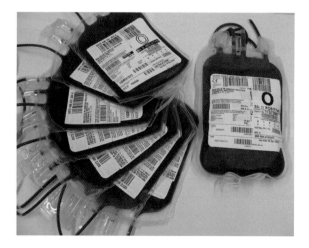

Figure 17.1 An adult pack of red cells and a set of paediatric packs divided from one adult pack, photographed by Jan Green (2009).

Red blood cells for transfusion are separated from anticoagulated whole blood, the white cells removed (leucodepletion) and an optimal additive solution is added to preserve and nourish them. These packed red cells have a haematocrit (Hct) of 57%, which is higher than whole blood. They have a shelf-life of 35 days and must be stored at between +2°C and +6°C. The blood transfusion department will keep supplies of all common blood groups, but patients with unusual RBC antibodies need specially selected blood that is supplied on demand.

Anaemia has many causes. See Table 17.3 and Section 2 on Anaemias.

Table 17.2   Normal haemoglobin levels.

Normal haemoglobin levels for an adult*	
Men	13.0–18.0 g/dL
Women	11.5–16.5 g/dL

*Reference ranges may differ between laboratories.

Table 17.3   Causes of anaemia.

Acute anaemia		Chronic anaemia	
Trauma	• Gunshot wounds • Stabbings	Nutritional anaemia This can occur due to poor diet or malabsorption	• Iron deficiency • B12 deficiency • folate deficiency
Acute surgical haemorrhage	• Major obstetric haemorrhage (MOH) • Liver surgery • Abdominal aortic aneurysm (AAA)	Anaemia of chronic diseases	• Rheumatoid arthritis • Long-term diabetes • Chronic renal failure
Acute gastrointestinal bleeding		Chronic blood loss	• Gastrointestinal tract bleeding • Heavy menstrual blood loss • Recurrent nosebleeds
		Anaemia in patients with cancer	• As a result of cancer affecting the bone marrow • Following chemotherapy or radiotherapy
		Bone marrow failure	• Leukaemia • Myelodysplasia • Aplastic anaemia
		Haemoglobinopathies	• Thalassaemia and sickle cell disease

Red cell transfusion triggers

The decision to give a blood transfusion is based on a detailed understanding of the cause of the anaemia, an assessment of the clinical condition of the patient and the level of haemoglobin. The level of Hb alone is not a sufficient justification. There should be a local strategy in place to ensure appropriate use of red blood cells, which should look at alternatives to transfusion and means of supporting the patient's requirements before instituting blood transfusion therapy, as advocated by James (2004). For example, consideration should be given for the use of intra- or post-operative cell salvage in surgery, oral or intravenous iron replacement therapy for iron deficient patients and the use of erythropoietin injections in patients with anaemia due to chronic kidney disease. These strategies may or may not be appropriate for haematology patients and patients should not be symptomatic due to any restrictive transfusion policies that may be in place. However, blood transfusion is a lifesaving treatment and of course should be given immediately in a life-threatening situation (Murphy *et al.* 2001).

Platelets

Platelets are small cell fragments produced in the bone marrow, that play an essential role in the blood clotting process and are necessary to stop bleeding and bruising. When, as a result of injury, blood comes into contact with any tissue other than the lining of the blood vessel, platelets stick together and form a plug that seals the wound. They then release chemicals, which assist in the coagulation cascade. The plasma releases fibrin which binds with the platelet plug and creates a secure mesh over the wound, allowing healing to take place. Platelet transfusions are indicated for not only the prevention, but also treatment of haemorrhage in patients with thrombocytopenia (low platelet count) or inherited or acquired platelet function defects. Anti-platelet drugs such as aspirin are the commonest cause of acquired platelet dysfunction.

Some causes of low platelet counts where platelet transfusion may be required:

- Leukaemia, myelodysplasia
- Cancer chemotherapy treatment, which affects the bone marrow function and thus platelet production
- Disseminated intravascular coagulation (DIC) following sepsis
- Massive red cell transfusion
- Alcoholic liver disease

Some situations where platelet count is low but platelet transfusion is not effective and may be dangerous (BCSH 2003):

- Idiopathic thrombocytopenia purpura (ITP)
- Thrombotic thrombocytopenia purpura (TTP)
- Heparin induced thrombocytopenia syndrome (HITS)

Platelets for transfusion contain at least 240×10^9/L platelets in anticoagulated plasma, derived either from the pooling of platelets from four whole blood donations or from a single apheresis donation collected on a cell separator machine (McClelland 2007). The

UK Blood Services are working hard to increase apheresis (single donor) collections in order to reduce donor exposure to patients, especially those who require multiple platelet transfusion support. Platelet concentrates are available on demand from NHSBT for named patients, as most hospitals do not keep platelets in stock. They should be ABO compatible if possible but do not need to be cross-matched. Platelets are leucodepleted but may contain some RBC, so Rh D negative women of childbearing potential should always be given Rh D negative platelets.

Platelet concentrates have a shelf-life of only five days and are stored at between +20°C to 24°C in a temperature controlled cabinet that constantly agitates the platelets to keep them viable. They should never be placed in a refrigerator as this will affect their survival and function. However, storage at this (room) temperature has the potential for allowing bacterial growth if the donation has been contaminated at any stage. The bag should always be inspected carefully for signs of discolouration or large clumps and if there are any concerns return to the transfusion department. As with all transfusions, observe the patient closely during and after the transfusion for any signs of infection (see Box 17.2).

Box 17.2   Normal platelet levels

Normal platelet levels for an adult are* 150–400 x 10^9/L
Spontaneous bleeding can occur if platelets are less than 10–20 x 10^9/L
Platelets should be kept above 50 x 10^9/L if the patient is bleeding
Platelets should be kept between 50 to 100 x 10^9/L before and after surgery
(*Reference ranges may differ between laboratories)

Indications for platelet transfusion

Guidelines for the use of platelet transfusions are produced by the British Committee for Standards in Haematology (BCSH 2003). As with red cell transfusion, the decision to give a platelet transfusion should be based on a detailed understanding of the cause of the low platelets and an assessment of the clinical condition of the patient, including the presence of bleeding, bruising or purpura (a pinpoint rash, usually on dependent parts of the body, caused by tiny haemorrhages from capillaries in the skin or mucosa). In stable patients with a platelet count above 10×10^9/L and no signs of bleeding, a platelet transfusion is not required.

Platelets can be given prophylactically to prevent bleeding. The list below gives the platelet count trigger for transfusion and the platelet count target to aim for (where appropriate):

- When the patient is actively bleeding or a count is below 10×10^9/L
- When the patient requires an invasive procedure such as insertion of a central line the platelet count should be above 50×10^9/L
- When the patient requires major surgery the platelet count should be above 100×10^9/L

Local policies may vary on the precise target platelet count, as dictated by the locally agreed clinic guidelines, with the final decision made by the clinician undertaking the procedure.

How many units to transfuse?

One unit of platelets is an adult dose and is usually sufficient to raise the count by 20–40 × 10⁹/L. Survival of transfused platelets varies from patient to patient. The lifespan of platelets is reduced in patients with infection, particularly if they are on high-dose antibiotics. Platelets are destroyed more quickly if the patient has HLA antibodies (from previous transfusions or pregnancy) or if they have an enlarged spleen. Two units of platelets may be needed if the incremental platelet count (on a blood count taken within 30 minutes of the transfusion) has not reached the target and the patient is bleeding or needs surgery or a central line insertion. Two or more units may be required in the case of massive haemorrhage. All hospitals should have a local 'massive haemorrhage' policy established.

Fresh frozen plasma

Plasma is the liquid component of blood and constitutes 55% of total blood volume. It contains:

- Clotting factors
- Plasma proteins, including immunoglobulins (antibodies) and enzymes
- Electrolytes, glucose and minerals
- Hormones
- The anticoagulant used to prevent the whole blood donation clotting
- Any drugs or other chemicals the donor may have ingested

Plasma is separated from whole blood and frozen to a core temperature of –30°C or below where it can be stored for up to 24 months. This is known as fresh frozen plasma (FFP) and contains active clotting factors.

Fresh frozen plasma contains the naturally occurring antibodies within the ABO system (anti-A and anti-B, depending on the blood group of the patient) but does not contain any red cell antigens. Fresh frozen plasma should be ABO compatible with the recipient but it does not have to be matched for the patient's D type (D negative women can have D positive FFP without risk of sensitisation).

Since 1999, the UK Blood Services ceased the use of UK plasma for fractionation and only FFP imported from areas where vCJD is not prevalent is processed into blood products or plasma derivatives. This is because the Advisory Committee on Microbiological Safety of Blood and Tissues for Transplantation, who advises on blood safety issues, made this recommendation to the Department of Health to reduce the possible risk of vCJD transmission. Additionally, from 2004, FFP for all recipients born after 1 January 1996 is sourced from accredited donors in the USA. This has since been extended to all patients under the age of 16. This single donor FFP for paediatric use is virally inactivated using methylene blue. Single donor adult FFP is not virally inactivated, although solvent detergent treated pooled FFP is available commercially. A special product called cryoprecipitate can be made from FFP which is rich in the specific clotting factors, factor VIII and von Willebrand factor, as well as fibrinogen. Although this is no longer used to treat haemophilia or von Willebrand's disease because specific clotting factor concentrates are available, it is very useful in severely ill patients with DIC who are bleeding and have a low fibrinogen level (BCSH 2004).

Indications for fresh frozen plasma transfusion

The indications are very limited. Fresh frozen plasma should be used to treat patients with abnormal coagulation screens who are bleeding or at risk of bleeding.

A clotting screen should be taken before and after transfusion of FFP (see Box 17.3).

Box 17.3 Reasons for giving fresh frozen plasma

FFP may be given if:

- APTR is greater than 1.5
- INR is greater than 1.5
- Fibrinogen is less than 1 g/dL

Consult local laboratory for reference ranges.

Indications for FFP transfusion:

- Disseminated intravascular coagulation (DIC) (also consider cryoprecipitate)
- Massive haemorrhage to replace clotting factors
- Fresh frozen plasma should only be used to replace single inherited clotting factor deficiencies for which no virus-safe fractionated product is available. Currently applies mainly to factor V deficiency

Fresh frozen plasma is not recommended for:

- Volume replacement, other colloids or crystalloids are more appropriate and safer
- Reversal of anticoagulation due to warfarin because FFP has only a partial effect, and is not the optimal treatment for over-anticoagulation
- Prothrombin complex concentrate, a freeze-dried concentrate, is better in patients who are bleeding
- Vitamin K is better in patients who need reversal of anticoagulation in the absence of bleeding

The guideline emphasises appropriate use of FFP by reiterating: 'the purpose of the (BCSH 2004) guidelines are to assist clinical decisions about the transfusion of FFP'. Many of the conventional and widely taught indications for the transfusion of FFP are not supported by reliable evidence of clinical benefit. The largest avoidable risk to patients from transfusion is probably due to the transfusion of FFP for inappropriate or unproven clinical indications (Cohen 1993).

How many units to transfuse?

The volume of each unit of FFP varies between 230 and 300 ml. A therapeutic dose of FFP is 12–15 ml/kg (rounded to the nearest unit). This means that a patient will need 3–4 units of FFP, or about one litre in an average sized person. The rate of infusion depends on the status of the patient, but rapid administration is associated with more adverse reactions and possible fluid overload. The dose of cryoprecipitate is 1–2 pooled units. Each unit contains the cryoprecipitate from five donors. Both FFP and cryoprecipitate have to be thawed before administration, so there will be a delay before this product can be issued by the transfusion laboratory. It has to be used as soon as possible after thawing.

Granulocytes

Granulocytes are the major phagocytic white cells in the blood and are crucial in the control of fungal and bacterial infections. These may be prepared either by apheresis collection or derived from whole blood. Volunteers or directed donors (family or friends of the patient) for apheresis require premedication with steroids and G-CSF to obtain a high cell count yield in the collection. Granulocyte concentrates prepared from whole blood donations yield a lower dose of active granulocytes. As the lifespan of a white cell is thought to be approx 7–10 hours they have to be collected and infused into the patient very quickly. The donor is screened prior to donation (Contreras 1998; McClelland 2007).

Indications for use

Indications for granulocyte infusions are limited to very selected cases where the possible unproven benefits are thought to outweigh the high risks. They include patients who have very low neutrophil counts with intractable severe sepsis which does not respond to standard antimicrobial drugs. Clinical trials have not so far established the effectiveness of this treatment, but some clinicians think it is life-saving. Though there are no established guidelines supporting the clinical use of granulocytes, it is thought reasonable to attempt a three-day course of granulocyte infusions. It is reported that a large randomised controlled trial is planned in the USA sometime in the future (Massey 2008).

The risks from granulocyte infusions for these severely immunocompromised patients include:

- Sensitising the patients and causing them to have a non-haemolytic febrile reactions
- Activating latent viruses, for example cytomeglovirus (CMV) or human T-lymphotropic virus type I (HTLV-1), which can conceal themselves in the granulocytes
- Transfusion associated graft versus host disease (TA-GvHD)

Special requirements

Due to the high risk of side effects, it is extremely important that the transfusion laboratory is informed of the patient's special requirement needs. SHOT (2006) reported that of 400 incorrect blood components transfused (IBCT) incidents, 27% (108) of them were of transfusion of blood of inappropriate specification that did not meet the patient's special requirements. The Medicines and Healthcare products Regulatory Agency

(MHRA) requires hospitals to ensure that a pathway of managing these patients' special requirements is integrated within local policies. This would go some way to prevent errors around the requesting and transfusing of incorrectly treated blood components for transfusion.

Irradiated blood components

The BCSH (1996) has produced *Guidelines on Gamma Irradiation of Blood Components for the Prevention of Transfusion Associated Graft-Versus-Host Disease* (TA-GvHD). This is a rare but usually fatal complication of transfusion of cellular blood components (red cells, white cells and platelets but not FFP).

Indications for use of irradiated components include:

- All transfusions received from first or second-degree relatives (directed donation), even if the recipient is immunocompetent
- All HLA selected platelets, even if recipient is immunocompetent
- All recipients of allogeneic stem cell transplant from time of initiation of conditioning until graft versus host disease (GvHD) prophylaxis is discontinued or lymphocytes are more than 1×10^6/L
- Any cellular blood products transfused to stem cell donors for seven days prior to, or during, stem cell harvest
- All patients undergoing autologous haemopoietic stem cell transplant (HSCT) or peripheral blood stem cell transplant (PBSCT) from initiation of conditioning until three months post-transplant or six months if total body irradiation (TBI) is used as conditioning
- All granulocyte transfusions
- All patients with Hodgkin's disease at any stage
- All patients treated with purine analogue drugs: fludarabine, cladribine or deoxycoformycin

Cytomegalovirus negative blood components

Cytomegalovirus is derived from the Greek *cyto*, 'cell', and *megalo*, 'large'. It is a viral subtype of the herpes viruses. All herpes viruses share a characteristic ability to remain latent or dormant within the body over long periods. Cytomegalovirus (CMV) infection can cause serious morbidity in immunocompromised CMV-negative patients. The risk can be minimised by the use of CMV-antibody-negative (seronegative) blood components. Leucodepletion also confers some protection since the virus is associated with white blood cells (McClelland 2007). The BCSH has not produced any guidelines for the use of CMV-negative components and their use is very much by consensus and monitoring the outcomes of various studies.

The following is from a consensus conference in 2001. However, some studies suggest that effective leucodepletion may confer as much protection as the use of CMV-negative components. It applies to cellular components including red cells, platelets and white cells, but not FFP. Indications for CMV negative use include:

- CMV antibody-negative pregnant women
- CMV antibody-negative recipients of allogeneic stem cell grafts
- Intrauterine transfusions (IUT)
- Neonatal transfusions
- Patients with HIV disease

Human leucocyte antigens matched platelets

Human leucocyte antigens (HLA) are found on most tissues in the body and some cellular blood components, including white cells and platelets but not red cells. Matching for HLA is important for some patients undergoing a stem cell or solid organ transplant. This is because HLA typing is a measure of the unique (genetic) tissue type. Patients exposed to tissues expressing 'foreign' HLA can form antibodies to these antigens. This can happen with non-leucocyte depleted transfusions or during pregnancy when a woman can be sensitised to the antigens from her baby.

Why are HLA matched platelets needed?

Human leucocyte antigen matched platelets are used to treat patients with HLA antibodies who have a poor response to 'standard' platelet transfusions. The presence of these HLA antibodies may affect the survival of platelets after transfusion. Human leucocyte antigen matching reduces the risk of the patient's HLA antibodies destroying the transfused platelets.

How are HLA matched platelets obtained?

The National Blood Service (NBS), a division of NHS Blood and Transplant searches its database for donors who match a specific patient's HLA type. A panel of HLA typed donors is coordinated to ensure a regular supply of matched platelets to meet hospital requests for an individual patient. Thus, several donors are required to support an individual patient.

Why is a blood test required after receiving an HLA matched platelet transfusion?

It is necessary to check that the transfused platelets have been effective in providing a rise in the platelet count post-transfusion as, in some cases, however closely matched, a response is not achieved, thus resulting in wasting that donor's time and the patient receiving an inadequate treatment. Therefore, informing the NBS of the patient's platelet count after each transfusion, helps ensure the most effective platelets are selected for subsequent transfusions. Failure to monitor a patient's response to HLA matched platelets may compromise their treatment. Nurses caring for multi-HLA platelet transfused patients must ensure that the NBS HLA selected platelets follow-up form is completed and returned to their local issue centre after each transfusion.

Blood products and plasma derivatives

Blood products or plasma derivatives (McClelland 2007), are defined as derivatives prepared from pooled human plasma.

Human albumin solution (4.5% and 20%)

Replacement of albumin when large volume ascites is drained is used to restore circulating blood volume, where volume deficiency has been demonstrated and where the use of a colloid is appropriate.

Anti-D immunoglobulin

This is:

- Used to prevent HDN in babies of Rh D negative women
- Given to Rh D negative women of childbearing age if Rh D positive products have been transfused to prevent sensitisation to the Rh D antigen

Clotting factors (recombinant factors are also available)

This is used for treating:

- Haemophilia A (factor VIII) and B (factor XI)
- Von Willebrand disease
- Factor XI deficiency
- Factor XIII deficiency
- Antithrombin deficiency

Human normal immunoglobulin is used in:

- Long-term replacement therapy for missing or defective immunoglobulin in patients with antibody deficiency disorders (primary or secondary immune deficiency)
- Much higher doses (usually in short courses), as immunomodulatory agents in patients with a range of autoimmune or inflammatory conditions.

Nursing care of the patient undergoing blood transfusion therapy

Hospital staff have a responsibility for many aspects of the transfusion processes. Many of the tasks involved with blood transfusion are supported by the National Patient Safety Agency (NPSA) (2006). Nurses may be involved in some or all of these processes, which include:

- Informing the patient
- Providing the written instruction for blood component transfusion

- Care pathways
- Patient identity
- Taking and labelling the blood sample correctly
- Collection of blood from the blood bank
- Checking and administering the transfusion
- Completing documentation clearly and correctly
- Monitoring of the patient during and after the transfusion
- Managing side effects
- Returning and completing traceability documentation

Informing the patient

The patient (or an appropriate responsible person), must be informed that a blood transfusion may be required as part of the treatment. This may not be possible if the patient is unconscious. Currently, written consent is not a legal requirement for blood transfusion (McClelland 2007). However, the BCSH guidelines currently state that: 'Blood transfusion must be treated like any other prescription, for example: patients should be informed of the indication for blood transfusion, its risks and benefits' (BCSH 1999).

Patients also have the right to refuse blood transfusion and therefore alternatives may well need to be considered and in fact should be considered for all patients if appropriate. The guidelines continue and state (BCSH 1999) that:

- 'The patient should be given information about alternatives to blood transfusion'
- 'It is helpful to provide patients with an information sheet outlining the risks and benefits of blood transfusion'

A patient leaflet is available from NHSBT National Blood Service detailing the risks and benefits of blood transfusion. These can be obtained from the hospital transfusion practitioner or downloaded from: http://hospital.blood.co.uk/library/patient_information_leaflets/leaflets/index.asp

Providing the written instruction for blood component transfusion

The BCSH (2009) guidelines state that blood components are excluded from the current legal definition of medicinal products and the requirement for prescription by a registered medical practitioner. This guideline emphasises the need for institutions to develop clear policies to extend the authorisation of administration of blood components safely and conveniently to other appropriately trained and competent practitioners. *Guidelines written to Support Nurses and Midwives Making the Clinical Decision and Providing the Written Instruction for Blood Component Transfusion* (Green and Pirie 2009) are available at: http://www.transfusionguidelines.org.uk/Index.aspx?Publication=BBT&Section=22&pageid=1298 (scroll down to the bottom of the page to download the whole document). Additionally there should be a signed entry in the patient's notes confirming the need for the transfusion.

The BCSH guidelines state: 'The rationale for the decision to transfuse and the specific components to be transfused should be documented in the patient's clinical records' (BCSH 2009).

Care pathways

Care pathways are a useful tool for ensuring the correct processes are followed in a consistent manner. Many hospitals have developed their own and there are examples of algorithms in the *Handbook of Transfusion Medicine* (McClelland 2007) which can be translated into care pathways for local use.

Patient identity

It is vital that the correct blood is given to the correct patient and therefore the patient must be identified. The patient must have a recognised correctly completed wristband *in situ* (NPSA 2007). It must detail:

- Full name (first name and surname)
- Date of birth
- Local hospital identifying number which is soon to be the national NHS ID number (DoH 2008).

Taking and labelling the blood sample correctly

It is important to only bleed one patient at a time to minimise risk of an error and mislabel the sample. Positively identify the patient by asking them for their demographic information rather than asking them if they are Mrs or Mr 'so and so' as anecdotal evidence suggests that patients have been known to respond 'yes' to anything. Immediately after the blood has been collected, label the sample tube *by hand* (unless the local system has a bedside printer incorporated into the process) with the patient's:

- Full name (first name and surname)
- Date of birth
- Local hospital identifying number or NHS ID number (DoH 2008)
- The date bled
- The signature of the person bleeding the patient

Check these details match those on the patient's identity wristband and the sample request form. Avoid taking samples from a patient's arm if they have an IV infusion running into that arm, as this could dilute a full blood count result, which may trigger a transfusion when one is not actually required.

Collection of blood from the blood bank

It is important that the member of staff collecting the blood component from the blood bank has documentation containing the patient's identification details (collection slip, prescription chart or patient's notes). The member of staff must:

- Check the details on the above document and ensure that they match the details on the compatibility label on the unit.
- Check that the blood group and unit number on the pack match those on the compatibility report form.

- When blood components are delivered to the ward or operating theatre a member of appropriately trained staff must be responsible for checking that the correct blood component has been delivered.
- The component must be used within the correct timeframe.
- If the component is not required for immediate transfusion it must be returned to the laboratory within 30 minutes to prevent its wastage.
- The component must not be stored on the ward under any circumstances.

Checking at the bedside

The unit must be inspected prior to administration to ensure it:

- Is not damaged in any way
- Shows no signs of leakage
- Has not passed its expiry date
- Is not an unusual colour
- Has not haemolysed (showing clumping or cloudiness in the case of platelet transfusions)

Local hospital policy will determine if there is a one or two person identity checking procedure in place. It is the responsibility of staff to follow local procedure. The identity check must take place at the patient's bed/chair side. Local policy must include:

- The patient must be positively identified by being asked their full name and date of birth, if they are capable of responding.
- Patients undergoing transfusion must have an identification wristband *in situ*, correctly completed. If there is no wrist band *in situ* then the patient must not be transfused.
- The details on the wristband must be checked and be identical with the details on the blood pack.
- The blood group on the unit must be compatible with the blood group of the patient as indicated on the blood pack label.
- The blood group may not be identical but it must be compatible and in cases where the blood groups may differ, a specific comment should have been made on the compatibility form to indicate that the blood is compatible.
- The unit must be checked for compliance with any special requirement on the prescription chart. For example if CMV seronegative or irradiated blood components have been requested and supplied.
- The person who has carried out the above checks must sign the blood transfusion compatibility form, although SHOT recommends dispensing with the use of the compatibility report for checking purposes (SHOT 2008) and the prescription chart.
- If any discrepancies are found during the bedside check the unit should not be transfused and the transfusion laboratory should be informed immediately. The unit and compatibility form should then be returned to the transfusion laboratory (BCSH 1999; McClelland 2007).

Completing the documentation

There must be a permanent record of the transfusion episode kept in the patient's notes. This must include any additional documentation including:

- The prescription chart
- The observation chart
- The compatibility report, although SHOT recommends dispensing with the use of the compatibility report for checking purposes (SHOT 2008) (see local policy for local practice)
- Any records of adverse events which may have occurred during or after the transfusion
- The management of those events
- A record of the reason for the transfusion
- The outcome of the transfusion (for example whether the transfusion achieved the desired result)

The Blood Safety and Quality Regulations (OPSI 2005) require vein-to-vein traceability of all blood components. The record of this audit trail needs to be kept for 30 years. Most transfusion departments have introduced a traceability system to record the fate of a blood transfusion which is either electronic or a paper based system. Either system requires the nurse administering the component to confirm transfusion as soon as the transfusion starts.

Blood administration

There are a variety of blood administration sets available. Red cells, plasma and platelets should be transfused through a giving set with an integral 170–200 micron filter (see Table 17.4). All blood components (excluding granulocytes) in the UK are leucodepleted so supplemental microaggregate filters are not required for any blood component transfusions (including granulocytes).

Priming the line

The line must be primed before attaching it to the patient. It is unnecessary to prime with anything other than the blood component, but 0.9% sodium chloride may be used for this purpose. Dextrose should never be used in a giving set before or after blood components, as it can cause haemolysis. Manufacturers' instructions for priming the line should always be followed.

Changing the administration set

If multiple units are being transfused, the administration set should be changed at least every 12 hours to prevent bacterial growth. Some administration sets may be supplied with different instructions, or local hospital policy may vary. In these cases you should follow the manufacturer's instructions or your hospital policy, as appropriate.

Table 17.4 Methods of administration.

Blood component	Instructions for adult administration
Red cells	• A 170–200 micron filter is required (standard red cell administration set) • Either gravity or electronic infusion pumps may be used • Electronic infusion pumps should only be used if the manufacturer verifies them as safe for that purpose and an approved and compatible giving set is used • A unit of red cells is usually administered over 2–3 hours and the transfusion must be completed no more than four hours after the product has been removed from temperature controlled storage
Platelets	• A 170–200 micron filter is required (either a blood or platelet administration set may be used) • Platelet concentrates should not be transfused through administration sets which have already been used for blood • Platelet administration sets have a smaller priming capacity than a blood administration set • A unit of platelets is usually administered over 30 minutes
Fresh frozen plasma (FFP)	• A 170–200 micron filter is required (standard red cell administration set) • Once thawed, FFP must not be re-frozen and should be transfused as soon as possible • Post-thaw storage will result in a decline in the activity of clotting factors • For products kept at 22°C post thawing, the transfusion must be completed within four hours of thawing • For products stored at 4°C post thawing, the transfusion must be completed within 24 hours of thawing • A unit of FFP is usually administered over 30 minutes
Granulocytes	• A 170–200 micron filter is required (standard red cell administration set) • The whole dose should be transfused over 1–2 hours
Cryoprecipitate	• A 170–200 micron filter is required (standard red cell administration set) • Once thawed cryoprecipitate must not be re-frozen and should be used immediately • If delay is unavoidable it can be stored only in the laboratory in a controlled environment for up to 24 hours

On completion of the transfusion

Flushing through the remainder of the blood in the line with 0.9% sodium chloride is unnecessary and is not recommended because it may result in particles being flushed through the filter. If another intravenous (IV) infusion is to take place after the blood transfusion, it is good practice to use a new administration set to reduce the risk of incompatible fluids or drugs causing haemolysis of any residual red cells which may be left in the administration set.

Drugs

Drugs must not be added to any blood component pack. An infusion line that is being used for blood should not be used to administer any other drugs as an interaction may occur causing damage to the component. For example dextrose solution (5%) can cause haemolysis and calcium-containing solutions may cause clotting of citrated red cells (McClelland 2007).

Blood warmers

Hypothermia impairs haemostasis and reduces red cell oxygen delivery to the tissues. Therefore rapid transfusion of red cells at 4°C can lower the patient's core temperature by several degrees. It has been reported that cold blood infused faster than 100 mL/minute can cause cardiac arrest in adults (McClelland 2007). Rapid infusion devices which usually incorporate a blood warming device may be used when large volumes have to be infused rapidly. Red cells should only ever be warmed using a specifically designed commercial device, which is CE marked with a visible thermometer and audible warning. The manufacturer's instructions must be strictly followed. Some blood warmers are designed to operate up to and including 43°C but are safe, provided they are used and maintained according to the manufacturer's instructions. Blood and blood components should not be warmed using improvisations such as putting the pack into hot water, in a microwave or on the radiator. Fatalities have occurred due to haemolytic transfusion reactions and/or bacterial contamination of the blood component following the use of inappropriate blood warming procedures.

Monitoring of the patient during and after the transfusion

Vital signs must be measured and recorded before the start of each unit of blood or component and at the end of each transfusion episode. These observations should be recorded separately from routine observations so that they are clearly related to the transfusion episode. The patient's temperature and pulse should be recorded 15 minutes after the start of each unit of blood or component. Further observations are necessary only if the patient becomes unwell or shows signs of a transfusion reaction. It is very useful to advise patients to alert ward staff if they experience any adverse effects (BCSH 1999; McClelland 2007).

Visual observation of the patient is the best way of assessing their condition during the transfusion. Unconscious patients are more difficult to monitor for signs of a transfusion reaction and should be observed frequently during their transfusion. Therefore it is vital that transfusions should take place in clinical areas where patients can be readily observed throughout the procedure. Routine observations should continue and transfusion reactions should be considered if there is a change or deterioration in the patient's condition. It is good practice, when possible, to avoid transfusing patients out of core hours (usually avoid transfusion between 8 pm and 8 am) unless clinically essential (BCSH 1999; McClelland 2007).

Returning and completing traceability documentation

The fate of the donation must be recorded (OPSI 2005). This is to ensure all components can be traced from donor to recipient and from recipient back to the donor. It is mandatory for hospitals to comply with this practice. The transfusion laboratory must have a system in place so they are informed. Hospital practice varies as to how this is achieved so it is important to check local policy.

Complications of blood transfusion

One of the most serious potential hazards of transfusion is a patient receiving blood which is incompatible with their own. In most cases these incidents are entirely preventable and are usually due to human error. Staff are fallible human beings and do not always follow the correct procedures laid down in locally approved policies, which are there to protect patients as well as themselves. SHOT (2008) is a UK-wide confidential, voluntary reporting system for serious adverse events and near misses associated with transfusion. In their Annual Report the category of 'incorrect blood component transfused' (IBCT) represented the highest proportion of all reports received. Examples include:

- Patient not wearing a wrist band, thus could be the wrong patient
- Not checking the patient identity and thus not the correct patient
- Commencing the transfusion on the wrong patient as patient's identity not checked
- Bleeding a patient and labelling the sample with incorrect details

A series of errors are a consistent feature of IBCT incidents, with more than one error reported in many cases. Errors occur at all stages of the transfusion process: in prescribing, taking of blood samples from the patient, in the transfusion laboratory, in the collection of blood from storage and at the bedside. By far the most common error contributing to IBCT was failure of the bedside checking procedure. The bedside check is the final chance to spot errors which may have occurred earlier in the transfusion process.

Transfusion reactions

Some reactions to the transfusion of blood components can be acute (by definition within 24 hours, although typically during the first few minutes of a transfusion) and life threatening; it is important to recognise these and know how to manage the patient in the emergency setting. It may not be obvious at the onset of the reaction what the cause is but this can be investigated after the initial resuscitation. Other reactions to blood components may be delayed for several days with immunological complications, to several months for transfusion transmitted infection. A history of transfusion should always be sought or the association with a previous transfusion may be overlooked. All serious adverse reactions and events related to blood transfusion should be reported, via the hospital transfusion team, to the SHOT and/or SABRE.

Symptoms/signs of acute transfusion reactions include:

- Fever
- Chills

- Tachycardia
- Hypertension
- Hypotension
- Rigor
- Collapse
- Flushing
- Urticaria
- Shortness of breath
- Bone, muscle, chest or abdominal pain
- Nausea
- Generally feeling unwell or anxious.

Iif you suspect a patient is having a transfusion reaction:

- Stop the transfusion.
- Call a doctor immediately.
- Keep the line patent with a new IV giving set and 0.9% sodium chloride infusion.
- Take and record temperature, pulse and blood pressure readings.
- Check and record respiration rate and oxygen saturation.
- Check the identity of the recipient against the details on the pack and on the compatibility report.
- Inform the blood transfusion laboratory.
- Be aware of, and refer to, local hospital policy for treatment protocol.

Recognition and management of acute transfusion reactions

In 1–2% of patients, particularly multi-transfused patients, minor non-haemolytic febrile transfusion reactions (FNHTRs) occur. These are characterised either by an isolated rise in temperature of more than 1°C or by minor rigors, chills or skin rash, such as urticaria. The patient may feel nauseated, become mildly tachycardic or hypotensive. The transfusion should be stopped and the patient treated with paracetamol. The antihistamine drug, chlorpheniramine, can be given if a rash is present. If the observations stabilise and symptoms settle the infusion can be started at a slower rate with more frequent observations. The majority of patients are able to complete their transfusions and no further investigation is required. If FNHTRs are a recurrent problem with subsequent transfusions, patients may be pre-medicated with paracetamol and chlorpheniramine although there is some debate about whether this is effective or not (Geiger and Howard 2007).

Acute haemolytic transfusion reaction

This occurs as a result of ABO incompatible red cells being transfused and can occur after a few millilitres have been given. Rapid onset of intravascular haemolysis is due to the recipient's anti-A or anti-B antibodies reacting with the donor A or B red cells. As well as developing the above symptoms, the patient may experience pain over the kidney area and dark brown urine. Always let the transfusion laboratory know as soon as possible – if there has been a mix-up between patients a second incompatible transfusion can be prevented.

Infusion of a bacterially contaminated unit

This is likely to cause a severe acute reaction similar to acute haemolytic transfusion reaction (ATR) with rapid onset of hypotension, rigors and collapse. It is fortunately a rare occurrence but it is more likely to occur in platelet components than red cells as they are stored at room temperature. If a contaminated unit is suspected, it is necessary to refer the blood component back to the blood collection facility for further testing as well as following the local protocols for culturing the patient and the unit and treating with antibiotics.

To prevent bacterial proliferation:

- Ensure components are not damaged.
- Store component correctly.
- Adhere to time limits for transfusion of each blood component.
- Visually inspect component for leaks, signs of contamination, clumps, discolouration or unusual appearance prior to transfusion.

If in any doubt about whether to transfuse the unit or not contact the blood transfusion department.

Severe allergic reaction or anaphylaxis is a rare but life-threatening complication of rapid onset which is again similar to ATR, but the patient is more likely to have urticaria and wheezing due to bronchospasm. It usually occurs in the early part of the transfusion episode. The risk is higher with the transfusion of components containing larger volumes of plasma, for example FFP or platelets. Transfusion associated circulatory overload (TACO) can occur when too much fluid is transfused or transfusion is too rapid. Patients, particularly the elderly, with chronic anaemia may have signs of cardiac failure prior to transfusion. They are typically normovolaemic and increase in their circulating volume results in acute onset of breathlessness due to left ventricular failure. This usually occurs later in the transfusion than other ATRs and may occur some hours after the transfusion has finished. If TACO is anticipated, each unit may be given more slowly, often with a diuretic, and the patient should be closely observed.

Transfusion related acute lung injury (TRALI) should be suspected when severe respiratory distress occur within six hours of a transfusion. It is thought to be caused by a reaction between white cell antibodies present in the plasma of the blood component and the patient's own white cells. It presents as acute onset of shortness of breath and hypoxia during or soon after a transfusion, occurring more commonly after the transfusion of plasma or platelets because most red cell components contain very little plasma.

Delayed transfusion reactions

These can be divided into immunological reactions, transfusion transmitted infection and iron overload. Only immunological reactions will be discussed here. For further reading, consult the *Handbook of Transfusion Medicine* (McClelland 2007).

Delayed haemolytic transfusion reactions (DHTRs) occur after 24 hours and are a result of a red cell antibody reacting with and damaging the donor cells. The RBC antibody may have been caused by a previous transfusion or in women, by a pregnancy. If the Hb fails to increase post-transfusion, or it increases and then drops quickly, then suspect a DHTR. Contact the transfusion laboratory who will investigate advice on selection of further blood products and report to SHOT.

Transfusion associated graft versus host disease (TA-GVHD) can occur in immuno-compromised patients if any immunocompetent lymphocytes are transfused that can then engraft and grow in the host, where they attack the tissues and cause a very serious and rapidly fatal multi-organ failure. To prevent this, cellular blood components are gamma irradiated for certain groups of vulnerable patients.

Governance, regulation and legislation

Blood component transfusion has become one of the most heavily regulated aspects of health care in the United Kingdom, with practice and compliance monitored by the NHS Litigation Authority (NHSLA) and the Care Quality Commission.

- The Department of Health (DoH) has issued three Health Service circulars promoting safe practice and appropriate use of blood:
  o *Better Blood Transfusion* (HSC 1998/224)
  o Better Blood Transfusion – Appropriate use of Blood (HSC 2002)
  o Better Blood Transfusion – Safe and Appropriate use of Blood (HSC 2007)
- The Medicines and Healthcare products Regulatory Authority (MHRA) has been designated the competent authority by the Department of Health to oversee compliance with the *Blood Quality and Safety Regulations* (OPSI 2005)
- The Serious Hazards of Transfusion reporting scheme (SHOT) together with Serious Adverse Blood Reactions and Events (SABRE) the reporting arm of MHRA, monitors adverse events
- The British Committee for Standards in Haematology (BCSH) has made recommendations for the administration of blood transfusion as well as the safe and appropriate use of blood components and products
- The National Patients Safety Agency (2006) in conjunction with the National Blood Transfusion Committee has made many recommendations regarding mandatory competency assessment of all staff involved in blood transfusion from venepuncture and sampling of the patient to administration of the actual transfusion.

For any further information please see www.transfusionguidelines.org (also Figure 17.2).

The National Blood Transfusion Committee (NBTC) for England and North Wales was established in 2001. There are similar structures covering the rest of the UK Blood Services. Its remit is to promote safe and appropriate transfusion practice and to work collaboratively to improve transfusion practice. The committee provides a forum to discuss national transfusion issues and to channel information to regional transfusion committees (RTCs) to share with hospitals in their region. The NBTC meets twice a year. The minutes from each meeting are sent to chairs of the regional transfusion committees and are subsequently disseminated to all hospital transfusion committees (HTCs).

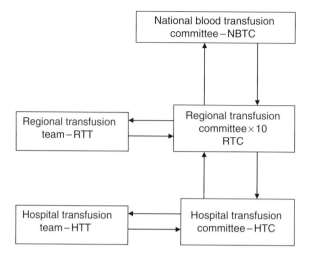

Figure 17.2 An overview of blood transfusion infrastructure in England and North Wales.

The regional transfusion committees (RTCs) are responsible for implementing actions of the NBTC in England. They oversee the activities of the local hospital transfusion committees (HTCs) and provide a link between the HTCs and NBTC.

The RTC is usually made up of representatives from:

- The region's hospital transfusion committees (including NHS and private hospitals)
- The NHS blood and transplant regional hospital liaison team
- Patient groups
- Strategic health authority

There are up to four meetings of the regional transfusion committees per year; minutes and actions are disseminated to chairs of all HTCs in the region. The work of the RTC is coordinated by the regional transfusion team.

The regional transfusion team

The regional transfusion team (RTT) is the working group of the RTC and consists of elected or nominated members. They usually meet around six to eight times per year to plan the agenda of the RTC, review workgroup outputs and plan education meetings.

The hospital transfusion committee

Every trust involved in blood transfusion should have a hospital transfusion committee (HTC) as stated by the DoH in the Health Service circular (2002): *Better Blood Transfusion – Appropriate use of Blood*. The HTC should have the authority to take the necessary actions to improve transfusion practice by promoting safe and appropriate use of blood. Although there are no definitive recommendations from the DoH guidance documents regarding actual HTC membership, the committee membership should include:

- Chair (often an anaesthetist)
- Transfusion laboratory manager
- Transfusion practitioner
- Haematologist in charge of blood transfusion department
- Senior nursing and midwifery representation
- Clinical representatives who are users of blood components
- Anaesthetist
- Member of risk management
- Representative from finance
- Representative from the primary care trust

The hospital transfusion team

The hospital transfusion team (HTT) is the working group of the HTC, monitoring day-to-day issues around blood transfusion and should report to the HTC. It should consist of:

- Transfusion laboratory manager
- Transfusion practitioner
- Haematologist in charge of blood transfusion department

Conclusion

As demonstrated, blood transfusion is a highly regulated aspect of health care. It is essentially a safe procedure but it is not without its risks, many of which can be avoided if correct procedures are followed.

References

British Committee for Standards in Haematology (1996) Guidelines for gamma irradiation of blood components for the prevention of transfusion-associated graft-versus-host disease. *Transfusion Medicine*, 6, 261–271.

British Committee for Standards in Haematology (1998) Guidelines for the administration of blood and blood components and the management of transfused patients. *BCSH Blood Transfusion Task Force. Transfusion Medicine*, 9, 227–239.

British Committee for Standards in Haematology (2003) Guidelines for the use of platelet transfusions. *British Journal of Haematology*, 122, 10–23.

British Committee for Standards in Haematology (2004) Guidelines for the use of fresh-frozen plasma, cryoprecipitate and cryosupernatant. *British Journal of Haematology*, 126, 11–28.

British Committee for Standards in Haematology Guideline on the Administration of Blood Components (Dec 2009) *British Society for Haematology* http://www.bcshguidelines.com/4_HAEMATOLOGY_GUIDELINES.html?dtype=Transfusion&dpage=0&sspage=0&ipage=0#gl.

Chohan, S.S., McArdle, F., McClelland, D.B.L., Mackenzie, S.J. and Walsh T.S. (2003) Red cell transfusion practice following the transfusion requirements in critical care (TRICC) study: prospective observational cohort study in a large UK intensive care unit. *Vox Sanguinis*, 84 (3), 211.

Cohen, H. (1993) Avoiding the use of FFP. *British Medical Journal*, 307, 395–396.

Contreras, M. (1998) *ABC of Blood Transfusion*, 3rd edition. BMJ Books, London.

Department of Health (2008) *Announcement Concerning the NHS Number Programme Subject. Professor Sir Bruce Keogh*, NHS Medical Director, Department of Health May 2008 (only published electronically) http://www.dh.gov.uk/en/Publicationsandstatistics/Lettersandcirculars/Dearcolleagueletters/DH_084729.

Geiger, T.L. and Howard, S.C. (2007) Acetaminophen and diphenhydramine premedication for allergic and febrile non-haemolytic transfusion reactions: good prophylaxis or bad practice? *Transfusion Medicine Reviews*, 21 (1), 1–12.

Green, J. and Pirie, L. (2009) A *Framework to Support Nurses and Midwives Making the Clinical Decision and Providing the Written Instruction for Blood Component Transfusion*. Transfusion Guidelines website: http://www.transfusionguidelines.org.uk/Index.aspx?Publication=BBT&Section=22&pageid=1298.

Hearnshaw, K. (2007) Transfusion matters. *British Journal of Anaesthetic and Recovery Nursing*, 8 (Spring) (3), 51–55.

James, V. (2004) *A National Blood Conservation Strategy for NBTC and NBS* http://www.dh.gov.uk/en/Publichealth/Healthprotection/Bloodsafety/Bloodsafetygeneralinformation/index.htm.

Massey, E. (2008) Granulocyte therapy. *Blood Matters* (Spring), NHSBT publication London: http://hospital.blood.co.uk/library/pdf/bm24.pdf.

McClelland, D.B.L. (2007) *Handbook of Transfusion Medicine*, 4th edition. The Stationery Office, London. http://www.transfusionguidelines.org.uk/index.aspx?Publication=HTM.

Murphy, M.F., Wallington, T.B., Kelsey, P. *et al.* (2001) Guidelines for the clinical use of red cell transfusions. *British Journal of Haematology*, 113 (1), 24–31.

National Health Service Blood and Transplant (NHSBT) National Blood Service (NBS) (2007) *Will I need a blood transfusion*. Patient information leaflet. http://www.blood.co.uk/pages/e34patnt.html.

National Patient Safety Agency (2006) Safer Practice Notice 14, *Right Patient, Right Blood*. http://www.npsa.nhs.uk/patientsafety/alerts-and-directives/notices/blood-transfusions/.

Nursing and Midwifery Council (NMC) (2008) *The Code – Standards of Conduct, Performance and Ethics for Nurses and Midwives*. NMC, London. http://www.nmc-uk.org/aArticle.aspx?ArticleID=3057.

Office of Public Sector Information (2005) *Blood Safety & Quality Regulations SI 2005/50*. The Stationery Office, London. http://www.opsi.gov.uk/si/si2005/20050050.htm.

Parris, E. and Grant-Casey, J. (2007) Promoting safer blood transfusion practice in hospital. *Nursing Standard*, 21 (41), 35–38.

Pirie, E. and Green, J. (2007) Should nurses prescribe blood? *Nursing Standard* (6 June), 21 (39), 35–41.

Serious Hazards of Transfusion Steering Group (2008) *Annual Report* http://www.shotuk.org/home.htm

Chapter 18

Venous access devices

Janice Gabriel

By the end of reading this chapter you will be able to:

* Identify the range of VADs
* Discuss the clinical indications for a specific group of VADs
* Summarise their care and management
* Identify their potential complications
* Discuss the importance of individual patient assessment

Introduction

The health care professional has access to a wide range of vascular access devices (VADs), including peripheral, midline and central venous access devices (CVADs). Each device has been carefully designed to meet both the clinical requirements and, where appropriate, the lifestyle needs of the individual patient.

It is rare for a haematology patient admitted to hospital not to become a recipient of a VAD. It should also be noted that increasing numbers of patients in the day care, outpatient and, indeed, community setting also require vascular access for a range of infusion therapies (Dougherty 2008; Kayley 2003). Knowledge of these devices, their indications and management, together with patient assessment are crucial to ensure safe, reliable and high quality care for the individual patients (Carrico 2006; Dougherty 2008; Ingram and Lavery 2005; Petersen 2002).

Classification of vascular access devices

Vascular access devices fall into three categories, for example:

* Peripheral
* Midline
* Central

Haematology Nursing, First Edition. Marvelle Brown and Tracey J. Cutler.
© 2012 Blackwell Publishing Ltd. Published 2012 by Blackwell Publishing Ltd.

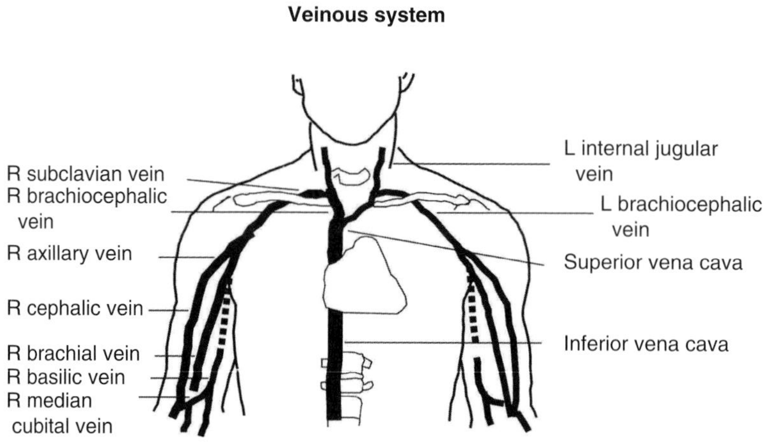

Veinous system

Figure 18.1 Venous circulation (Dougherty 2006). Reprinted with permission of John Wiley & Sons, Inc.

Peripheral

Peripheral cannulae are available in a variety of gauge sizes and lengths. Some have integral stabilisation wings and some injection ports – often referred to as 'ported' cannulae. These are short devices which are placed into a peripheral vein (see Figure 18.1) (Dougherty 2008; RCN 2010). Selection of veins in areas of flexion in the upper limbs, for example the wrist and antecubital fossa, should be avoided whenever possible, as the movement of these joints can result in the cannula puncturing the wall of the vein. This can result in infiltration of the infusate to surrounding tissues, or extravasation if a vesicant agent is being administered (Dougherty 2008; Hadaway 2006; RCN 2010). Cannulation of veins in the lower limbs should also be avoided, if at all possible, due to the increased risk of thrombophlebitis and also pulmonary embolism. If the patient has no accessible veins elsewhere and the lower limbs have to be considered, the dorsum of the feet and the saphenous veins should be the sites of first choice. If one of these sites is selected, the cannula should be re-sited at the earliest opportunity (Dougherty 2008).

Midline

Midline catheters, or peripherally inserted catheters (PICs), are inserted into a vein in the antecubital area (cephalic, median cubital or basilic) (Figure 18.1). The catheter is then advanced along the vein, but due to its overall length (20–25 cm) does not extend beyond the axillary vein (Griffiths 2007). These devices have been confused with peripherally inserted *central* catheters (PICCs). PICCs are *central* venous access devices, and as such their tips terminate in the central venous circulation (Dougherty 2006; Gabriel 2006; RCN 2010; Vesley 2003). Midline catheters can remain *in situ* for several weeks, and offer a more comfortable alternative to peripheral cannulae for patients requiring shorter term parenteral therapies, but who do not require a central venous access device (Dougherty 2008).

Central venous access devices

Central venous access devices (CVADS) are a group of catheters whose tip terminates in the central venous circulation, for example superior vena cava (SVC), inferior vena cava (IVC) or right atrium (RA) (Figure 18.1) (RCN 2010; Vesley 2003). Following placement of any CVAD, the tip location should be confirmed by chest X-ray (CXR) prior to first use and recorded in the patient's notes (RCN 2010).

There are four types of CVADs:

- Non-tunnelled catheters
- Skin tunnelled catheters
- Implantable injection ports
- Peripherally inserted central catheters (PICCs)

CVADs are available in a range of gauge sizes and can have up to five lumens (Dougherty 2006; Gabriel 2006; RCN 2010).

Non-tunnelled catheters

Non-tunnelled catheters are commonly used for short-term central venous access. Access can be achieved from a number of approaches, including the internal and external jugular, femoral and subclavian veins (Figure 18.1) (Scales 2008).

Skin-tunnelled catheters

Skin-tunnelled catheters are tunnelled under the patient's skin, usually on the chest wall, where they access the central venous circulation via the external/internal jugular or subclavian veins (Figure 18.1). The portion of catheter in the skin tunnel incorporates a 'Dacron' cuff which encourages the growth of tissue. This cuff not only helps to stabilise the device, but also provides an additional barrier to minimise the potential for infection (Dougherty 2006).

Implantable injection ports

Implantable injection devices consist of a subcutaneous injection port attached to a central catheter. The injection port can be placed under the patient's skin peripherally (on an arm), or centrally (on the chest). Once the port is placed under the patient's skin, it is anchored to underlying muscle with sutures, and the catheter tunnelled under the skin until the desired venous access point is reached. The catheter is then advanced along the vein until its tip reaches the central circulation (Dougherty 2006) (Figure 18.1). (Ports are available as two-part devices, for example the injection port requires connection to the catheter during insertion, or as a complete unit where the port is already connected to the catheter during the manufacturing process.)

Peripherally inserted central catheter

For peripherally inserted central catheter (PICC) placement venous access is achieved by cannulation of the median cubital, cephalic or basilic vein (Figure 18.1). The PICC is then passed through the cannula and advanced along the vein until the tip reaches the central venous circulation. The cannula is then removed and the PICC secured to the patient's skin (RCN 2010).

Gauge sizes

The size of a VAD will be described by the various manufacturers in terms of length and gauge size. The length will be expressed in either millimeters or centimeters, for example 36 mm or 60.0 cm. The gauge size will refer to the external diameter of the device and not the internal diameter. The external diameter can be expressed in either 'French' (Fr) or 'gauge' (ga) size, for example 4.0 Fr or 18 ga. With multi-lumen devices it is the overall diameter of the device which is stated, for example 5 Fr (16 ga) (Gabriel *et al.* 2005). The flow rate through a VAD will depend upon the internal diameter of the particular device and its overall length. (Individual manufacturers will be able to provide specific information on their products regarding the gravity flow rates and rates achieved by the use of a pump.)

Valved and non-valved devices

Central venous access devices (CVADs) are available as valved or non-valved (open-ended) catheters. The purpose of the valve is to remain closed when the catheter is not being used. When positive pressure (injecting) is applied to the catheter, the valve will open outwards, thereby allowing infusion. When negative pressure (aspiration) is applied, the valve will open inwards. The valve can be incorporated into either the distal or proximal end of the catheter, depending on individual manufacturer design (Gabriel 2006) (Figure 18.2).

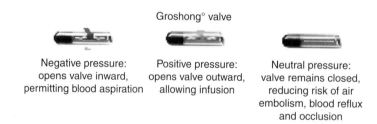

Groshong° valve

Negative pressure: opens valve inward, permitting blood aspiration

Positive pressure: opens valve outward, allowing infusion

Neutral pressure: valve remains closed, reducing risk of air embolism, blood reflux and occlusion

Figure 18.2   Valved catheter.

Construction material

The construction material of midline devices and CVADs can either be polyurethane, polyvinyl or silicone rubber (Scales 2008). Devices constructed from polyurethane or polyvinyl tend to be more rigid than those manufactured from silicone rubber, but they do become softer at body temperature. They also have the advantage of facilitating the manufacture of thinner walled devices, which are able to deliver high flow rates as a consequence of their larger internal lumen. Their main disadvantage, especially if used for longer term therapies, is that there is the potential for irritation to the tunica intima (the inner lining of the vein), which may slightly increase the potential for phlebitis (Dougherty 2006). Devices constructed from silicone rubber have thicker walls than those made from polyurethane or polyvinyl, which results in slower flow rates due to a smaller internal lumen. As silicone rubber is softer than polyurethane or polyvinyl, it is less of an irritant to the tunica intima and is associated with a lower incidence of phlebitis and thrombosis (Dougherty 2006). All three materials are radio opaque, allowing clear visualisation of the device under fluoroscopy or when X-rayed (Dougherty 2006).

Clinical indications

The choice of VAD should take into consideration the diagnosis, or suspected diagnosis of a patient. For many haematology patients, the requirement for a VAD will be inevitable as they will receive a protracted course of treatment. For some patients this may be intermittent treatment spread over many months/years. For others it may be for multiple therapies over a number of weeks, for example a patient with acute myeloid leukaemia (AML) undergoing a haemopoietic stem cell transplant (HSCT).

A patient requiring venous access for a few hours to a few days, with a non-irritant/ non-vesicant medicine/infusate, may well have their clinical needs met with a peripheral venous access device, for example a cannula. For patients requiring longer term therapy, again with non-irritant/non-vesicant substances, a midline catheter may be the solution (Dougherty 2008; Griffiths 2007). For patients requiring multiple therapies, which will include vesicant and/or highly irritant substances, a CVAD would be the solution (Dougherty 2006). The particular choice of CVAD will depend on the individual requirements of the patient. For those requiring short-term central venous access, such as in the emergency setting or for a major surgical procedure, a non-tunnelled catheter would probably suffice (Gabriel *et al*. 2005; Scales 2008).

Non-tunnelled catheters do carry an increased potential for infection the longer they are left *in situ*, and would not be suitable for the longer term needs of a haematology patient, or indeed any patient who may be potentially immunocompromised. Patients requiring intermittent, long-term parenteral therapy may prefer to have an injection port, such as a patient with thalassaemia who may require intermittent therapy. For the patient with acute leukaemia, including those undergoing HSCT, a tunnelled catheter would be the device of choice, as the device provides ready venous access with easily accessible injection hubs (Dougherty 2006; Gabriel 2006).

Care and management

Infection

Insertion of any VAD, whether peripheral, midline or central, is an invasive procedure and therefore has the potential to result in infection, especially in patients who are immunocompromised or have the potential to become so. To reduce the risk of infection to both patient and health care worker a few simple, but effective steps can be taken.

Health care professional

- Washing of hands with soap and water before and after procedure
- Appropriate use of alcohol hand rubs
- Use of well fitting sterile gloves
- Wearing of disposable plastic aprons
- Use of sterile, single use equipment
- Appropriate disposal of equipment immediately following the procedure

Patient

- Ensure the patient is comfortable.
- Removal of any *excess* hair with scissors/electric shaver if necessary prior to insertion of VAD.
- Clean the intended venepuncture site with an antimicrobial solution (preferably 2% chlorhexidine in 70% isopropyl alcohol) and allow it time to dry.
- Never attempt reinsertion of a 'used' cannula/needle.
- Remove any blood on the patient's skin prior to stabilisation of cannula/catheter.
- Apply an appropriate dressing to cannula/catheter.
  (Casey and Elliott 2007; Epic2 2007; Gabriel 2006; Lavery and Ingram 2006; RCN 2010)

For insertion of CVADs maximum sterile precautions should be used, with the health care professional wearing sterile gloves and gown, and use of large sterile drape(s) to cover the patient. If there is a possibility that there could be the risk of blood splashing onto the face of the health care worker, mask and goggles/facial visor should also be worn (Dougherty 2006; Epic2 2007; RCN 2010).

Dressings

Research supports the use of moisture permeable transparent dressings (Dougherty 2006; Gabriel 2006; Hart 2008; RCN 2010). They allow easy observation of the insertion site for peripheral VADs, midline devices, PICCs and other types of CVADs, but also provide a waterproof barrier to minimise the potential for infection. Such dressings used on peripheral VADs can remain *in situ* until the device is removed/re-sited (72–96 hours), unless its integrity is compromised, or there is moisture/blood observed under the dressing. In these circumstances the dressing should be removed, the insertion site cleaned and a new dressing applied (RCN 2010). For midline devices, PICCs and non-tunnelled catheters, there is usually some slight oozing of blood during the first few hours following the insertion procedure. In this case a small piece of sterile gauze can be placed directly over the insertion site and the moisture permeable dressing applied. This dressing should then be changed the following day, or sooner if the gauze becomes contaminated. Following this first dressing change and, providing the integrity of the dressing is not compromised, or there is no further exudate, it can be left *in situ* for up to seven days, for example, when it should next be routinely changed. The 'routine' dressing change should include the removal of the stabilisation device, cleansing of the insertion site, reapplication of a new stablisation device and dressing (Gabriel 2006; Epic2 2007; RCN 2010). If gauze and sterile tape dressings are used, they will require a 24–48 hour routine dressing change, or more frequently if they become soiled (RCN 2010). Skin tunnelled catheters do not require a dressing once the skin tunnel and insertion wounds are healed.

Stabilisation of venous access devices

For the majority of patients, careful application of an appropriate dressing will be sufficient to stabilise their cannula. However, stabilisation can be greatly increased, together with minimising the potential for resulting complications associated with an inadequately stabilised device, for example mechanical phlebitis, premature loss of the cannula, infiltration/extravasation, by the use of a dedicated IV stabilisation device (Figure 18.3). Such devices are recommended for midlines, PICCs and non-tunnelled CVADs. Not only are they more comfortable for the patient than suturing, but they also minimise further the potential for infection by eliminating the need for suturing, and also eliminate the risks associated with needlestick injuries, again associated with suturing (Gabriel 2006).

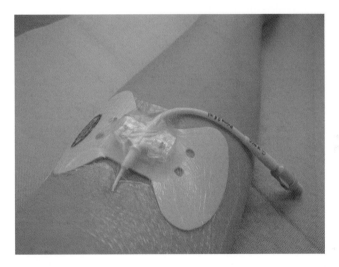

Figure 18.3 Stablisation device.

Maintaining patency

A non-patent VAD is one of the commonest causes of premature device removal. Appropriate care of a patient's VAD will not only add to the longevity of their device, but also help to ensure the patient's parenteral therapy is not delayed. Dougherty (2006) defines patency as:

- 'Ability to infuse through a catheter
- Ability to aspirate blood from a catheter'

Prior to administration of any parenteral medicine, or commencement of any infusion, the patency of the VAD should be checked with 0.9% sodium chloride. If the health professional is unable to 'flush' the VAD, or resistance is encountered, the device should not be used until a further assessment has been made. This assessment should be as outlined in the next two sections.

Peripheral venous access devices

- How long has the VAD been *in situ*?
- Is the patient complaining of any discomfort arising from the VAD?
- What does the insertion site and surrounding area look like?
- When was the device last used and were there any documented problems/does the patient recall any problems?
- What medication/infusions were last administered – could they have resulted in precipitation, for example blockage of the internal lumen of the VAD?
- Is there any external kinking/pressure to connecting IV tubing?
- Can the patient's prescribed therapy now be given orally instead of intravenously?

If the answer(s) to the above do not resolve the problem, then it would be appropriate to re-site the cannula so the patient's treatment can continue. To minimise the potential for occlusion, a peripheral cannula should be flushed with 0.9% sodium chloride directly following the administration of medicines/infusions and at regular intervals when the device is not in use (Dougherty 2006). The frequency of 'routine' flushing of peripheral cannulae to minimise the risk of occlusions is still undetermined. However, a 'flushing' technique that has been demonstrated to be highly effective is a positive pressure/turbulent flush (positive pressure flushing is achieved by maintaining pressure on the plunger of the syringe as it is removed from the injection cap). This will minimise the potential for reflux of blood into the lumen of the VAD. Turbulent flushing is achieved by a rapid push/pause technique when injecting the 0.9% sodium chloride (Dougherty 2006; Gabriel 2006; RCN 2010).

Midline and central venous access devices

Midline catheters and CVADs should be flushed with 0.9% sodium chloride, using a positive pressure/turbulent flush technique, with twice their prime volume (the capacity of the internal lumen) directly following the administration of drugs and/or infusions. If the device has more than one lumen, each lumen will require positive pressure/turbulent flushing to ensure its potential for occlusion is minimised. While it is generally accepted that 0.9% sodium chloride is the acknowledged flush solution for peripheral cannulae when they are not in continual use, there is still no conclusive evidence to support the use of either 0.9% sodium chloride or heparinised saline for CVADs. However, Epic2 (2007), who have looked at the risks and benefits associated with the use of heparinsed saline, recommend the use of 0.9% sodium chloride. Manufacturers of valved catheters recommend the use of 0.9% sodium chloride to be used on a weekly basis for each lumen of their CVADs when not in continual use. The manufacturers of open-ended (non-valved) devices will be able to supply specific product information relating to flush solution and frequency of flushing for their own products (Dougherty 2006; RCN 2010). For implantable injection ports, individual manufacturers will also be able to provide specific information on the flush solution to be used and its frequency.

Phlebitis

Richardson and Bruso (1993) identified three types of phlebitis: chemical, mechanical and infective.

Chemical phlebitis

As the tip of a CVAD terminates in the SVC/IVC/RA, it would be rare to see this type of phlebitis in recipients of skin tunnelled catheters, non-tunneled catheters, implantable injection ports or PICCs. This is because the devices terminate in a large blood vessel, and the infusates are quickly diluted by the volume of blood flowing, so they have little opportunity to irritate the lining of the vein wall (Figure 18.1).

Mechanical phlebitis

Mechanical phlebitis is more likely to occur within the first seven days following insertion of the VAD (peripheral cannula, midline or PICC). It is commonly a consequence of too large a device being placed into an individual with small blood vessels. This causes the blood to be restricted from flowing around the VAD, which can result in mechanical phlebitis. It can usually be resolved within 48 hours by the application of heat to the upper arm, for 20 minutes three times a day for recipients of PICCs and midlines. For recipients of a peripheral cannula it would be more appropriate to re-site the cannula with a smaller size, or consider an alternative VAD, for example a midline catheter (Richardson and Bruso 1993).

Infective phlebitis

If phlebitis presents more than seven days after insertion of a VAD (peripheral cannula, midline or PICC), or if a suspected case of mechanical phlebitis is not resolved by the application of heat, infection could be the cause (Richardson and Bruso 1993). A swab should be taken from the insertion site and sent to microbiology for culture and sensitivity. If considered appropriate, blood should also be aspirated from the lumen(s) of the CVAD and sent for culture and sensitivity (Hart 2008).

Thrombosis

Patients with certain types of malignancies, for example mucin-secreting adenocarcinomas, promyelocytic leukaemia and myeloproliferative disorders, are more at risk of thrombosis as a result of CVAD placement than other groups (Brothers *et al.* 1988;

Wickham *et al.* 1992). Camp-Sorrell (1992) highlighted a study which recorded a 40% risk of thrombosis in patients with adenocarcinoma of the lung that had a CVAD, compared with 17% in patients with small-cell lung cancer or squamous cell carcinoma.

The process of developing a thrombosis related to CVADs is believed to be linked to a series of events (Dougherty 2006; Ryder 1995; Wickham *et al.* 1992). The process of introducing the catheter into the vein causes trauma, which results in thromboplastic substances and platelets collecting at the site of venepuncture. The larger the size of the venepuncture, the greater the injury to the vein. This trauma to the vein may result in the development of small thrombi which can adhere to the wall of the damaged vein, or possibly migrate, increasing in size and leading to occlusion of a larger vessel (Camp-Sorrell 1992; Wickham *et al.* 1992).

The size and rigidity of the CVAD can also cause further trauma to the vein. Large, rigid catheters are associated with a higher risk of thrombosis than finer, more supple devices (Camp-Sorrell 1992; Gabriel *et al.* 2005; Ryder 1995; Wickham *et al.* 1992). The rapid administration of vesicant/highly irritant drugs or infusates can lead to chemical phlebitis, which may result in the development of thrombosis (Ryder 1995; RCN 2010; Wickham *et al.* 1992).

The clinical features of thrombosis formation are variable and may not become apparent until there is total occlusion of the blood vessel. Early symptoms may include erythema of the skin overlying the CVAD, oedema, discomfort, pyrexia and pain radiating down the arm on the side the device has been placed. Later symptoms tend to be more indicative of the underlying problem, with facial swelling, neck vein distension and/or arm swelling; this could be expanded as superior vena cava thrombosis can lead to superior vena cava obstruction which is an emergency situation. Diagnosis is usually confirmed by cathetergram or ultrasound examination (Dougherty 2006; Wickham *et al.* 1992).

It is possible to treat a patient's thrombosis without removing the CVAD, but this depends upon the severity of the symptoms and the patient's general condition (Dougherty 2006; Wickham *et al.* 1992). Management of the thrombosis is more effective if treatment is initiated early. Treatment can include the surgical removal of the clot, but more commonly urokinase, heparin or tPA is administered as a continuous infusion through the CVAD. A review of the literature has identified that although these agents have been used with varying degrees of success, there are no uniform doses or lengths of infusion (Brothers *et al.* 1988; Dougherty 2006; Gabriel *et al.* 2005; Wickham *et al.* 1992). Brothers *et al.* (1988) highlighted that, once the patient's thrombosis has resolved, parenteral therapy can be resumed through the original CVAD. Initiation of such treatments should be discussed on an individual basis with the consultant in charge of the patient's care.

Pinch-off syndrome

Hinke *et al.* (1990) first described pinch-off syndrome (POS) as a condition which can arise when the CVAD is compressed between the clavicle and the first rib. When the arm moves, the movement of the clavicle can cause the CVAD to be compressed, which can ultimately result in the shearing of the device and lead to catheter migration (Figure 18.4).

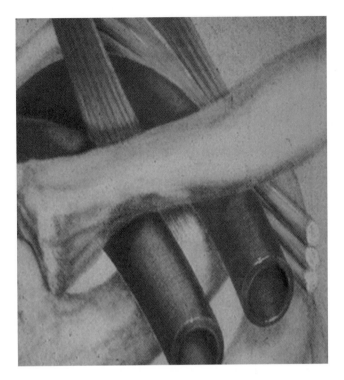

Figure 18.4   Pinch-off syndrome.

Clinical indications of POS can include:

- Inability to infuse fluids
- Difficulty in aspirating blood

If these signs are ignored, the catheter can go on to rupture and migrate through the blood vessels and into the heart.

Patient assessment

Prior to placing any VAD (peripheral cannula, midline or central) it is important that the patient's clinical condition and, where appropriate for recipients of longer term devices, their lifestyle is assessed. This will help to ensure that the patient will 'accept' the device, and complications are minimised (Chernecky 2002; Gabriel 2006). The patient should receive written and verbal information about the device, its insertion procedure, potential complications, care and management and who to contact if they have any concerns about the device. This is especially important if the patient will be 'living' with their VAD away from the hospital environment as they will almost certainly not have immediate access to a health care professional who is familiar with their particular type of VAD.

Before the patient consents to the procedure the health professional must ensure that the patient has had sufficient opportunities to ask any questions, to seek clarification on any aspect of the procedure, and what the after care of the particular VAD may entail (Dougherty 2008). Prior to the placement of a CVAD the patient's blood count should be checked to ensure that the platelet and WBC counts are adequate for the procedure (Gabriel *et al.* 2005). If appropriate, a clotting screen should also be undertaken. Where necessary, a thrombocytopenic patient can have the CVAD placed whilst receiving a platelet infusion. Patients with an elevated INR can have their anticoagulant therapy adjusted accordingly if considered appropriate by the clinician in charge of their care (Gabriel 2006; Richardson and Bruso 1993). CVADs should not be placed in patients who are experiencing neutropenic sepsis, as there is a potential for the device itself to become infected and therefore contribute further to the patient's problems.

For all insertions in the patient's upper body, except in the case of a PICC, the patient should be placed in the Trendelenburg position. This will ensure that the venous access point is below the level of the heart and therefore minimizes the risk of an air embolus. As PICCs are placed in an arm vein, the Trendelenburg position can be dispensed with, providing the health professional placing the device ensures that the patient's arm remains below the level of the heart (Dougherty 2006; Gabriel 2006; Richardson and Bruso 1993).

Central venous access devices can be placed under either local or general anaesthetic in order to minimise the discomfort of the procedure for the patient. Peripherally inserted central catheters can be successfully placed using a topical anaesthetic ointment. This is because the procedure involves accessing an arm vein with a conventional wide gauge cannula, or using the Seldinger technique (Griffiths 2007; RCN 2010). (The Seldinger technique involves using a hollow bore needle to access the vein, passing a wire through the needle, withdrawing the needle and then threading the catheter over the wire to gain access to the vein.) Midline placements can also be successfully placed using topical anaesthetic cream, and by using the Seldinger technique (Griffiths 2007). The use of ultrasound guidance is recommended for placement of all CVADs where placements are undertaken without the assistance of imaging, for example outside the radiology department or theatre (NICE 2002; RCN 2010).

Device removal

Once the decision has been made to remove the VAD the procedure should be discussed with the patient. For peripheral cannulae the dressing and, if used, securement device, should be removed. Gentle traction should be applied to the cannulae to remove it, and sterile gauze immediately applied over the insertion site with firm pressure. The gauze should then be secured with tape. The cannula and any dressing, should be immediately and appropriately disposed of in line with individual organisational policies/procedures, and the procedure recorded in the patient's notes.

Midline and PICCs should also be removed by using gentle traction, but if any resistance is encountered the procedure should be immediately stopped. The commonest reason for encountering resistance is venospasm, and allowing time for the muscles and valves to relax (20–30 minutes), often resolves the problem (RCN 2010). The application of a warm compress to the upper arm can also help to relax the muscles. Immediately the device is removed, sterile gauze should be used to cover the insertion site using firm pressure. The device should be inspected to ensure that it is intact, for example all of it has been withdrawn, and the procedure recorded in the patient's notes (Gabriel 2006; Griffiths 2007). When removing PICCs, the patient's arm should be kept below the level of their heart to minimise the risk of air embolism.

Removal of skin tunnelled catheters and implantable injection ports are more involved and invasive procedures, requiring the use of local anaesthetic agents, or indeed sedation/general anaesthetic for nervous patients and children. For ports, the tissue surrounding the injection port will require dissection to enable the catheter to be removed. For tunnelled catheters, the 'Dacron' cuff in the skin tunnel itself will require dissection to enable the catheter to be removed, especially if the device has been in place for a considerable period of time (Dougherty 2006).

Conclusion

With the range of VADs now available, individual patient assessment is crucial in order to ensure that patients are offered the most appropriate device to meet their clinical needs and, where appropriate, their lifestyle away from the hospital environment. The potential for complications associated with any vascular access device has to start with the assessment process, but is augmented through both staff and patient education and by careful management of the chosen device. This is not only beneficial to the individual patient, but will also be advantageous to the organisation by ensuring that valuable resources are used appropriately.

References

Brothers, T.E., Von Moll, L.K., Arbor, A. *et al.* (1988) Experience with subcutaneous infusion ports in three hundred patients. *Surgery, Gynaecology and Obstetrics*, 6 (4), 295–301.

Camp-Sorrell, D. (1992) Implantable ports: everything you always wanted to know. *Journal of Intravenous Nursing*, 15 (5), 262–272.

Carrico, R. (2006) Preventing catheter-associated bloodstream infection: changing practice in a complex environment. *Oral presentation 20th Annual Conference of Association of Vascular Access (AVA)*, Indianapolis, USA. September.

Casey, A. and Elliott, T. (2007) The usability and accessibility of needleless connector systems. *British Journal of Nursing*, 16 (5), 267–271.

Chernecky, C., Macklin, D., Nugent, K. and Waller, J.L. (2002) The need for shared decision making in the selection of vascular access devices: an assessment of patients and clinicians. *Journal of Vascular Access Devices*, 7 (3), 34–39.

Dougherty, L. (2006) *Central Venous Access Devices Care and Management*. Blackwell Publishing Ltd, Oxford.

Dougherty, L. (2008) Obtaining peripheral venous access. In: *Intravenous Therapy in Nursing Practice*, 2nd edition (eds L. Dougherty and J. Lamb). Blackwell Publishing Ltd, Oxford.

Epic2 (2007) National evidence-based guidelines for preventing healthcare-associated infections in NHS hospitals in England. *Journal of Hospital Infection*, 65 (Suppl 1).

Gabriel, J. (2006) Vascular access. In: *Nursing in Haematological Oncology* (ed. M. Grundy). Baillière Tindall Elsevier, Edinburgh.

Gabriel, J., Bravery, K., Dougherty, L. *et al.* (2005) Vascular access: indications and implications for patient care. *Nursing Standard*, 19 (6), 45–54.

Griffiths, V. (2007) Midline catheters: indications, complications and maintenance. *Nursing Standard*, 22 (11), 48–57.

Hadaway, L. (2006) Infiltration and extravasation from vascular access devices. *Oral Presentation 20th Annual Conference of Association of Vascular Access (AVA)*, Indianapolis, USA. September.

Hart, S. (2008) Infection control in intravenous therapy. In: *Intravenous Therapy in Nursing Practice*, 2nd edition (eds L. Dougherty and J. Lamb). Blackwell Publishing Ltd, Oxford.

Hinke, D.H., Zandt-Stastny, M.D., Goodman, L.R., Quebbeman, E.J., Kyzywda, E.A. and Andris, D.A. (1990) Pinch-off syndrome: a complication of implantable subclavian venous access devices. *Radiology*, 177, 353–335.

Ingram, P. and Lavery, I. (2005) Peripheral intravenous therapy: key risks and implications for practice. *Nursing Standard*, 19 (46), 55–64.

Kayley, J. (2003) An overview of community intravenous therapy in the United Kingdom. *Journal of Vascular Access Devices* (Summer), 22–26.

Lavery, I. and Ingram, P. (2006) Prevention of infection in intravenous devices. *Nursing Standard*, 20 (49), 49–56.

National Institute for Clinical Excellence (NICE) (2002) *Ultrasound Imaging for Central Venous Catheter Placement*. NICE, London.

Petersen, B. (2002) Stepping into the future: who will care for healthcare? *Oral Presentation National Association of Vascular Access Networks (NAVAN) Conference*. San Diego, CA. September.

Richardson, D. and Bruso, P. (1993) Vascular access devices – management of common complications. *Journal of Intravenous Nursing*, 16 (1), 44–49.

Royal College of Nursing (RCN) (2010) *Standards for Infusion Therapy*, 3rd edition. RCN, London.

Ryder, M. (1995) Peripheral access options. *Surgical Clinics of North America*, 4 (3), 395–427.

Scales, K. (2008) Vascular access in the acute care setting. In: *Intravenous Therapy in Nursing Practice*, 2nd edition (eds L. Dougherty and J. Lamb). Blackwell Publishing Ltd, Oxford.

Vesley, T. (2003) X-ray interpretation: theory to practice. *Presentation 17th National Association of Vascular Access Networks (NAVAN) Conference*, Atlanta, GA. September.

Wickham, R., Purl, S. and Welker, D. (1992) Long-term central venous catheters: issues for care. *Seminars in Oncology Nursing*, 2 (8), 133–147.

Chapter 19

Chemotherapy and monoclonal antibodies

Alison Simons and Tracey Cutler

This chapter aims to provide an overview of chemotherapy and monoclonal antibodies. By the end of the chapter you will:

- Have an insight into the rationale behind the use of these treatments
- Have an awareness of the methods of administration
- Be aware of the side effects of these treatments

What is cytotoxic chemotherapy?

Cytotoxic chemotherapy is a group of drugs that are used to treat many conditions. They are, however, predominately used in the treatment of malignant disorders including haematological disorders. But in the haematology setting they are used in both malignant and non-malignant disorders. 'Cytotoxic' is derived from 'cyto' meaning 'cell', and 'toxic' meaning 'poison'. Chemotherapy means chemical therapy.

How does chemotherapy work?

Chemotherapy drugs act on all rapidly dividing cells, including malignant cells that are rapidly proliferating, and either stops the cells being able to divide or causes apoptosis; either action prevents cell replication. Cytotoxic chemotherapy drugs are designed to interfere with the cell cycle during cell division to induce apoptosis (Wilkes *et al.* 2007).

Chemotherapy drug classification

There are many different chemotherapy drugs widely available, and a number of methods used to classify these drugs. However, for the purpose of this chapter it will focus on the most common classification groups of chemotherapy drugs. This is not

Haematology Nursing, First Edition. Marvelle Brown and Tracey J. Cutler.
© 2012 Blackwell Publishing Ltd. Published 2012 by Blackwell Publishing Ltd.

an exhaustive list, and with new developments and research many other types of drugs are being discovered.

Alkylating agents

These are non-cell cycle specific, so will act on any stage of the cell cycle. These drugs alter DNA by adding an alkyl bond onto the DNA bases, causing cross links to form, and double strand breaks, destroying the DNA template (Baquiran 2001). The DNA is unable to separate during the synthesis phase, which leads to cell death (Wilkes *et al* 2007). Examples include cisplatin, oxaliplatin, carboplatin, chlorambucil, cyclophosphamide and melphalan.

Antimetabolites

These drugs have a structure that is very similar to naturally occurring metabolites; the cell mistakes them and incorporates them into the DNA strand (Wilkes *et al.* 2007). This stops essential enzymes that are needed for DNA and RNA synthesis, causing cell replication to stop and cell death occurs (Brighton *et al.* 2005; Wilkes *et al.* 2007). These drugs act predominately in the S phase but also in G1. Examples include 5Fu, methotrexate, gemcitabine, fludarabine, capecitabine and cytarabine.

Anti-tumour antibiotics

These drugs are non-cell cycle specific, and cause intercalation, adding a group or molecules, between base pairs of the DNA (Baquiran 2001), which then leads to single and double DNA breaks. Examples include dactinomycin, danorubicin, epirubicin, mitomycin C, bleomycin.

Topoisomerase inhibitors

These drugs are S phase and early G2 phase specific. Topoisomerase is an enzyme that allows the DNA double helix to unwind during cell division, and then realign following cell division. These drugs stop this from happening and cause irreparable nicks/ breaks in the DNA strand, thus preventing the realignment of the DNA double helix (Brighton *et al.* 2005). Examples include etoposide, anthracyclines, doxorubicin, epirubicin, topotecan, camptothecin, irinotecan.

Mitotic inhibitors (plant alkaloids)

This group contains two subgroups, Vinca alkaloids (made from periwinkle plant) and taxanes (made from pacific yew bark). These drugs stop mictrotubules that are involved in mitotic spindle formation, which enable the chromosomes to migrate during mitosis. This is predominately during metaphase (M phase specific) but also acts on G2, and results in stopping mitosis (Skeel 2003). Examples include vinblastine, vincristine and paclitaxel.

Combination chemotherapy

Each disorder has a gold standard treatment. This has been proven by clinical trials to be the most effective for that type of disorder. Chemotherapy treatment is often given in a regimen/protocol consisting of a combination of two or more drugs (although single agent chemotherapy can be used). This is done to maximise the chance of causing the most cell death with the least toxicity (Brighton *et al*. 2005) and therefore increases the overall survival for that patient. Each of the different drugs in the regime may act differently on different phases of the cell cycle. Also, if each drug has different toxicities it means we can give as close to the maximum dose as possible, without causing too severe side effects (Baquarin 2001).

Chemotherapy cycles

Chemotherapy regimes are given in cycles, and are delivered to patients over regular periods of time, with a specific gap between each cycle. This is done in order to allow normal cells to recover, including the bone marrow. The drugs used within the regimen depend on the rest period, but usually 21–28 days, in order to allow enough time for normal cells to recover but not enough time to allow malignant cells to start to grow again (Brighton *et al*. 2005).

Drug dosage

The dose of each chemotherapy drug within the regime is carefully calculated based on the individual about to receive the drug. The maximum tolerated predefined dose has been developed from clinical studies. Each drug has a specific maximum tolerated dose in order to be able to give the highest dose possible to maximise efficacy, but be safely administered and tolerated by the patient (Brighton *et al*. 2005).

The drugs used determine what method or formula is used to calculate the maximum tolerated dose; the most common method used is patient's body surface area multiplied by the predefined dose. This highlights the importance of accurate recording of a patient's height and weight prior to chemotherapy treatment and before subsequent courses as it may result in a dose alteration of the chemotherapy drugs in the regimen. However, there are some chemotherapy agents which have a maximum life time dose, which also needs consideration when dose calculations are made.

Routes of administration

Chemotherapy can be administered via a number of different routes. It can be given via the blood supply, systemically or locally (see Table 19.1).

Table 19.1 Routes of administration.

Route	Method
Intravenous	This is the most common way of chemotherapy delivery, via a cannula or central venous access device, it provides rapid dilution and rapid reliable delivery of the drug but is not without risks of infiltration and extravasation.
Oral	In the form of tablets or capsules, this can be an economical non-invasive way of administering chemotherapy but relies on a functioning gastrointestinal tract, swallowing ability and compliance of the patient (Brighton *et al.* 2005).
Subcutaneous and intramuscular	Given as an injection, this method of administration can result in incomplete absorption. Some chemotherapy drugs can be an irritant, and cause discomfort from regular injections.
Topical	Creams and ointments containing cytotoxic agents, applied superficially.
Intrapleural	Introduction of chemotherapy drugs into the pleural cavity.
Intravesical	Bladder instillation via a urinary catheter.
Intraperitoneal	Introduction of cytotoxic drugs into peritoneal cavity following drainage of ascites.
Intra-arterial	Introduction of chemotherapy directly to the tumour via arterial blood supply.
Intrathecal	Administration of chemotherapy into cerebral spinal fluid. This can be fatal if intravenous Vinca alkaloids are injected intrathecally. There have been recorded incidents of this, and as a result numerous safety measures are now in place. This is comprehensively outlined in the Department of Health (2008) document entitled *Updated National Guidance on the Safe Administration of Intrathecal Chemotherapy*.

Health and safety

All chemotherapy agents in whatever form, are potentially hazardous substances and are classed as carcinogenic (cancer producing), mutagenic (DNA damaging) and teratogenic (produce malformations in the foetus) (Allwood *et al.* 2003). There are three main routes of exposure to chemotherapy, inhalation (via splash or spillage), absorption (via splash, spillage or needlestick injury) and ingestion (via poor hand hygiene, eating, drinking or smoking in contaminated areas) (Health and Safety Executive 2003). Acute effects such as irritation of skin, eyes and mucous membranes, light headedness and nausea may be experienced. More chronic mutagenic, carcinogenic and teratogenic effects have been shown (from data in animals) (HSE 2003).

Under the Control of Substances Hazardous to Health (Health and Safety Executive 2002) guidelines, employers have a legal duty to protect the staff and the public, undertaking risk assessment, controlling that risk and protecting against exposure. Staff also need to be informed, instructed and trained about the risks of chemotherapy and the precautions required to be in place and observed; this is outlined by Management and Awareness of Risks of Cytotoxic Handling (MARCH 2008). Health and safety policies with regard to cytotoxic chemotherapy handling and administration must be in place (Health and Safety Executive 2002). Equally, employees must utilise the measures put in place by the employer.

In order to control exposure of chemotherapy, preparation should take place in a central pharmacy (DoH 2003); this should be done in a closed system with adequate ventilation using a laminar flow cabinet. Personal Protective Equipment at work regulation (MARCH 2008b) should be observed. Transporting chemotherapy needs to be done in sealed bags or rigid containers (HSE 2003) to reduce the risk of leaks or spillage during transit. Chemotherapy should be stored in a designated locked fridge or cabinet, depending on which drug is being stored (MARCH 2008a). Areas that store and administer chemotherapy drugs should be clean and prohibit eating drinking and smoking.

Some form of protective clothing should be worn at all times when dealing with chemotherapy equipment, depending on what activity and drug is being used (MARCH 2008b). The equipment should meet minimal legal safety requirements, and be stored and maintained appropriately. The clothing should be suitable for the task, suited to the wearer and the environment and compatible with other PPE in use. The equipment needs to be in good condition and be worn correctly. There is some argument that staff should also be given training on how to use these correctly (MARCH 2008b). The balance of being able to protect staff from exposure and not frightening patients and their family is a difficult one to achieve and should be assessed on an individual basis. Policies and guidelines should be in place in areas preparing and administering chemotherapy on what to do if contamination or spillage should occur and this must be in line with MARCH (2009) and Health and Safety Executive (2002) guidelines.

Side effects

As cytotoxic chemotherapy affects all rapidly dividing cells, including healthy normal cells, this can result in many side effects (Allwood *et al.* 2003; Baquirin 2001; Skeel 2003). These can be either temporary or long term. Each cytotoxic drug has specific side effects; collectively there are numerous side effects that can be classified in different ways. For the purpose of this chapter the more common side effects will be discussed, but this is by no means an exhaustive list (see Table 19.2).

It is important to assess the patient's potential of developing side effects on an individual basis, in order to be able to identify and implement management of these side effects promptly and reduce severity. The use of performance status and Common Toxicity Criteria Assessment (Allwood *et al.* 2003; National Chemotherapy Advisory Group (NCAG) 2008) is advised to monitor side effects and their severity, and also to monitor the effectiveness of any intervention. This should be done prior to subsequent courses of treatment and appropriate action taken such as dose reduction, stopping treatment and decision to treat (NCAG 2008).

Table 19.2   Side effects of chemotherapy.

Classification	Side effect	Explanation
Emergency	Anaphylaxis	Acute systemic reaction to the drug being administered (Allwood *et al.* 2003)
	Extravasation and infiltration	Inappropriate or accidental administration of chemotherapy into the subcutaneous or subdermal tissue rather than intravenous (Allwood *et al.* 2003)
	Tumour lysis syndrome	Rapid cell death due to therapy resulting in metabolic abnormalities (Skeel 2003)
General	Metabolic/ strange tastes	Due to alterations in the oral mucosa (Baquiran 2001) and use of platinum based drugs
	Chemical phlebitis and venous irritation	Reactions within the vein due to chemical properties of the drug (Allwood *et al.* 2003)
	Fatigue	As a result of disease process, aggressive therapy used and/or bone marrow suppression (Baquiran 2001)
	Alopecia	Hair loss
Toxicity	Haematological – due to drugs affecting rapidly dividing cells	Myelosuppression (bone marrow suppression) Anaemia (reduction of red blood cell production) Neutropenia (reduction of neutrophil production) Thrombocytopenia (reduction of platelets)
	Gastrointestinal – due to drugs affecting rapidly dividing cells	Nausea and vomiting Anorexia Mucositis Constipation Diarrhoea
	Dermatological	Hyper-pigmentation Nail changes Photosensitivity Hand foot syndrome/plantar palmer syndrome
	Organ toxicity	Hepatoxicity Nephrotoxicity Pulmonary toxicity Cardiotoxicity
	Neurological	Peripheral neuropathy Cerebella toxicity/encephalopathy Cranial neuropathy Autonomic neuropathy
	Sexuality and fertility changes	Gonadal dysfunction Infertility Testicular dysfunction Teratogenicity

Communication and information giving

It is vital that patients have information regarding their proposed treatment so that they can make an informed consent (DoH 2009). This information should be tailored to their individual disorder type, treatment regimen and drug side effects (DoH 2004).

Patients' expectations have risen, resulting in increasing demands for accurate information concerning treatments and their side effects (Verity 2005). This is currently being addressed by the DoH (2007) in the Cancer Reform Strategy, which recognised the need for good quality information to be provided. It is good practice to provide written information for patients (DoH 2009) This must include what type of chemotherapy they are receiving, what likely side effects they may experience and contact details of health care professionals should they experience any problems (NCAG 2008).

Monoclonal antibodies

Paul Ehrlich, the German Nobel prize winner in 1908, first proposed the idea of a 'magic bullet' which could treat infectious disease and cancer cells. In 1975 Kőhler and Milstein describe the methodology for the production of monoclonal antibodies, which won them the Nobel prize in 1986. This allowed the start of large-scale clinical testing of antibodies, leading to the first published report of a treatment in lymphoma with a monoclonal antibody in 1980 (Dillman 2001): 'Since 1975, the pharmaceutical industry has been engaged in using Biotechnology to produce these drugs with precise targets and low toxicity' (Capriotti 2001, p. 89).

What are monoclonal antibodies?

As discussed in Chapter 2, any antigen which is recognised as foreign, for example viruses or transplanted tissue, will be recognised and destroyed by the immune system.

The body's natural defences against these foreign agents are antibodies (produced by B-cells), these antibodies are specific to one particular antigen and once activated will enlist the immune system to destroy the antigens and can also provide ongoing resistance to future infection. Antibodies are proteins produced by activated B-cells (plasma cells). The activation occurs after the first exposure to a specific antigen. These Y-shaped structures are found on the surface of B-cells or circulating in the blood stream after secretion from a plasma cell (Modjtahedi 2007). The basic structure of an antibody is composed of two heavy and two light polypeptide chains further divided into variable or constant regions (see Figure 19.1). The variable portion of both the heavy and light chains forms the two identical antigen-binding fragments (Fab). The constant portions of the heavy chains are called crystallisation fragments (Fc).

Fab – is the antigen binding site
Fc – activation of the complement system and alert of the immune system for cellular attack

Monoclonal antibodies are synthesised antibodies which target specific antigens; these antibodies activate the immune system, leading to the destruction of the specified target and limited damage to healthy cells. The original methodology for producing monoclonal antibodies described by Kőhler and Milstein in 1975 is to immunise a mouse (murine) with the antigen. The mouse will then produce antibodies which can be seen as immunoglobulins in the blood serum; the spleen is then removed and cells from the spleen are fused with myeloma cells (these cells are used as they are B-tumour cells which are constantly dividing 'immortal' cells). The cells are now called hybridomas. Each

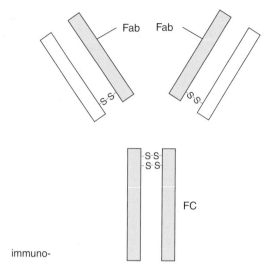

Figure 19.1 Antibody (from Coico *et al*. 2003).

hybridoma is then tested individually to assess which antibody is being secreted. Once the antibody of choice is produced the hybridomas are cloned in a culture vessel allowing the production of large numbers of monoclonal antibodies specific to one antigen. Monoclonal antibodies can also be produced by combining murine and human antibodies. These are: chimeric, humanised and human (see Table 19.3). You will be able to ascertain which type of monoclonal antibody by the name.

Table 19.3 Identification of origin (adapted from Schmidt and Wood 2003).

Type	Name	Percentages	Gene	Example
Murine	'Momab'	100% mouse	Mouse	90Y Ibritumomab tiuxetan (Zevalin)
Human	'Umab'	100% human	Human	In trial
Chimeric	'Xmab'	65–95% human	Human	Rituximab (Rituxan)
Humanised	'Zumab'	95–98% human	Human	Gemtuzumab Ozogamycin (Myelotarg)

A transgenic (genetically modified) animal will have been used to produced 100% human monoclonal antibodies (see Table 19.3). The cloned gene (where the mouse immunoglobulin gene is replaced by a human immunoglobulin gene) is injected into a fertilised mouse egg and implanted into a surrogate mouse (Coico *et al*. 2003); the offspring are then screened for expression of the antibody.

Classifications of monoclonal antibodies

There are two classifications of monoclonal antibodies, unconjugated and conjugated. Unconjugated antibodies are pure antibody and not modified in any way. They are effective cytotoxic and regulatory agents and have been studied in multiple malignant and non-malignant diseases. They can be used to target specific anti-tumour antigens and depend on the immune system to destroy the targeted cell. Conjugated antibodies combine antibody structure with radioimmunoconjugates (α, β, γ, emitting particles), chemoimmunoconjugates or immunotoxins. When the antibody attaches, the radionucleotide, toxin or chemotherapy is released, destroying the cell and in some cases the surrounding cells (Schmidt and Wood 2003) (Table 19.4).

How do monoclonal antibodies work?

Monoclonal antibodies have both diagnostic and therapeutic actions; diagnostic actions detect medical conditions and therapeutic actions, for example, are purging bone marrow and treatment. They can be used as a single or combination therapy. An example of this is the analysis of the human leukocyte membrane antigens (CD numbers). These were all identified with the use of monoclonal antibodies. Also the CD34 pluripotent stem cell can be identified and harvested at time of collection and T-cell depletion can be undertaken (Zola 2000b).

As stated earlier monoclonal antibodies rely on the ability of the immune system to destroy the target antigen; ideally the target antigen must demonstrate specificity, meaning that the antigen should be present only on the malignant cells. This specificity determines the extent of the toxicity to the cell and the recipient.

Rituximab was the first monoclonal antibody to gain NICE approval and is the treatment practitioners are most familiar with. This monoclonal antibody is specific to the CD20 protein which is present on both malignant and normal B-cells (Capriotti 2001).

The antigen-binding fragment (Fab) of the antibody attaches itself to any CD20 receptor it finds. Once attached, activation of the complement system begins, which in turn alerts the immune response leading to antibody-dependent, cell-mediated cytotoxicity (ADCC). Ultimately death of the cell will occur (Medical News Today 2009).

What are the side effects of monoclonal antibodies?

Each different monoclonal antibody has a specific action, therefore each one will elicit differing side effects. The most common to all of the current therapies is the risk of the patient recognising the murine element (no matter how small) of the treatment as foreign and developing human anti-chimeric antibodies (HACA). If these do develop then the risk of reaction to the infusion is more likely (Capriotti 2001).

Baseline observations of temperature, manual pulse, blood pressure and respiratory rate are essential nursing procedures prior to the commencement of the infusion. The first infusion will be given slowly, with incremental increases and vigilant observation; if the patient shows signs of fever or flu-like symptoms reduction of the infusion rate may be necessary whilst symptoms settle or are managed. There is also a risk of tumour lysis syndrome, especially if the patient has bulky disease. Close monitoring of urea, potassium, calcium and fluid balance prior to administration and post-infusion is required in patients at high risk.

Table 19.4 Monoclonal antibodies currently in use or in trial for haematological disorders.

Name	Classification	Conjugate used	Cell target	Haematological disorder
Rituximab (Rituxan)	Unconjugated	None	B-cell CD20	Non-Hodgkins Lymphoma (NHL)
Gemtuzumab Ozogomycin (Myelotarg)	Conjugated	Calicheamin – antitumour antibiotic	Myeloblasts CD33	Acute myeloid leukaemia (AML)
Alemtuzumab (MabCampath 1-H)	Unconjugated	None	T-cell and B-cell CD52 and CD25	Chronic lymphocytic leukaemia (CLL)
90 Y – Ibritumomab tiuxetan (Zevalin)	Conjugated	Tiuxetan (yttrium 90) radioisotope	B-cell CD20	Rituximab resistant NHL
131 I – Tositumomab (Bexxar)	Conjugated	Iodine – 131	B-cell CD20	Refractory NHL
Daclizumab (Zenapax)	Unconjugated	None	T-cell CD25	T-cell leukaemia
Epratuzumab (LymphoCide)	Unconjugated	None	CD22	Relapsed NHL (trial)

Conclusion

It is apparent that chemotherapy treatment has many issues to consider for both the patient receiving the drugs and the health care staff that are administering the treatment. Education, knowledge skills and training are paramount in ensuring that cytotoxic chemotherapy is administered safely and best practice and high care standards are achieved. Ongoing regular training and updates are important in an area that is frequently changing, and new treatments are being developed. Monoclonal antibodies appear to be one of the treatments destined to become 'gold standard' therapy within the field of haematology, both in the diagnostic and therapeutic setting.

However, there is little data on the long-term effects of these treatments and therefore the issue of informed consent will always remain a challenge to the practitioner.

References

Allwood, M., Stanley, A.S. and Wright, P. (2002) *The Cytotoxics Handbook*, 4th edition. Radcliffe, Oxford.

Baquiran, D.C. (2001) *Lippincotts Cancer Chemotherapy Handbook*. 2nd edition. Lippincott, Williams and Wilkins, Philadelphia.

Barton-Burke, M., Wilkes, G.M. and Ingwersen, K.C. (2001) *Cancer Chemotherapy Care Plans Handbook*, 3rd edition. Jones Bartlett, London.

Brighton, D., Wood, M., Johnston, S. and Ford, H. (2005) *The Royal Marsden Hospital Handbook of Cancer Chemotherapy: A Guide for the Multidisciplinary Team*. Churchill Livingstone, London.

Capriotti, T. (2001) Monoclonal antibodies: drugs that combine pharmacology and biotechnology. *MEDSURG-Nursing*, 10 (30), 89–95.

Coico, R., Sunshine, G. and Benjamini, E. (2003) Antigen-antibody interactions, immune assays and experimental systems. In: *Immunology*, 5th edition (eds R. Coico, G. Sunshine and E. Benjamini). Chapter 5, pp. 59–78. Wiley, Oxford.

Department of Health (2000) *Cancer Information Strategy*. DoH, London.

Department of Health (2001) *Good Practice in Consent Implementation Guide: Consent to Examination or Treatment*. DoH, London.

Department of Health (2004) *Better Information, Better Choices, Better Health*. DoH, London.

Department of Health (2008) *HSC2008/001 Updated National Guidance on the Safe Administration of Intrathecal Chemotherapy*. DoH, London.

Department of Health (2009) Reference guide to consent for examination of treatment. 2nd edition. DoH, London.

Dillman, R.O. (2001) Monoclonal antibody therapy for lymphoma: an update. *Cancer Practice*, 9 (2), 71–80.

Health and Safety Executive (2002) *Control of Substances Hazardous to Health*. Stationery Office, London.

Health and Safety Executive (2003) *Safe Handling of Cytotoxic Drugs (MISC615)*. HSE, London.

Management and Awareness of Risks of Cytotoxic Handling (MARCH) (2008a) *Responsibilities of Employers and Practitioners*. Available from http://www.marchguidelines.com/members/guidelines/ResponsibilitiesOfEmployersAndPractitioners.aspx. Accessed on 6 August 2009.

Management and Awareness of Risks of Cytotoxic Handling (MARCH) (2008b) *Personal Protective Equipment (PPE): Selection and Use*. Available from http://www.marchguidelines.com/members/guidelines/PNF1_PersonalProtectiveEquipment.aspx. Accessed on 6 August 2009.

Management and Awareness of Risks of Cytotoxic Handling (2009) *Administration of Anticancer Drugs: Safe Practice*. Available from http://www.marchguidelines.com/members/guidelines/AdministrationOfAnticancerDrugs.aspx. Accessed on 6 August 2009.

Medical News Today (2009) *Monoclonal Antibody Drugs For Cancer Treatment*. http://www.medicalnewstoday.com/articles/145092.php. Accessed 7 August 2009.

Modjtahedi, H. (2007) Monoclonal antibodies. In: *The Biology of Cancer*, 2nd edition (ed. J. Gabriel). Chapter 10, pp. 111–124. Wiley-Blackwell, Oxford.

National Chemotherapy Advisory Group (2008) *Chemotherapy Services in England: Ensuring Quality and Safety*. National Cancer Action Team: London.

Personal Protective Equipment at Work Regulations (PPE 1992). Available at: http://www.opsi.gov.uk/SI/si1992/Uksi_19922966_en_1.htm. Accessed on 6 August 2009.

Roitt, I.M. and Delves, P.J. (2003) Immunochemical techniques. In: *Roitt's Essential Immunology*, 10th edition (eds I.M. Roitt and P.J. Delves). Chapter 6, pp. 108–128. Blackwell Publishing Ltd, Oxford.

Schmidt, K.V. and Wood, B.A. (2003) Trends in cancer therapy: role of monoclonal antibodies. *Seminars in Oncology Nursing*, 19 (3), 169–179.

Skeel, R.T. (2003) *Handbook of Cancer Chemotherapy*, 6th edition. Lipincott, London.

Verity, R. (2005) Mastering chemotherapy. *Cancer Nursing Practice*, 4 (3), 2.

Wilkes, G.M. and Barton Burke, M. (2007) *Oncology Nursing Drug Handbook*. Jones and Bartlett, London.

Zola, H. (2000a) Antibodies as laboratory and therapeutic reagents. In: *Monoclonal Antibodies: The Basics from Background to Bench* (ed. H. Zola). Chapter 1, pp. 1–15. BIOS Scientific, Oxford.

Zola, H. (2000b) Applications of monoclonal antibodies to the study of cells and tissues. In: *Monoclonal Antibodies: The Basics from Background to Bench* (ed. H. Zola). Chapter 6, pp. 127–143. BIOS Scientific, Oxford.

Chapter 20

Haemopoietic stem cell transplant

Tracey Cutler

The aim of this chapter is to provide an overview of haemopoietic stem cell transplant (HSCT), current procedures and developmental treatments. After reading this chapter you will:

- Have an overview of the types of transplant available
- Have an understanding of the rationale behind conditioning and mobilization regimens
- Have an overview of the early and late complications associated with HSCT
- Be familiar with the nursing care required by a patient undergoing HSCT

The utilisation of HSCT is increasing, with a number of developmental treatments allowing for a larger number of diseases to be treated which were previously excluded from standard therapy. Haemopoietic stem cell transplant (HSCT) is now indicated as standard therapy for a number of malignant and non-malignant conditions. The type of HSCT performed depends on the diagnosis, prognosis and performance status of the individual. The nursing care of a patient undergoing HSCT is considered to be specialist. However, many transplant patients are cared for prior to and post-transplant in non-specialist haematology units. Therefore, professionals working in these units need to have an understanding of the therapies and long-term side effects in order to provide good quality supportive care.

Bone marrow transplant is an umbrella term used to classify a number of procedures. These transplants utilise stem cells from bone marrow, peripheral blood or cord blood and more recently the procedure has been termed haemopoietic stem cell transplantation (HSCT): 'HSCT refers to any procedure where haemopoietic stem cells of any donor type and any source are given to a recipient with the intention of repopulating and replacing the haemopoietic system in total or in part' (Ljungman *et al.* 2006, p. 2). The type of procedure is then classified based on the origin of the stem cells, autologous being derived from the recipient, allogeneic and donor lymphocyte infusions from a donor who is related or unrelated to the recipient.

Haemopoietic stem cells

As highlighted in Chapter 1, haemopoiesis occurs in the bone marrow (red marrow), which is present in many bones of the skeleton at birth. As humans age the activity of this red marrow reduces and the main areas of activity are the pelvis, the sternum and the vertebrae (Ososkie and O'Riley 2007).

Haemopoietic stem cells (HSC) are also known as pluripotent stem cells as they have the ability to divide by proliferation and can differentiate into all blood cell lines depending on the body's need. This ability of the HSC to proliferate and differentiate can be manipulated, allowing mobilization, growth stimulation and harvest of these cells. The HSC is identified by the expression of a protein CD34+ which is present on the surface of all HSC and is the target used to monitor and harvest the cells.

Sources of stem cells and the importance of tissue typing

The HSC can be from three main sources: the patient (autologous), a donor (allogeneic) or donated umbilical cord blood (cord blood transplant) (Powell 2009). If the cells are to be collected from a donor, then tissue type will need to be ascertained. Tissue typing is the process of matching the donor and recipient tissue. Potential donors can be family members, most commonly siblings, or they can be matched unrelated donors (MUD). The donor and the recipient's blood is tested to match the major histocompatibility complex (MHC) or human leucocyte antigens, which are found on the surface of all nucleated cells. Forman (2008, p. 697) states that: 'a match is found when the MHC I antigens (A and B loci), as well as the MHC II antigens (DR), are the same as those of the donor'. There is approximately a 25–30% chance of having a familial match, if no sibling match is found there are international registries which can be searched to try to find an unrelated donor. The major concern with any donated HSC is the risk of graft rejection by the recipient or graft versus host disease (GVHD). This is due to the infusion of immunocompetent donor T-cells which recognise the recipient (host) as foreign. For this reason, conditioning regimens are tailored to the source of the HSC.

Mobilisation of haemopoietic stem cells

Originally HSC were physically harvested from the pelvis under general anaesthetic (Figure 20.1). A large aspiration needle is inserted into the posterior iliac crests and liquid bone marrow is removed repeatedly with a syringe. The National Institute for Health (2001) states that approximately 1 in 100,000 cells in the bone marrow is CD34+. This equates to approximately 15–20 mL/kg of liquid bone marrow (Damon *et al.* 2008). Therefore, specific cell harvesting was impossible and the collection contained HSC, stromal cells, precursor cells and maturing white and red blood cells.

Consideration of the weight of the recipient is needed to ensure enough cells are collected to repopulate the bone marrow.

Currently the preferred method of harvesting HSC is via the peripheral blood; the HSC are mobilized from the bone marrow into the peripheral blood and then collected via apheresis (Powell *et al.* 2009). This mobilisation is enabled by the subcutaneous administration of granulocyte colony stimulating factor (G-CSF, filgrastim (Neupogen))

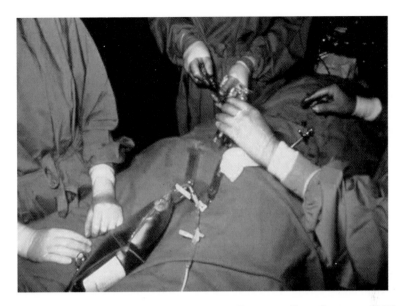

Figure 20.1 Harvesting bone marrow from posterior iliac crests (from Contreras 2007).

to cause proliferation of the HSC prior to apheresis procedures. The amount of HSC is assessed by ascertaining the number of CD34+ cells collected. This, as stated by Forman (2008), is a minimum of 2 x 10^6 CD34+ cells/kg of body weight of the recipient.

This is an important issue as the donor will receive double the dose of G-CSF to obtain enough cells for the recipient. Therefore side effects such as fatigue and long bone pain are usually more severe.

Once collected, the HSC are processed at the National Blood Service, this entails dilution in plasma (which is also collected as part of the apheresis procedure). If the HSC are to be stored prior to reinfusion di-methyl sulphoxide (DMSO) is added to protect the cells, which are then frozen to minus 160°C, in liquid nitrogen. If the HSC are donor cells they are given to the recipient within 48 hours and do not require DMSO.

Conditioning

The days prior to the actual infusion are numbered in countdown fashion, so that the week leading up to the transplant is numbered -7 to 0 (0 being the day of the transplant (infusion). Post day 0 the days are numbered upward for example 30 days after the infusion would be day +30 (Léger and Nevill 2004). Between days -7 and -1 all of the conditioning treatment will be given.

High dose therapy

Prior to receiving HSC, patients will need to undergo high dose therapy (HDT) the regimen utilized will be dependent on the patient's disease status and type of transplant. 'The intention of high dose therapy (HDT) is to eliminate malignant disease by myeloablation of the rapidly dividing cells in the bone marrow, often termed as "conditioning" this can be achieved with high dose chemotherapy or total body irradiation' (NICE 2003).

Total body irradiation

Total body irradiation (TBI) is a supralethal dose of irradiation which immunosuppresses the recipient prior to infusion of the HSCT. It also destroys any remaining malignant cells and can penetrate sanctuary sites (Bensinger and Spielberger 2004). It can be given as a single treatment or the dose can be fractionated over a number of days (allowing a higher dose to be administered). The most common delivery is by linear accelerator. This method allows higher doses to be administered and shielding can be used to reduce pulmonary toxicity (Bensinger and Spielberger 2004).

Tumor lysis syndrome is a potential complication at this stage due to the lysis of cells. Analysis of serum urea, potassium, calcium, creatinine and liver function should be undertaken twice a day. Allopurinol is prescribed and intravenous (IV) hydration may be required to ensure pH of the urine remains at neutral, this should be monitored by urinalysis. Diuretics and supplemental infusions of calcium and potassium may be required.

Types of haemopoietic stem cell transplant

The current opinion regarding indication for type of transplant is shown in Table 20.1.

Table 20.1   Classification of indications for blood and marrow transplants adapted from Murphy M.F, Pamphilon D.H (2009).

Degree of consensus	Allogeneic HSCT	Autologous HSCT
Very high level of agreement	Poor risk AML CR1	Multiple myeloma first response
	AML other than CR1	Relapsed Hodgkin disease
	Adults <35 years with ALL CR1	Relapsed aggressive NHL
	ALL other than CR1	
	CML CP1 if poorly responsive to TKI	
	CML other than CP1	
	Poor risk myelodysplasia	
	Very severe aplastic anaemia in children and young adults	
Some variation in practice between BMT units/nations	Multiple myeloma	AML CR1
	Chronic lymphocytic leukaemia	AML other than CR1
	Low-grade NHL	
Little consensus as to evidence in support of indication. Clinical trials highly appropriate in these conditions	Hodgkin's disease	CML CP1
		CML other than CP1
		Myelodysplasia
		Chronic lymphocytic Leukaemia

Autologous haemopoietic stem cell transplant

This is the use of the patient's own HSC which have been mobilised, harvested and cryopreserved. These CD34+ cells are then used as either: a 'rescue' therapy following ablation of existing bone marrow or to return remission cells to restore a functioning haemopoiesis. Autologous HSC are defrosted in a water bath at the bedside and re-infused following high dose therapy to re-establish haemopoiesis (Forman 2008). The most common side effect at the time if re-infusion is nausea, the patient needs to be informed that they may experience a strange taste in their mouth which can make them feel nauseous. This is caused by the DMSO which the patients will excrete in their breath and body fluids over the next 2–3 days. Prior to administration the patient needs to be well hydrated and a strict fluid balance should be maintained as any red cells collected at the time of harvest will have been damaged during cryopreservation. This cellular damage will cause the release of free haemoglobin which can be monitored in the urine output and can indicate renal damage (Craddock and Chakraverty 2005).

Donor haemopoietic stem cell transplant

These types of HSCT are the infusion of donor cells into a recipient. The purpose is to replace non-functioning, diseased or suppressed bone marrow and restore normal haemopoiesis. As these cells are 'foreign' to the recipient there is a need for tissue typing. The conditioning in preparation for a donor HSCT is given for two purposes; the first is to ablate the marrow and remove any residual cells the second reason is to immunosuppress the recipient. As stated earlier the infused HSC are 'foreign' to the recipient and the body's natural defence is to destroy foreign invaders, therefore an immunosuppression treatment is given to prevent rejection of the new marrow and suppress the donor marrow.

Graft versus disease effect

This is an important factor in the choice of HSCT. Patients who experience graft versus host disease have a lower risk of relapse, due to the donor T-cells (CD8 cells) recognizing any residual recipient cells as foreign and mounting an immune response against them. This effect is often termed graft versus leukaemia (GVL) or graft versus tumour (GVT) (Craddock and Chakraverty 2005).

Standard allogeneic haemopoietic stem cell transplant

High dose therapy with or without total body irradiation is the standard therapy. Commonly used conditioning regimens include: cyclophosphamide and TBI, fludarabine and busulfan or cyclophosphamide and busulfan (Damon *et al.* 2008). After the conditioning is completed and just prior to the donor HSC infusion the recipient begins immunosuppressive therapy which will continue for 9–18 months post transplant. The medication is used to suppress the donor HSC and reduce the effects of graft versus host disease (GVHD). This medication is either cyclosporin or tacrolimus combined with four post-transplant doses of methotrexate (Damon *et al.* 2008).

Syngeneic allogeneic haemopoietic stem cell transplant

This form of HSCT utilises HSC from an identical twin; as the cells are genetically identical the conditioning is similar to autologous HSCT as the risk of GVHD and rejection is minimal.

Standard matched unrelated donor haemopoietic stem cell transplant

Although the cell collection and dose are similar the recipient will require a different conditioning regimen. This is due to the genetic differences between donor and recipient; this difference increases the risk of both graft rejection and GVHD.

The conditioning is high dose therapy with or without total body irradiation, but there is also the addition of T-cell depletion, for example CAMPATH-1H.

Reduced intensity conditioning haemopoietic stem cell transplant

This type of HSCT uses lower doses of chemotherapy with or without TBI. There is usually the addition of a T-cell depletion agent such as CAMPATH-1H. These regimens cause immunosuppression not ablation and rely on the donor cells to destroy any residual recipient cells (graft versus tumour (GVT). The toxicity is less, with reduced intensity conditioning (RIC); therefore older patients, patients with co-morbidities and slower growing malignancies can be treated (Powel *et al*. 2009).

Cord blood haemopoietic stem cell transplant

Umbilical cord blood contains high numbers of haemopoietic stem cells which can be used as donor HSCT; however, there is only a small amount of blood which has limited the use to children and small adults (Hoffbrand *et al*. 2001). The expansion and pooling of donated HSC is currently being studied to widen the application (Powell *et al*. 2009).

Complications of haemopoietic stem cell transplant

There are a number of side effects which can be experienced, these can be short and/or long term, the majority of the short-term side effects are due to the chemotherapy and total body irradiation, which are discussed in Chapter 19.

Early effects

These effects are seen between day 0 and +90 days post transplant (Craddock and Chakraverty 2005).

Graft failure

Bone marrow ablation post HDT and/or TBI will be seen on approximately day +7–+10. Full blood counts will show anaemia and thrombocytopenia, which can be treated with irradiated (25 Gy) and filtered red blood cell and platelet transfusions. White cell counts will also reduce with a differential neutrophil count of 0.0 x 10⁹/L. If neutrophils are not above 0.5 x 10⁹/L by day +29 graft failure is suspected; this can be due to graft rejection, drug toxicity or infection. The treatment recommended may be second transplant from the original donor or autologous rescue (Craddock and Chakraverty 2005).

Acute graft versus host disease

Graft versus host disease (GVHD) is classified into two types: acute and chronic. Acute GVHD occurs in the first 100 days post donor HSCT (Balsdon and Craig 2003). As stated earlier, prophylaxis against severe GVHD is administered prior to the infusion of HSCs. This medication is either cyclosporin or tacrolimus combined with four post-transplant doses of methotrexate (Damon *et al.* 2008). Patient's serum levels of cyclosporin will be monitored at least three times per week. Sub-therapeutic levels would put the patient at risk of severe GVHD and overdosing can cause severe hepatic and renal toxicity.

The primary organs affected by acute GVHD are the skin, the gastrointestinal tract and the liver. Symptoms of GVHD usually appear about three weeks post transplant (Forman 2008). Skin GVHD presents as a rash on the palms of the hands, soles of the feet, face and ears (Hoffbrand *et al.* 2001). Patients will often complain that their sensitivity to cold and hot water is affected. In severe cases the whole body can be affected and this grade of skin GVHD can be life threatening. Gastrointestinal GVHD presents as diarrhoea which has a typical appearance and is often referred to as 'mince meat stool', the diarrhoea is very loose and contains blood and mucus. It is important to maintain strict fluid balance as severe cases can cause over two litres of diarrhoea per day. Liver GVHD is indicated by rising bilirubin and alkaline phosphatase. As these increase, jaundice in the sclera and skin may be noted (see Table 20.2 for clinical staging of acute GVHD).

Treatment is with high doses of steroid, which is reduced until an oral dose can be maintained. Blood sugar monitoring is required throughout this course of treatment and vigilance of surveillance for infection due to the masking effects of the steroid.

Table 20.2 Acute graft-versus-host disease: clinical staging (Seattle system) (from Hoffbrand *et al.* 2001).

Stage	Skin	Liver (bilirubin, mmol/L)	Gut (diarrhoea, L/day)
I	Rash <25%	20–35	0.5–1.0
II	Rash 25–50%	35–80	1.0–1.5
III	Erythroderma	80–150	1.5–2.5
IV	Bullae, desquamation	>150	>2.5; severe pain, ileus

Infection-related complications

Infection-related complications require strict attention, as the patients are immunosuppressed due to the conditioning regimen and the prophylaxis against GVHD. There is ongoing debate about how to protect these patients and no definitive answer has been given. However, it is thought that protective isolation is good practice especially if patients have received TBI (NICE 2003). Prophylactic antibacterial, antifungal and antiviral medications may be given during the transplant itself and some areas will also include a low microbial diet. Constant monitoring for early signs of infection is the mainstay of nursing care. Temperature, pulse, blood pressure and respiratory rate should be recorded 4–6 hourly and more regularly if an abnormal reading is found. Weekly routine surveillance is often practiced (MSU, stool specimen, vascular access device swabs, blood cultures and chest X-ray) to assist in the early recognition of infection. Allogeneic HSCT presents more of a problem with infectious complications as the risks continue until the patient is off all immunosuppressive therapy.

Neutropenic sepsis

Irrespective of the type of transplant, nearly all patients undergoing HSCT will develop a fever, often of unknown origin. The longer the patient is neutropenic, the higher the risk of neutropenic sepsis. As stated above, early identification of infection is the key. This can be relatively well controlled whilst the patient is in hospital; however, this is not as well regulated when the patient is discharged home. Patients need to be educated in looking for early signs of infection and each department will have a neutropenia policy in place which covers outpatient reporting of a fever and the policy on the use of antipyretics at home (DoH 2004). Standard practice when a patient has pyrexia is shown in Figure 20.2.

Cytomegalovirus

This viral infection was historically one of the most feared infections, which accounted for approximately 20% of transplant related mortality (Forman 2008), causing pneumonia and requiring intensive care and respiratory ventilation. Prior to conditioning treatment recipients and donors are tested by polymerase chain reaction (PCR) for their viral status (CMV IgG positive or IgG negative). If either of the matches are positive there is a risk of reactivation of the virus. Throughout the HSCT the recipient will have routine PCR blood tests to identify early reactivation. If a positive result returns the recipient will receive a course of ganciclovir or one of the derivatives. This will continue until the recipient receives three clear PCR results. This new testing has enabled early identification and treatment prior to the recipient becoming symptomatic.

Gastrointestinal toxicity

Mucositis

This complication of HSCT is also seen in patients receiving chemotherapy and head and neck radiotherapy. Due to the high doses of conditioning and TBI the severity is increased and up to 80% of the patients receiving HSCT will be affected (Finley *et al.* 2003; Fulton and Treon 2007). The mucositis experienced can affect any part of the gastrointestinal

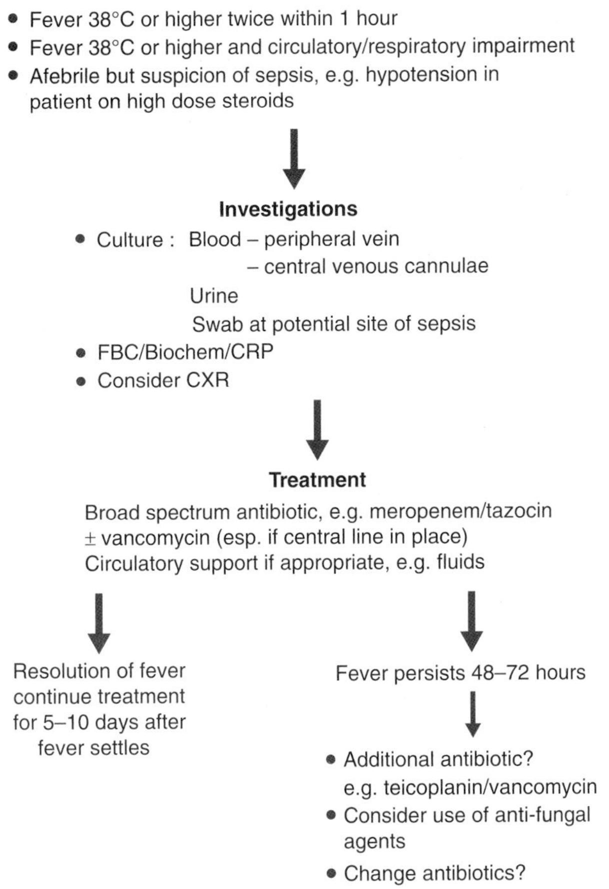

- Fever 38°C or higher twice within 1 hour
- Fever 38°C or higher and circulatory/respiratory impairment
- Afebrile but suspicion of sepsis, e.g. hypotension in patient on high dose steroids

↓

Investigations

- Culture : Blood – peripheral vein
  – central venous cannulae

  Urine

  Swab at potential site of sepsis
- FBC/Biochem/CRP
- Consider CXR

↓

Treatment

Broad spectrum antibiotic, e.g. meropenem/tazocin
± vancomycin (esp. if central line in place)
Circulatory support if appropriate, e.g. fluids

↓   ↓

Resolution of fever   Fever persists 48–72 hours
continue treatment
for 5–10 days after   ↓
fever settles
                             - Additional antibiotic?
                               e.g. teicoplanin/vancomycin
                             - Consider use of anti-fungal
                               agents
                             - Change antibiotics?

Figure 20.2 Management of pyrexia in a neutropenic patient (from Hoffbrand *et al.* 2006). Reprinted with permission of John Wiley & Sons, Inc.

tract, causing mucositis, oesophagitis and gastroduodenitis. This damage to the mucosa causes severe pain, reduction in nutritional intake and increased risk of infection (Balsdon and Craig 2003). Assessment is the key nursing role, as early identification and intervention will reduce the risk of systemic infection and prevent unnecessary suffering. There are a number of assessment tools available. However, as Finley *et al.* (2003) state, ideally a tool should be used daily by all members of the team, be easy to use, be objective, assess all areas of the oral cavity and lips, and also consider the patient's level of pain. Grading of the severity is often recorded within documentation; the two commonly used tools are the World Health Organisation and the National Cancer Institute's grading scale (see Table 20.3).

Treatment is with regular mouth wash and analgesia, often requiring opioids. Pain will be assessed and analgesia utilised according to the WHO analgesic ladder (Spathis 2003).

Table 20.3   Grading tools (adapted from WHO and NCI).

WHO grading scale	
Grade 0	None
Grade 1	Soreness with or without erythema, no ulceration
Grade 2	Erythema and ulcers; patients can swallow solid diet
Grade 3	Ulcers, extensive erythema, patients cannot swallow solid food
Grade 4	Oral mucositis to the extent that eating is not possible
NCI scale	
Grade 0	None
Grade 1	Painless ulcers, erythema or mild soreness, no ulcers
Grade 2	Painful erythema, swelling or ulcers, but the patient can swallow solid food
Grade 3	Painful erythema, swelling or ulcers, patient needs IV hydration
Grade 4	Severe ulceration, unable to eat, requiring parenteral or enteral feeding
Grade 5	Death related to toxicity

Nutrition

Recipients may require enteral or parenteral nutrition (TPN) post transplant due to nausea and mucositis. Collaboration with the pharmacy and dietetic service prior to conditioning will enable planning to take place based on assessment of the individual's needs. If the recipient is prescribed TPN they are at a higher risk of sepsis due to the rise in blood glucose. For this reason TPN is always the last option.

Haemorrhagic cystitis

High doses of cyclophosphamide are commonly the standard conditioning chemotherapy. Acrolein is a metabolite of cyclophosphamide which is excreted via the urine. This metabolite can cause bleeding of the bladder wall (Hoffbrand *et al.* 2006). Mesna is given to prevent this. Recipients need to receive at least three litres of fluid per day and they should pass urine every two hours. Fluid balance and urinalysis should be undertaken to identify any blood present. A side effect of mesna is ketones in the urine. By ensuring ketones are present the practitioner can monitor that a high enough dose of mesna has been given.

Veno-occlusive disease of the liver

This is caused by damage to the hepatocytes (causing micro-thrombi in the liver) during HDT and occurs in 5–20% of recipients. The clinical signs are jaundice, hepatomegaly and ascites (Hoffbrand *et al.* 2001). Within two weeks of starting conditioning patients will gain weight and present with oedema and eventually ascites.

Strict fluid balance must be maintained; weight and girth measurements are a useful method of monitoring. There are currently trials into the use of thrombolytic agents to reverse veno-occlusive disease (VOD) (Forman 2008).

Late complications

Pneumocystis carinii pneumonia

Once haemopoiesis has been restored recipients will be prescribed co-trimoxazole and possibly acyclovir. This medication will continue whilst the recipient remains on cyclosporin. If the recipient cannot tolerate this regimen nebulised pentamidine can be used.

Chronic graft versus host disease

Chronic GVHD occurs post 100 days (Balsdon and Craig 2003); this may be preceded by acute GVHD but can be *de novo*. The organs affected continue as before (skin, gastrointestinal tract and liver). However, the joints, oral mucosa and lacrimal glands also become involved (Forman 2008). Chronic GVHD resembles other autoimmune connective tissue diseases, for example scleroderma, Sjögren's syndrome and biliary cirrhosis. Treatment is with steroids, cyclosporine, azathioprine and thalidomide. All of these medications will suppress the recipient's immune system; therefore prophylactic medication will need to be given to protect against bacterial, fungal and viral infections. Skin changes which take place can psychologically affect recipients as scarring (similar to a burn) can occur. As it scars the skin can contract, reducing movement in the limbs, skin pigment changes and bodily hair may thin or fall out. Nutrition is also affected as malabsorption of nutrients occurs; dietary supplements are recommended.

Endocrine dysfunction and infertility

High dose therapy and TBI will cause infertility in the recipient, azoospermia in males and menopause in females. Males should be offered semen storage prior to any chemotherapy regimen; females may be offered embryo-cryopreservation but this requires time to undertake treatment (Balsdon and Craig 2003). Hormone replacement therapy will be offered to the female patients after discharge to reduce the menopausal symptoms and protect them against osteoporosis. Rarely post-transplant male patients can present with gynacomastia. Endocrine function should be monitored post transplant as thyroid function can also be affected by TBI, causing hypothyroidism.

Relapse post transplant

Donor lymphocyte infusions

Donor lymphocytes (DL) can be collected from the donor, and stored in several incremental doses (aliquots – this is a term used to describe a small portion of solution). If the recipient shows signs of early relapse DL can be infused in incremental doses (smallest first) to try to induce graft versus disease effect. Craddock and Chakraverty (2005) state that 80% of patients with early relapse of chronic myeloid leukaemia regain remission. However, this percentage is greatly reduced in other haematological malignancies.

Secondary malignancy

High dose therapy and TBI cause mutation of cellular DNA, which leads to apoptosis; this mutation of DNA is the rationale behind HSCT. However, the risk of secondary malignancy is increased six or seven-fold compared to the general population risk (Hoffbrand *et al.* 2006).

Conclusion

This chapter has given an overview of HSCT. The current procedures and developmental treatments have been discussed and the nursing care issues considered. As stated earlier, many HSCT donors and recipients are cared for prior to and post transplant in non-specialist haematology units; therefore, professionals working in these units need to have an understanding of the therapies and long-term side effects in order to provide good quality supportive care.

References

Balsdon, H. and Craig J.I.O. (2003) Bone marrow and peripheral stem cell transplantation. In: *Palliative Care Consultations in Haemato-oncology* (eds S. Booth and E. Bruera), Chapter 5, pp. 61–73. Oxford University Press, Oxford.

Bensinger, W.I. and Spielberger, R. (2004) Preparative regimens and modification of regimen-related toxicities. In: *Thomas' Hematopoietic Cell Transplantation*, 3rd edition (eds K.G. Blume, S.J. Forman and F.R. Appelbaum) Blackwell Publishing Ltd, Oxford.

Contreras, M. (2007) *ABC of Transfusion*, 4th edition. Blackwell, Oxford.

Craddock, C. and Chakraverty, R. (2005) Stem cell transplantation. In: *Post Graduate Haematology* (eds A.V. Hoffbrand, D. Catovsky and E.D.G. Tuddinham). Chapter 25. Blackwell Pubslishing Ltd, Oxford.

Damon, L., Wolf, J. and Linker, C. (2008) *Bone Marrow Transplantation.* http://knol.google.com/k/lloyd-damon-m-d/bone-marrow-transplantation/IYUvigG-/cFXSLw# (updated 30 July 2008, accessed 6 October 2009).

Department of Health (2004) *Manual of Cancer Standards.* DoH, London.

Finley, I., Amsler, P. and Wade, R. (2003) Mouth care for haematology patients. In: *Palliative Care Consultations in Haemato-oncology* (eds S. Booth and E. Bruera). Chapter 7, pp. 89–109. Oxford University Press, Oxford.

Forman, S.J. (2008) Haematopoietic cell transplantation. In: *Cancer Management: A Multidisciplinary Approach. Medical, Surgical and Radiation Oncology*, 11th edition (eds R. Pazdur, L.D. Wagman, K.A. Camphausen and W.J. Hoskins). CMPmedica, New York.

Fulton, J.S. and Treon, M.L. (2007) Oral mucositis. In: *Oncology Nursing*, 5th edition (eds M.E. Langhorne, J.S. Fulton and S.E. Otto). Chapter 29, pp. 505–523. Mosby, Missouri.

Hoffbrand, A.V., Moss, P.A.H. and Pettit, J.E. (2006) *Essential Haematology*, 5th edition. Blackwell Publishing Ltd, Oxford.

Hoffbrand, A.V., Pettit, J.E. and Moss P.A.H. (2001) Stem cell transplantation. In: *Essential Haematology*, 4th edition. Chapter 8, page 98–112. Blackwell Publishing Ltd, Oxford.

Léger, C.S. and Nevill, T.J. (2004) Hematopoietic stem cell transplantation: a primer for the primary care physician. *CMAJ*, 170 (10).

Ljungman, P., Urbano-Ispizua, A., Cavazzana-Calvo, M. *et al.* (2006) Allogeneic and autologous tranaplantation for haematological diseases, solid tumours and immune disorders: definitions and current practice in Europe. *Bone Marrow Transplantation*, 1–11, www.nature.com/bmt.

Mehta, A. and Hoffbrand, A.V. (2009) *Haematology at a Glance*. Wiley-Blackwell, Oxford.

Murphy, M.F. and Pamphilon, D.H. (2009*) Practical Transfusion Medicine*, 3rd edition. Wiley-Blackwell, Oxford.

National Institute for Clinical Excellence (2003*) Improving Outcomes in Haemato-oncology Cancers*. NICE, London.

National Institute for Health (2001) Stem Cell Information. http://stemcells.nih.gov/info/scireport/chapter5.asp (accessed 23 September 2009).

Ososki, R.E. and O'Riley, K. (2007) Leukaemia. In: *Oncology Nursing*, 5th edition (eds M.E. Langhorne, J.S. Fulton and S.E. Otto). Chapter 13, pp. 232–257. Mosby, Missouri.

Powell, J.L., Hingorani, P., Grupp, S.A. and Anders Kolb, E. (2009) Haematopoietic stem cell transplantation. http://emedicine.medscape.com/article/991032-overview (updated 11 September 2009, accessed 23 September 2009).

Richardson, C. and Atkinson, J. (2006) Blood and marrow transplantation. In: *Nursing in Haematological Oncology*. 2nd edition (ed. M. Grundy). Chapter 13, pp. 265–291. Baillière Tindall, Edinburgh.

Spathis, A. (2003) The essentials of symptom control in haemato-oncology. In: *Palliative Care Consultations in Haemato-oncology* (eds S. Booth and E. Bruera). Chapter 8, pp. 110–135. Oxford University Press, Oxford.

Chapter 21

Palliative care in haematology

Dion Smyth

This chapter aims to examine and discuss the principles and practice of palliative care, with particular reference to the real relevance of this caring approach, which is appreciated and highly esteemed by patients and their families (Conner et al, 2008). By the end of reading this chapter you will have an:

- Overview of the principles of palliative care
- Understanding of the challenges faced by nurses when caring for these patients

---

Introduction

Whenever palliative care is discussed for and about patients with blood disorders, 'haematologists don't "do" palliative care' is a not uncommon refrain. Various research papers, reports and recollections from practice would seem to support this rejoinder. A peculiar, particular and conceivably controversial example of this professional distancing from the principles and practice of palliative care is, perhaps, seen in the morbid and mordant black humour of the following 'joke':

Q: Why are haematology patients buried with a hole in the coffin lid?
A: So the Hickman line can be passed through and the haematologist can prescribe just *ONE* more course of chem. ...

I use the term 'joke' advisedly, as the wordplay employed at once highlights the defining features of the material to follow – in an attempt to be amusing the punch-line of the anecdote also shows up the complete absurdity and inadequacy of that care being delivered and the incomplete acceptance of palliative care into routine practice.

And yet, palliative care can be characterised simply by the sympathetic desire to prevent and relieve suffering (Sepulveda *et al.* 2002), and this philosophy and practice is centred not only on the physical body processes but 'whole person' or holistic principles (Kahn and Steeves 1995), which are common to nursing. Alleviating suffering has been identified as one of the fundamental responsibilities of nursing (ICN 2006), whilst the

---

need to protect and promote the well-being of the individual, and their families, is enshrined in the recent Nursing and Midwifery Council (NMC 2008) *Standards of Conduct, Performance and Ethics for Nurses and Midwives*. So, it might be considered surprising, therefore, that palliative care is not always and immediately considered an obvious element of haematology nursing and medical practice. The experience of suffering may be an often intangible and inadequately understood phenomenon but it may also, nevertheless, be frequently associated with the individual, subjective and complex attributes of loss (Rodgers and Cowles 1997). The patient with a blood disease suffers many objective, observable and imperceptible subjective circumstances that can often be viewed as significant, sorrowful, miserable or distressing events, all requiring the support and direct intervention of a suitably trained nurse.

An overview of the clinical context

Cancer is a considerable cause of morbidity and mortality in the UK; approximately 288,000 cases are diagnosed annually, with 154,000 deaths recorded each year (Westlake 2008). The four most common cancers: breast, lung, prostate and colorectal cancer accounted for over 50% of both cases and deaths from cancer (CRUK 2008). Haematological malignancies are a disparate assortment of diseases with varying prevalence, clinical presentation, disease trajectories, treatments and care measures, and outcomes. Whilst the frequency of blood disorders may be fewer in number compared to the solid tumours they nevertheless constitute a small but significant proportion of the overall cancer incidence in the UK. Non-Hodgkin's lymphoma is the fifth most commonly diagnosed cancer, with over 10,000 new cases per annum; the leukaemias constitute the twelfth most common type of cancer, whilst multiple myeloma is the seventeenth most common form of this disease, accounting for just less than 4000 cases.

Advances in cell and molecular biology, cytogenetics and immunotherapy have broadened our understanding of the haematological cancers and the potential for treatment. This scientific laboratory progress, when translated into clinically viable therapies, as will be explored later, may, in part, complicate or contribute to the apparent lack of specialist palliative care provision in patients with haematological malignancies. As we will see in the next section, palliative care originally developed from cancer services but is being extended into the care of other conditions; however, there is increasing evidence that despite being presently free at the point of delivery in the UK via either the statutory National Health Service provision or voluntary charitable establishments, various groups of people are not receiving adequate palliative care services (Koffman *et al.* 2007). Read and Thompson-Hill (2008) describe, for example, the discrepancies with accessibility and availability of palliative care services for patients with learning disabilities, whilst patients from other populations such as the elderly (Jones 2005), rural populations (Evans *et al.* 2003), black and minority ethnic populations (NCPC 2006) are in the same way amongst those groups disadvantaged by inequitable access and utilisation of palliative care services. It is obvious that patients with a blood disorder may also belong to one of the social groups or circumstances described above or any of the other similarly disadvantaged groups and therefore be correspondingly denied access to services on those grounds;

nonetheless, there is also evidence that the diagnosis of a haematological malignancy is in itself liable to increase the likelihood of being deprived of access to appropriate specialist palliative care services. In the UK, Grande *et al.* (1998) and Addington-Hall and Altmann (2000) described how patients with a haematological malignancy were less likely to receive palliative home support. McDonnell and Morris (1997) found a striking difference in the perceptions about the involvement of palliative care practitioners in bone marrow transplant (BMT) for haematological disease. In this study, 73% of nurses thought that greater patient involvement in decision making was required, which contrasted markedly with the 8% response of doctors. In the same study, almost half of the doctors surveyed felt that patients were involved enough, compared to less than one-tenth of the nurses questioned. Kelly *et al.* (2000) proposed that palliative care provision in some bone marrow transplant (BMT) centres might not have been perceived as relevant, with possible consequences on the quality of care and the emotional well-being of the professional nursing staff. Assorted papers and studies from Australasia present findings comparable to the UK situation, namely that haematological practice does not readily incorporate specialist palliative care services (McGrath 1999; 2002a; 2002b; McGrath and Holewa 2006; 2007).

To address some of the reported deficiencies in palliative and supportive care provision in patients with haematological malignancies, in 2003 the UK National Institute for Clinical Excellence (NICE 2003) proposed that there should be more active involvement of palliative care in haematology services, with more effective collaboration to improve patients' quality of life. The guidance paper: *Improving Supportive and Palliative Care for Adults with Cancer* (NICE 2004) consequently spelt out that specialist palliative care and advice should be available to all, nationwide, 24 hours a day, 7 days a week. A recent exploratory research paper from the UK that examined the frequency and features of patients with haematological malignancies who were, or were not, referred to specialist palliative care found that less than a third of the patients were referred to specialist services and only a quarter of the patients dying in the hospital received specialist palliative care involvement or intervention (Ansell *et al.* 2007). Equally, an American study found that the diagnosis of a haematological malignancy was, with admission to the intensive care unit, associated with low rates of referral to palliative care consultants (Fadul *et al.* 2007), possibly suggesting that the problem of unequal access to services persists.

So far, we have determined that there is possibly little integration between specialist palliative care services and haematology, or certainly less than may be desirable in some circumstances. The next section explores the defining characteristics of palliative care, specialist palliative care and some of the potential reasons why this approach is apparently not readily assimilated into haematology.

Defining and delivering palliative care

The word 'palliative' is derived from the Latin *pallium* and originally referred to a woollen cloak worn as an ecclesiastical vestment (see Figure 21.1). This source is apposite as much of the care that we presently associate with palliative care derives from hospice care, which in itself shares a common heritage and history with the various religious

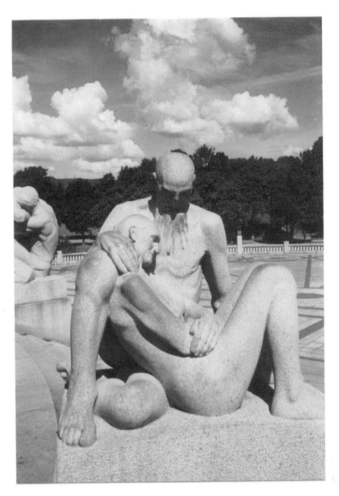

Figure 21.1 A graphic illustration of the literal meaning of pallium – to cloak, as in swaddle or envelop.

orders that cared for the sick and dying (Clark 2004). The Latin word *hospes*, from which we get the word 'hospice', actually means stranger or guest and also forms the root of words such as hospital and hospitality. Thus, from a Judeo-Christian injunction of 'love thy neighbour' and the ethic recorded in the Christian Gospel of St Matthew (25: 34–44): 'When did we see you sick and go to see you? I tell you solemnly when you did this to the least of these brothers of mine, you did it to me', the compassion expressed in palliative care is continuing a tradition of ministering to the needy, whether to a weary fourth century pilgrim or worried twenty-first century patient (Beuken 2003).

The modern hospice movement developed during the 1960s, as a response to public and professional dissatisfaction with the end of life care of patients dying from cancer, and that afforded their carers (Craven 2000). The overt medicalisation of dying allied to the depersonalisation of the increasingly technological health care environment, as evident by the increasingly apparent professional inability to accept death, and associated concerns about the futility of aggressive treatments when death was inevitable, also triggered disquiet (Clark 2002; Tinnelly *et al.* 2000; White 1999).

Contemporary clinical haematology may be associated with rigorous and exhausting invasive interventions, high technology and aggressive cutting edge treatments such as chemotherapy, biotherapy and haemopoietic stem cell transplant. The seeming surfeit of options for patients with blood cancers is, according to McGrath and Holewa (2007), seen to contribute to 'therapeutic optimism', in both the patient and the haematologist, so that a sanguine hope for always being able to provide further life prolonging treatment exists. What has been described as the 'treatment [of cancer] agenda' with the attendant potential prolongation of quantity of life, may often precipitate an intensification of possible treatments (Willard and Luker 2005; 2006). As such, many haematology patients are most likely to die with insufficient knowledge of or referral to palliative care (McGrath and Joske 2002) in the acute hospital institutional setting (McGrath 2002b).

The timely referral to palliative care services is influenced by the practitioner's acceptability of palliative care to the referring physician (Costantini *et al.* 1999) and also the clinician's knowledge of palliative care services and their ability to recognize and accept that the patients will not benefit from further anti-cancer treatment (Bestall *et al.* 2004). This understanding needs to be communicated sensitively to the patient and their family; hospital palliative care teams have been shown to play a vital role in facilitating the development of the patient's perception of their diagnosis and prognosis (Jack *et al.* 2004). Where patients are not fully apprised of their situation and involved in the decision-making process, and lack the necessary and correct information about what palliative care entails, the transition to palliative care can be confusing and distressing (Ronaldson and Devery 2001). This distress may be exacerbated by the sense of 'abandonment' upon cessation of disease modifying treatment and referral to services such as hospice care without an appropriate consideration of the patients, professionals and, in the case of the patient's death, the bereaved families need for closure (Back *et al.* 2009).

The utility or futility of treatment is dependent upon a host of individual circumstances; however, the use of treatments burdensome to the patient because the health care team are reluctant to or refuse to, or are otherwise unable to discuss or disclose the reality of the situation for want of effective communication skills, is clearly undesirable and inappropriate. Nevertheless, Audrey *et al.* (2008) found, in their recent examination of UK medical oncologists communication with patients about the survival benefits of palliative chemotherapy that most patients were not given clear information and may have been denied this from the well-intentioned but incorrect purpose of protecting the patient from psychological harm, which raises concerns about decision making and informed consent. It also conflicts with findings from McGrath (2002), which established that patients and their families required openness about death and often regretted the pressure and real cost of a much reduced quality of life for minimal quantity of life but would nevertheless comply with the offers of treatment and technological intercession. The desire to protect the patient is, perhaps, understandable; even so patients have been found to be more robust than the professionals' fears would initially suggest. Patients in a UK study were found to be willing and able to estimate their own life expectancy and did not take exception to questions about end of life care (Shah *et al.*

2006). The frequency and duration of treatments, let alone the toxicity experienced, denies the patient and their family time together and means that referral to palliative care services, if at all, may be too late to be effective. It also means that patients may be denied any opportunity to decide upon their own place of death, which is partly reflected in the fact that most patients want to die at home but most will die in an institutional setting (NCPC 2006).

The development of the hospice movement and the improvement in care for the terminally ill within the UK has since progressed into a worldwide programme of person-centred care that aims to achieve a 'good death'; however, the initial emphasis on terminal cancer care has meant that palliative care was, and to many still is, reserved for the dying (DoH 2000; Roy 2000) or may even be associated with decreasing the patient's life expectancy (Morita *et al.* 2005). A distinction between discrete phases of illness and treatment, namely curative, palliative and terminal, has been promoted for patients with cancer where disease progression clearly defined the transition of care approaches (Roy 2000) This ostensibly had support from haematologists; Laussaniere and Auzanneau (1995) suggested that due to the chemosensitivity of most malignant diseases it was 'difficult to define the boundaries of palliative care in this field'. Despite the fact that Jeffrey (1995) considered that the boundaries between curative, palliative and terminal care are frequently blurred, a rigid, dichotomous, philosophical and professional stance between active curative and active palliative care that contradicts the current ethos that conventional care alone is inadequate for patients with incurable forms of malignant or non-malignant disease, thus developed. This perception that palliative care was synonymous with terminal care and a separate specialist activity rather than a specific approach or resource, which could be integrated early into oncology practice, was subsequently found in other studies at that time (Lowden 1998), including patients requiring haemopoietic stem cell transplant (McDonnell and Morris 1997) and also patients with haematological malignancies not requiring HSCT as a treatment modality (National Cancer Alliance 2001). More recently, Randall and Wearn (2005) found that patients with leukaemia and lymphoma continued to have false impressions regarding the function of Macmillan nurses and hospices, which prevented them from better exploiting these resources. The participants in their study understood these services as something set aside specifically and exclusively for patients with advanced disease in the terminal stages of their life. This view persists for various reasons, including the dissimilar interpretations of the definition of palliative care. Farquahar *et al.* (2002) found that GPs and medical oncologists described palliative care differently. Reasons for the discrepancy related, in part, to inadequate communication from the hospital team that subsequently rendered the GP assessment invalid – they were seemingly more reluctant to determine and define a patient's status as 'palliative'. However, Farquhar *et al.* (2002) suggest that this may be because professionals make distinctions between 'palliative' and 'palliative care', giving the example that palliative chemotherapy may not be considered palliative care even though it is both 'palliative' and 'care'. Van Kleffens *et al.* (2004) similarly argue that the term 'palliative' in clinical oncology is problematic, confusing to both professional and patient and not always appropriate in clinical oncology. They suggest that anti-cancer treatment should be clarified and described as curative and non-curative and that the idiom 'palliative', when used, should be used in the context of 'palliative care' and should be reserved for patients requiring interventions such as symptom relief.

What we now consider to be palliative care, although seemingly contrived out of professional and social concern to counter the mistreatment or lack of care for dying cancer patients, should not necessarily be restricted to a particular group of malignant diseases or essentially to the discrete and definite end of life period. The need for an integrated, collaborative interdisciplinary approach that incorporates the best practices of hospital, hospice and home services has been acknowledged as not only required but possible and likely to be beneficial to patients and their families (Byock 2009; DoH 2000). As a result, over the past few decades, health care policy and professional practice has seen the development of a distinct specialty and specific services to achieve the best quality of life, and death, for all patients with a long-term, progressive and incurable illness, that is applicable much earlier in the disease trajectory (DoH 2005; 2006; NICE 2004).

The developments in care practices are predicated on the fact that the improvement of quality of life is integral to palliative care (World Health Organisation 2006). The WHO (2006) defines palliative care as an approach that improves the quality of life of patients and their families facing the problems associated with life-threatening illness, through the prevention and relief of suffering by means of early identification and impeccable assessment and treatment of pain and other problems, physical, psychosocial and spiritual. Additionally, other fundamental facets of palliative care are outlined in Box 21.1.

Box 21.1   Principles of palliative care practice.

- Provides relief from pain and other distressing symptoms
- Affirms life and regards dying as a normal process
- Intends neither to hasten nor postpone death
- Integrates the psychological and spiritual aspects of patient care
- Offers a support system to help patients live as actively as possible until death
- Offers a support system to help the family cope during the patient's illness and in their own bereavement
- Uses a team approach to address the needs of patients and their families, including bereavement counselling, if indicated
- Will enhance quality of life, and may also positively influence the course of illness
- Is applicable early in the course of illness, in conjunction with other therapies that are intended to prolong life, such as chemotherapy or radiation therapy, and includes those investigations needed to better understand and manage distressing clinical complications.

Considering the definition above it is easy to see why Jeffery (1995) noted that much of palliative care is nursing care. Florence Nightingale, in her *Notes on Nursing: What it is and What it is not* suggested that 'what nursing has to do ... is to put the patient in the best condition for nature to act upon him', which could in this context be considered to emphasise and employ a more humanistic approach alongside traditional measures rather than exercise purely or solely mechanistic, aggressive technological biomedical interventions.

The National Institute for Health and Clinical Excellence (NICE 2004) correspondingly defines palliative care as:

> The active holistic care of patients with advanced, progressive illness. Management of pain and other symptoms and provision of psychological, social and spiritual support is paramount. The goal of palliative care is achievement of the best quality of life for patients and their families. Many aspects of palliative care are also applicable earlier in the course of the illness in conjunction with other treatments.

Both of these definitions consider that palliative care assesses and manages pain and other symptoms. NICE (2003) acknowledged that the majority of the long-term treatment provided for patients with haematological cancers is essentially palliative in nature. The provision of blood product support to palliate the symptoms of anaemia, for example, is now an accepted practice in some hospices and specialist palliative care units (Brown and Bennett 2007). Consequently, haematology practitioners often become expert at managing the symptoms associated with the presenting disease or the adverse effects associated with the treatments; they may be less competent or confident with less common symptoms. Fadul *et al.* (2008) examined the symptom experience of patients with haematological malignancies and found an increased incidence of delirium and drowsiness amongst the sample, as well as noting that the patients received a later referral to palliative care services. Homsi and Luong (2007) had previously found that delirium acted as a poor prognostic marker in most studies and was associated with a much reduced survival. This would suggest that anything less than 'impeccable' assessment and management could have distressing consequences for the family that does not have time to achieve all that they hope for before the patient loses mental capacity or dies.

Palliative care is conventionally considered to be delivered by two discrete categories of health and social care professionals: generalists and specialists. The generalist provides routine care to patients and carers in their homes, and in hospitals, and would be able to assess and address the holistic care needs commonly associated with their clinical domain. The specialist services differ in the level of knowledge and expertise, as well as qualification; those who concentrate in palliative care also work within specialist multidisciplinary palliative care teams and deal primarily with the more complex cases, as well as advising, supporting and educating the generalist team members (NICE 2003; 2004).

Increasingly, palliative care is being linked with supportive care, which aims to provide emotional, spiritual and physical support to the patient and their family throughout the illness trajectory, from pre-diagnostic investigations to cure, progressive illness or death and bereavement (NICE 2003; 2004) (see Figure 21.2). Psychological, social, and spiritual support are emphasised and it is in these domains that specialist services perhaps provide more input than generalist. Psychosocial distress is commonly experienced in advanced cancer, but there is evidence to suggest that elements remain under-reported, under-detected and under-treated, which results in a considerable burden for the patient and their family (Thekkumpurath *et al.* 2008). The study by Botti *et al.* (2006) also revealed that providing for this care can place a significant burden on the clinically experienced haematology nurses caring for adult patients. Their findings suggested that the transition from active curative to active palliative intent and the end of the patient's life

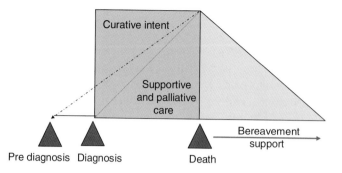

Figure 21.2 Relationship between supportive and palliative care with curative treatment.

were occasions that were associated with an increased need or demand for involvement, but also difficulty for the staff, meaning that patients may have experienced suboptimal care. As a result, the demands of and dissatisfaction with care had an impact on the nurses' quality of life as evidenced by the reduced level of satisfaction with their own personal lives. The need to develop more knowledge and skill in providing psychosocial care was acknowledged, as was the need for more effective intra- and inter-professional communication.

There is a significant stress associated with being involved in palliative care situations in which the practitioner feels ineffectual and engaged in futile activity that results in the patient experiencing unremitting and unnecessary suffering (White *et al.* 2004). Ultimately, burnout, typified by emotional fatigue and depersonalisation, where the person cuts themself off from the reality and anxiety associated with their actions, can result from such stress in the context of professional caring (Medland *et al.* 2004).

In 1964, the French intellectual, existentialist philosopher and novelist Simone de Beauvoir published the novella *A Very Easy Death*, an eloquent, elegiac and profound description of the death of her mother from bowel cancer. She also provides a powerful depiction of the various attitudes of the involved medical staff and how a patient and her family reacted to such a difficult situation. Thus, she writes about how, when her mother develops acute obstruction and the doctor advocates intervention, she ultimately acquiesces to the unpalatable situation of her mother attached to 'complicated apparatus' and necessarily detached from them, even after asking the doctor 'Why this tube? Why torture Maman, since there is no hope?' She is met by a 'withering look' and the rejoinder 'I am doing what has to be done' and later the doctors admonition that he has 'brought her [Maman] back to life'; de Beauvoir ponders why 'I did not venture to ask him "For what?"' and notes that when the situation is desperate and distressing and likely to be recognised as a 'long martyrdom', relatives and patients can be 'caught up in the wheels and dragged along, powerless in the face of specialists' diagnoses, their forecasts, their decisions. The patient becomes their property.' The palpable and painful sense of complicity is complicated and described later in this short book when she and her sister collude with the decision not to divulge the diagnosis or disclose the prognosis. She writes about the 'odious deception' and how they were confining their mother to a room that was analogous to a 'death chamber' and 'condemning her to silence; we forced her to say nothing about her anxieties and to suppress her doubts'. Arguably, and contentiously, this may be both exactly how some haematology practitioners feel and what they see when there is a lack of openness with their patients.

In the poem 'Wants' Philip Larkin talks about the 'costly aversion of the eyes from death' and perhaps this poetic observation, together with de Beauvoir's narrative, reflects the prevailing sense of responsibility and regret that we, our patients, and their families can feel about the denial of death and the delivery of care at this time. These erudite observations, both de Beauvoir's and Larkin's, were published at a time that preceded the modern hospice movement, which has undoubtedly influenced present palliative care and also before the major technological advances in medical and nursing care. Equally, one might argue that the society in which these historical literary documents were presented has changed in all matter and manner, where the relationship between patient and professional is appreciably, actually, and attitudinally different and arguably better. And yet, evidently, we still see and hear instances where medical and nursing practice suggest we can still be less than candid with patients about their status and real care needs, always with no little consequence to the practitioners sense of well-being too.

Implications for practice and conclusions

The philosophy of palliative care and supportive care in the UK is to enable people to live as well as possible, maximising the benefits of treatments and to live as well as possible with the effects of the disease (NICE 2003). To facilitate this process, health care provision has undergone a remarkable period of restructuring to improve equality of access, acceptability of services, the efficiency of services and effectiveness of interventions. Over the last decade, much emphasis has been placed on the end of life care agenda, specifically the patient's choice over place of death. The *End-of-Life Strategy* (DoH 2008) reported that patients still suffer unnecessary symptom distress or do not die in a place of their choosing. It also recognised the vital role that informal carers, such as the family of the patient, play in the care of the patient and it should no longer be taken advantage of, or their input and impact disregarded.

Nurses play an important role in the realisation of the various 'end of life care' initiatives such as the Liverpool Care Pathway, Gold Standards Framework or Preferred Priorities of Care documents and programmes. That said, the impetus of this chapter has been to establish that an important development is the drive to ensure that many aspects of palliative care are applied earlier in the course of the illness in conjunction with other treatments.

Good communication – a requisite skill, and between clinical team members – is key to the successful implementation of the principles and practices of palliative care. Noting the stress that can be engendered in the relationship between the nurse and a patient with an incurable haematological disease would indicate that clinical supervision and support is an important tool in ensuring the well-being of staff and optimising the care they are able to provide.

A sensible and pragmatic acceptance of the inevitability of death that is discussed openly and honestly with the patient, their family and all the members of the team is crucial. This needs to be combined with the sympathetic assurance that patients will not be neglected or forsaken and that attempts to ensure their comfort will need to be made. This dialogue should be ongoing, but those markers that indicate a worsening condition should be explained early in the diagnosis so that the patient and their family have a practical appreciation of what is reasonable and realistic from their treatment.

The concept and knowledge of palliative care should be addressed, including a clarification of the patient's preferred place of care, and possibly eventual death, and an explanation that measures to facilitate this would be explored. McGrath and Joske (2002) describe how in the care of a patient dying at home 'an orientation to living, rather than dying pervaded the experience', which clearly asserts the affirmation of the normality and commonality of death but not necessarily the need to be pre-occupied with it to the extent that a life is not lived fully and fruitfully. A primary feature of good clinical practice is recognising the responsibility of every health care professional to practice the palliative care approach, and to refer to specialist palliative care services if the need arises; as Becker (2011, p. 3) suggests, 'the skills of caring for someone at the end of life are not specialist in themselves and we need to remember that'. He further suggests that providing human contact and holistic care and not merely the mechanical tasks and procedures is the challenge to be met.

Palliative care addresses the principles and practicalities of providing a patient with a positive opportunity to exert their personal choices and preferences, and promotes and preserves the ability to better exercise it, at arguably the most important stage of their life.

References

Addington-Hall, J. and Altmann, D. (1998) Which terminally ill cancer patients in the UK receive care from community specialist palliative care nurses? *Journal of Advanced Nursing*, 32 (4), 799–806.

Ansell, P., Howell, D., Garry, A. *et al.* (2007) What determines referral of UK patients with haematological malignancies to palliative care services? An exploratory study using hospital record. *Palliative Medicine*, 21, 487–492.

Audrey, S., Abel, J., Blazeby, J.M. *et al.* (2008) What oncologists tell patients about survival benefits of palliative chemotherapy and implications for informed consent: qualitative study. *BMJ*, 337. a752 doi:10.1136/bmj.a752.

Back, A., Young, J.P., McCown, E. *et al.* (2009) Abandonment at the end of life from patient, caregiver, nurse, and physician perspectives: loss of continuity and lack of closure. *Archives of Internal Medicine*, 169 (5), 474–479.

Becker, B. (2011) Valuing patient contact and nursing skills. *International Journal of Palliative Nursing*, 17 (1), 3.

Bestall, J.C., Ahmed, N., Ahmedzai, S. *et al.* (2004) Access and referral to specialist palliative care: patients' and professionals' experiences. *International Journal of Palliative Nursing*, 10 (8), 381–381.

Beuken, G. (2003) Palliative care: a theological foundation. The spiritual dimension of palliative care in the local Christian community. *Scottish Journal of Healthcare Chaplaincy*, 6 (1), 44–46.

Botti, M., Endacott, R., Watts, R. *et al.* (2006) Barriers in providing psychosocial support for patients with cancer. *Cancer Nursing*, 29 (4), 309–316.

Brown, E. and Bennett, M. (2007) Survey of blood transfusion practice for palliative care patients in Yorkshire: implications for clinical care. *Journal of Palliative Medicine*, 10 (4), 919–922.

Byock, I. (2009) Palliative care and oncology: growing better together. *Journal of Clinical Oncology*, 27 (2), 170–171.

Cancer Research UK (2008) UK cancer incidence statistics for common cancers http://info. cancerresearchuk.org/cancerstats/incidence/commoncancers/ (page updated November 2008, accessed April 2009).

Clark, D. (2002) Beyond hope and acceptance: the medicalisation of dying. *British Medical Journal*, 324, 905–907.

Clark, D. (2004) History, gender and culture in the rise of palliative care. In: *Palliative Care Nursing: Principles and Evidence for Practice* (eds S. Payne, J. Seymour and C. Ingleton). OUP, Maidenhead.

Connor, A., Allport, S.,Dixon, J. *et al.* (2008) Patient perspective: what do palliative care patients think about their care? *International Journal of Palliative Nursing*, 14 (11), 546–552.

Costantini, M., Toscani, F., Gallucci, M. *et al.* (1999) Terminal cancer patients and timing of referral to palliative care: a multi-centre prospective cohort study. *Journal of Pain and Symptom Management*, 18 (4), 243–251.

Craven, O. (2000) Palliative care provision and its impact on psychological morbidity in cancer patients. *International Journal of Palliative Nursing*, 6 (10), 501–507.

De Beauvoir, S. (1985) *A Very Easy Death* (translated by Patrick O'Brien). Andre Deutsch, London.

Department of Health (2000) *NHS Cancer Plan*. DoH, London.

Department of Health (2005) *The National Service Framework for Long Term Conditions*. HMSO, London.

Department of Health (2006) *Our Health, Our Care, Our Say: a New Direction for Community Services*. HMSO, London.

Department of Health (2008) *End-of-Life Strategy*. DoH, London.

Evans, R., Stone, D. and Elwyn, G. (2003) Organizing palliative care for rural populations: a systematic review of the evidence. *Family Practice*, 20 (3), 304–310.

Fadul, N., Elsayem, A., Palmer, J.L. *et al.* (2007) Predictors of access to palliative care services among patients who died at a comprehensive cancer centre. *Journal of Palliative Medicine*, 10 (5), 1146–1152.

Fadul, N.A., El Osta, B., Dalal, S. *et al.* (2008) Comparison of symptom burden among patients referred to palliative care with haematologic malignancies versus those with solid tumours. *Journal of Palliative Medicine*, 11 (3), 422–427.

Farquhar, M., Grande, G., Todd, C. *et al.* (2002) Defining patients as palliative: hospital doctors versus general practitioners perceptions. *Palliative Medicine*, 16, 247–250.

Ferrell, B. (2005) Late referrals to palliative care. *Journal of Clinical Oncology*, 23 (12), 2588–2589.

Grande, G.E., Addington-Hall, J.M. and Todd, C.J. (1998) Place of death and access to home care services: are certain patient groups at a disadvantage? *Soc Sci Med*, 47, 565–579.

Homsi, J. and Luong, D. (2007) Symptoms and survival in patients with advanced disease. *Journal of Palliative Medicine*, 10 (4), 904–909.

International Council of Nurses (2006) *Code of Ethics for Nurses*. ICN, Geneva.

Jack, B., Hillier, V., Williams, A. *et al.* (2004) Hospital based palliative care teams improve the insight of cancer patients into their disease. *Palliative Medicine*, 18, 46–52.

Jeffrey, D. (1995) Appropriate palliative care: when does it begin? *European Journal of Cancer Care*, 4, 122–126.

Jones, R. (2005) Acute hospital-based palliative care services for the older person. *British Journal of Nursing*, 14 (11), 596–600.

Joske, D. and McGrath, P. (2007) Palliative care in haematology (Editorial) *Internal Medicine Journal*, 37 (9), 589–590.

Kahn, D.L. and Steeves, R.H. (1995) The significance of suffering in cancer care. *Seminars in Oncology Nursing*, 11 (1), 9–16.

Kelly, D., Ross, S., Gray, B. *et al.* (2000) Death, dying and emotional labour: problematic dimensions of the bone marrow transplant nursing role. *Journal of Advanced Nursing*, 32 (4), 952–960.

Koffman, J., Burke, G., Dias, A. *et al.* (2007) Demographic factors and awareness of palliative care and related services. *Palliative Medicine*, 21, 145–153.

Larkin, P. (1955) Wants. In *The Less Deceived*. The Marvell Press, Hessle.

Laussaniere, J. M. and Auzanneau, G. (1995) The quality of terminal care in haematology. *European Journal of Palliative Care*, 2 (4), 169–172.

Lowden, B. (1998) Introducing palliative care: health professionals' perceptions. *International Journal of Palliative Nursing*, 4 (3), 135–142.

McDonnell, T. and Morris, M. (1997) An exploratory study of palliative care in bone marrow transplant patients. *International Journal of Palliative Nursing*, 3 (2), 111–117.

McGrath, P. (1999) Palliative care for patients with haematological malignancies – if not, why not? *Journal of Palliative Care*, 15 (3), 24–30.

McGrath, P. (2002a) Are we making progress? Not in haematology! *OMEGA-Journal of Death and Dying*, 45 (4), 331–348.

McGrath, P. (2002b) End of life care for haematological malignancies; the 'technological imperative' and palliative care. *Journal of Palliative Care*, 18 (1), 39–47.

McGrath, P. and Holewa, H. (2006) Missed opportunities: nursing insights on end-of-life care for haematology patients. *International Journal of Nursing Practice*, 12 (5), 295–301.

McGrath, P. and Holewa, H. (2007) Special considerations for haematology patients in relation to end-of-life care: Australian findings. *European Journal of Cancer Care*, 16 (2), 164–171.

McGrath, P. and Joske, D. (2002) Palliative care and haematological malignancy: a case study. *Australian Health Review*, 25 (3), 60–66.

Medland, J., Howard-Reuben, J. and Whitaker, E. (2004) Fostering psychosocial wellness in oncology nurses: addressing burnout and social support in the workplace. *Oncology Nursing Forum*, 31 (1), 47–54.

Morita, T., Akechi, T., Ikenaga, M. *et al.* (2005) Late referrals to specialized palliative care service in Japan. *Journal of Clinical Oncology*, 23, 2637–2644.

National Cancer Alliance (2001) *Haematological Cancers: Patients Views and Experiences*. NCA, London.

National Council for Palliative Care (2006) *Ethnicity, Older People and Palliative Care*. NCPC, London.

National Institute for Clinical Excellence (NICE) (2003) *Improving Outcomes in Haematological Cancers: the Manual*. NICE, London.

National Institute for Clinical Excellence (NICE) (2004) *Improving Supportive and Palliative Care for Adults with Cancer*. NICE, London.

Nursing and Midwifery Council (2008) *The Code – Standards of Conduct, Performance and Ethics for Nurses and Midwives*. NMC, London.

Randall, T. C. and Wearn, A. M. (2005) Receiving bad news: patients with haematological cancer reflect upon their experience. *Palliative Medicine*, 19, 594–601.

Read, S. and Thompson-Hill, J. (2008) Palliative care nursing in relation to people with intellectual disabilities. *British Journal of Nursing*, 17 (8), 506–510.

Rodgers, B. L. and Cowles, K. V. (1997) A conceptual foundation for human suffering in nursing care and research. *Journal of Advanced Nursing*, 25 (5), 1048–1053.

Ronaldson, S. and Devery, K. (2001) The experience of transition to palliative care services: perspectives of patients and nurses. *International Journal of Palliative Nursing*, 7 (4), 171–177.

Roy, D.J. (2000) The times and places of palliative care. *Journal of Palliative Care*, 16, s3–s4.

Sepulveda, C., Marlin, A., Yoshida, T. and Ullrich, A. (2002) Palliative care: The World Health Organisation's Global Perspective. *Journal of Symptom Management*, 24, 91–96.

Shah, S., Blanchard, M., Tookman, A. *et al.* (2006) Estimating needs in life-threatening illness: a feasibility study to assess the views of patients and doctors. *Palliative Medicine*, 20 (3), 205–210.

Thekkumpurath, P., Venkateswaran, C., Kumar, M. *et al.* (2008) Screening for psychological distress in palliative care: a systematic review. *Journal of Pain and Symptom Management*, 36 (5), 520–528.

Tinnelly, K., Kristjanson, L., McCallion, A. *et al.* (2000) Technology in palliative care: steering a new direction or accidental drift. *International Journal of Palliative Nursing*, 6 (100), 495–500.

Van Kleffens, T., Van Baarsen, B., Hoekman, K. *et al.* (2004) Clarifying the term 'palliative' in clinical oncology. *European Journal of Cancer Care*, 13, 254–262.

Westlake, S. (2008) *Report: Cancer Incidence and Mortality in the United Kingdom and Constituent Countries, 2003–05. Office of National Statistics Health Statistics Quarterly*, 40, 91–97.

White, K. (1999) Increased medicalisation within palliative care. *International Journal of Palliative Nursing*, 5 (3), 108–109.

White, K., Wilkes, L., Cooper, K. and Barbato, M. (2004) The impact of unrelieved patient suffering on palliative care nurses. *International Journal of Palliative Nursing*, 10 (9), 438–444.

Willard, C. and Luker, K. (2005) Supportive care in the cancer setting: rhetoric or reality? *Palliative Medicine*, 19, 328–333.

Willard, C. and Luker, K. (2006) Challenges to end of life care in the acute hospital setting. *Palliative Medicine*, 20, 611–615.

World Health Organization (WHO) (2004a) *The Solid Facts: Palliative Care*. WHO, Geneva.

World Health Organization (WHO) (2004b) *Better Palliative Care for Older People*. WHO, Geneva.

World Health Organisation (WHO) (2006) *Definition of Palliative Care* http://www.who.int/cancer/palliative/definition/en/ (accessed 8 April 2009).

Glossary of terms

Acute haemolytic transfusion reaction (ATR)	This occurs as a result of ABO incompatible red cells being transfused.
Arthralgia	Joint pain.
Autosomal recessive	The gene carrying the mutation is located on one of the chromosome pairs. This means that males and females are equally affected. 'Recessive' means that both copies of the gene must have a mutation in order for a person to have the trait. One copy of the mutation is inherited from the mother, and one from the father.
BCSH	British Committee for Standards in Haematology.
Biofeedback system	In this instance it sustains iron regulation and balance within the storage and circulatory systems.
Blood components	These consist of: • Red blood cells • Platelets • Plasma • Cryoprecipitate • Fresh frozen plasma (FFP)
Blood products	These are any therapeutic products derived from plasma (Blood Safety & Quality Regulations SI 2005/50). These are: • Human albumin solution • The various clotting factor concentrates • Anti-D • Therapeutic immunoglobulins
BQSR	Blood Quality & Safety Regulations (SI 2005/50).
Cardiomyopathy	Disease of the heart muscle, making it abnormal, with no obvious cause.
Care Quality Commission	Government body that replaced the Healthcare Commission.
CMV neg	Cytomegalovirus negative.
Colloid	Intravenous plasma expanders such as Hartmann's solution.
Cryo	Cryoprecipitate.

Haematology Nursing, First Edition. Marvel Brown and Tracey J. Cutler.
© 2012 Blackwell Publishing Ltd. Published 2012 by Blackwell Publishing Ltd.

Crystalloid	Intravenous saline.
DHTRs	Delayed haemolytic transfusion reactions.
DoH	The Department of Health.
FFP	Fresh frozen plasma.
FNHTRs	Febrile transfusion reactions.
Genetic counselling	This is not primarily counselling in the psychological sense, but counsellors or indeed the GP or nurse specialist in the context of GH, can provide information and support to families who may be at risk, interpret information about the disorder, analyse inheritance patterns and review available testing options with the family.
Gonads	The ovaries and testes.
Granulocytes	These are the major phagocytic white cells.
Haemochromatosis (GH)	This is also known as iron overload disease or iron storage disease (BCSH 2000 p. 3) and is a genetic disorder.
Hb	Haemoglobin.
Hepatic fibrosis	Liver tissue damage caused in this case by the accumulation of iron deposits.
Heterozygous	An organism is referred to as being heterozygous when it carries two different copies of the gene affecting a given trait.
Homozygous	An organism is referred to as being homozygous when it carries two identical copies of the gene affecting a given trait.
HTC	The Hospital Transfusion Committee should have the authority to take the necessary actions to improve transfusion practice by promoting safe and appropriate use of blood.
HTT	The Hospital Transfusion Team is the working group of the HTC.
Liver cirrhosis	Liver scarring.
MHRA	Medicines and Healthcare products Regulatory Authority.
Magnetic resonance imaging (MRI)	This is a non-invasive imaging technique.
NBTC	National Blood Transfusion Committee.
NPSA	The National Patients Safety Agency.
Platelets	Small cell fragments produced in the bone marrow that play an essential role in the blood clotting process.
Red blood cells	Red blood cells are bi-concave, disc-shaped cells without a nucleus. They contain haemoglobin (Hb) which carries oxygen to the tissues.
RTCs	The Regional Transfusion Committees are responsible for implementing actions of the NBTC in England.
RTT	The Regional Transfusion Team is the working group of the RTC.
SABRE	Serious Adverse Blood Reactions and Events the reporting arm of MHRA.
Serum ferritin	Serum ferritin indicates the amount of iron stored in the body.
SHOT	Serious Hazards of Transfusion reporting scheme.
Special requirements	Blood components that are:

- Irradiated
- CMV negative
- Platelets that are HLA matched

TACO	Transfusion associated circulatory overload – can occur when too much fluid is transfused or transfusion is too rapid.
TA-GvHD	Transfusion Associated Graft-versus-Host Disease.
Therapeutic venesection	Transferrin saturation is the ratio of two simple blood tests, which indicates iron accumulation.
Transferrin saturation	Transferrin saturation is the ratio of two simple blood tests, which indicates iron accumulation.
TRALI	Transfusion related acute lung injury – should be suspected when severe respiratory distress is observed.
Universal leucodepletion	White cell removal – implemented in 1999, across the UK blood services, as a precautionary measure to minimise the risk of vCJD.

Index

Locators in **bold** refer to figures/diagrams
Locators for headings which also have subheadings refer to general aspects of the topic

Haematology Nursing, First Edition. Marvelle Brown and Tracey J. Cutler.
© 2012 Blackwell Publishing Ltd. Published 2012 by Blackwell Publishing Ltd.